Infection Protection

Also by the Authors

R. Klatz, *New Anti-Aging Secrets for Maximum Lifespan,*
STL, 2000

R. Klatz, *Ten Weeks to a Younger You,*
STL, 1999

R. Goldman with R. Klatz (and Lisa Berger), *Brain Fitness,*
Doubleday, 1999

R. Klatz, *Hormones of Youth,*
STL, 1998

R. Klatz with Carol Kahn, *Grow Young with HGH,*
HarperCollins, 1998

R. Klatz and R. Goldman, *Stopping the Clock,*
Bantam Books, 1996

R. Klatz and R. Goldman, *7 Anti-Aging Secrets,*
ESM Publishers, 1996

HOW TO FIGHT THE GERMS
THAT MAKE YOU SICK

Infection
Protection

RONALD M. KLATZ, M.D., D.O., AND

ROBERT M. GOLDMAN, M.D., D.O., PH.D.

WITH CATHERINE CEBULA

HarperResource

An Imprint of HarperCollins*Publishers*

FIRST EDITION

Designed by Ellen Cipriano

Library of Congress Cataloging-in-Publication Data has been applied for.

ISBN 0-06-018408-6

02 03 04 05 06 QW 10 9 8 7 6 5 4 3 2 1

Dedication

Discovery consists of seeing what everybody has seen and
thinking what nobody has thought.

—*American biochemist and Nobel Prize winner Albert von Szent-Gyorgyi*

This work pays tribute to the thousands of medical innovators who,
despite the harshest of circumstances and intellectual climates, perse-
vered to accomplish some of the greatest advancements through
which medicine has evolved for the betterment of its patients.

Take the example of the now obvious recommendation that to
avoid spreading infectious diseases, physicians wash their hands and
medical instruments between patient examinations. In the 1850s,
Hungarian physician Dr. Ignas Semmelweiss noticed that fewer of his
patients were dying since he had adopted this procedure. Year after
year, Semmelweiss held steadfastly to the notion that his colleagues
follow his advice. He was called all sorts of names for what was
branded a strange and preposterous theory. In an ironic twist, Semmelweiss died of an infectious disease contracted as a patient in a local
hospital. Today we owe a great debt to Dr. Semmelweiss for maintaining an unwavering commitment to his beliefs—beliefs that ultimately
improved medical care for every man, woman, and child in every
nation across the globe.

The great leap in health care of the twenty-first century is offered by antiaging medicine. A patient-centric, wellness-based model that delivers life-enhancing and life-extending medical care, antiaging medicine is a medical specialty that applies advanced scientific and medical technologies for the prevention, early detection, treatment, and reversal of age-related diseases. It is a health care model promoting innovative science and research to prolong the healthy life span in humans. As such, antiaging medicine is based on principles of sound and responsible medical care that are consistent with those applied in other preventive health specialties.

As Dr. von Szent-Gyorgyi intimated, the success of antiaging physicians, health practitioners, and scientists is in their ability to see what everyone else has seen but to think anew with this evidence. To this spirit of unbridled creativity and relentless pursuit of the same, the authors pay tribute and dedicate this work. May each of us alive today, and the generations to follow, reap the life-enhancing, life-extending benefits of the seeds that the innovative science of antiaging medicine is sowing today.

With our most sincere wishes for your personal longevity.

RONALD M. KLATZ, M.D., D.O., PRESIDENT
ROBERT M. GOLDMAN, M.D., D.O., PH.D., CHAIRMAN
AMERICAN ACADEMY OF ANTI-AGING MEDICINE
A nonprofit medical society of 10,000 physicians,
health practitioners, and scientists hailing from
60 countries worldwide who believe,
"Aging is not inevitable."

They're everywhere on us, in us, around us; they are a life force without which humans could not survive. We are as whales floating in a sea of microorganisms, most of which ignore us, some of which sustain us, and a few of which would like to eat us.

Contents

Preface

As a ten-year old, I'd often return home after the final school bell of the day to prepare a hot dog for a tasty snack. One evening, to pay tribute to the mad scientists in sci-fi movies I'd find myself cheering on, I dropped one of the hot dogs into a jar filled only with some flat cola. Screwing on the lid tightly, I let this experiment take its course overnight on the kitchen counter.

The next morning, I removed the hot dog from the soda and found it crawling with little, soft, pudgy white worms. But instead of losing my breakfast, I was captivated. What were these creepy things? Where did they come from? Those worms were parasites, which were drawn out of the hot dog by the sugar in the cola.

I look back on the hot-dog incident as the birth of my fascination with the highly adaptable and tenacious creatures called parasites. Eventually, my investigations branched out to include other pernicious invaders as well—viruses, bacteria, and fungi.

As I read more and more and eventually began my formal medical training, I saw just how destructive some microbes are and how little most people know about them. The statistics are sobering. Infectious diseases are the third leading cause of death in the United States after heart disease and cancer claiming more than 100,000 lives annually and costing more than $30 billion in direct treatment expenses alone. Infectious diseases are responsible for a quarter to a third of the 54 million deaths globally each year and are the world's leading cause of death among children and young adults.

We may think we have infectious disease under control, but we don't. Yes, we have made tremendous progress against these diseases, including smallpox, diphtheria, pertussis, tetanus, polio, measles, mumps, and rubella. But we can't afford to be complacent.

Since the eighteenth century, seven recorded pandemics of influenza have occurred worldwide. Perhaps the most alarming incident was the three waves of highly virulent strains of flu between 1918 and 1919 that spread aggressively to every nation on the planet, killing 20 million people. During the fall of 1918, 20,000 people in New York City alone died from influenza, while Western Samoa saw 20% of their population die from it. Medical science blamed the epidemic on everything from dirt and dust to closed windows and cosmic factors. Each year, infectious disease–related deaths in the United States nearly double, standing at approximately 170,000 for the 1990s. In fact, influenza kills more than 30,000 Americans each year, and epidemiologists agree that it is not a question of *if* but rather *when* the next killer flu pandemic will occur.

Twenty well-known diseases—including tuberculosis (TB), malaria, and cholera—have reemerged or spread geographically since 1973, often in more virulent and drug-resistant forms. At least 30 previously unknown disease agents have been identified since 1973, including human immunodeficiency virus (HIV), Ebola, and hepatitis C (of which an estimated 4 million people are carriers), and there is no known cure for any of these.

While improvements in sanitation and infection control since the early 1900s have substantially restrained widespread outbreaks of contagious diseases, you will see that evidence supports the suggestion that the degenerative diseases of aging—namely, heart disease, cancer, stroke, and mental decline—may be adverse effects of infectious disease, rather than illnesses in and of themselves.

As a physician, not a day goes by that I fail to read a shocking scenario of someone who has suffered with infections for years without his or her doctor ever discovering the source of the problem. Today, as the president of the American Academy of Anti-Aging Medicine, I recognize that immunity is one of the pillars of life-enhancing, life-extending medical care. Our immune system keeps us healthy. When it fails, we start coming down with aging-related disorders. You may be one of the thousands of people suffering from undiagnosed maladies overlooked by traditional medicine. *Infection Protection* shares important insights into diseases that could needlessly reduce the length and quality of your life. This book shows you how to recognize situations that may put you at risk and discusses the preventive measures you should follow.

There is no end to the damage parasites and other microorganisms can wreak on the human body. These bugs will weaken you physically and mentally, suck the life out of healthy cells, nibble your liver for lunch, gnaw at your kidneys and brain, blast your immune system to smithereens, and cause you to become terribly old before your time. By reading this book, I hope you begin to understand the profound importance of strengthening the immune, respiratory, reproductive, and digestive systems, each of which are integral defenders from infectious disease. In fact, the knowledge you glean from *Infection Protection* may be all you need to start feeling like your young self again.

RONALD M. KLATZ, M.D., D.O.
CHICAGO, ILLINOIS

Please Read—Important Notice

The content in this book is for educational purposes only, and is not intended to prevent, diagnose, treat, or cure disease or illness contracted in any way, including via biological attack. While potentially therapeutic nutraceuticals (dietary supplements such as vitamins, minerals, herbal products, hormone supplementation, and similar preparations) and interventions (processes such as lifestyle changes, dietary modifications, bodywork, prescription medications, and others) are mentioned in the course of this book, you are urged to seek the advice of a medical professional to make the appropriate selection for your particular medical situation.

With nutraceuticals, dosing is highly variable. Proper dosing is based on parameters including sex, age, and whether you are well or ill (and whether your illness is chronic or acute). Additionally, efficiency of absorption of a particular type of product and the quality of its individual ingredients are two major considerations for choosing appropriate agents for your medical situation.

Just because a product is natural doesn't mean it's safe for you. A small portion of the general population may react adversely to components in nutraceuticals (especially herbal products). Make your physician aware of any and all "natural" interventions you use regularly, and seek medical consultation before starting any others.

Caveat emptor: Investigate the vendors of the products before you buy them. Do they make third-party research on the efficacy of the product freely available? Is the company run by scientists, physicians, or health professionals—not marketers looking to turn a quick buck? Do they have any outstanding consumer complaints with the Better Business Bureau or state attorney general's office? An educated consumer will be less susceptible to being scammed.

Our best advice for infection-proofing yourself: Find a doctor who is open to new and innovative therapies and utilizes up-to-the-minute, state-of-the-art diagnostics to pinpoint disease as early as possible. Make this individual your partner in your program for optimal health

Buyer Beware
How Quackery Sells

- Fear: One of the most insidious forms of fear-mongering is the invented disease. Virtually everyone has minor aches and pains of one kind or another. These ups and downs are usually not symptoms of a disease needing "treatment."
- Hope: Common claims based on false hope fall into four categories: aphrodisiacs, fountains of youth, cure-alls, and athletic superperformance. Creating false hope for the seriously ill is quackery in its cruelest form.
- Clinical tricks: Combining a proven treatment with a quack treatment is a common trick. Then, when the proven treatment works, the quack remedy is given the credit. If the regimen doesn't work at all, the proven treatment is blamed for the failure.
- Disclaimers: Claiming that a product cleanses or detoxifies, rather than cures a specific condition, gets the purveyor off the hook because such processes are difficult, if not impossible, to measure. These claims also make the product sound "medical" without actually making a medical claim.
- Conspiracy theories: Charging that reputable public and private organizations are part of a conspiracy to suppress information or withhold treatment from the public is a popular ploy among quacks. Yet, be mindful that big business and government may not be exempt from withholding or restricting the privilege of treatments that may threaten their control. Such abuses of power have unfortunately and repeatedly burdened the science of medicine, and you are urged to seek objective information from trusted sources motivated by academics and not finances.

care. The American Academy of Anti-Aging Medicine (A4M) maintains a directory of physicians and health practitioners in this elite group. To obtain a referral to a qualified medical professional nearby, visit the World Health Network at www.worldhealth.net and select the interactive search feature, or call the A4M at (773) 528-4333.

The Authors and the Publisher disclaim all liability for any damage that may occur as a result of following the advice contained in this book.

Acknowledgments

The authors would like to acknowledge the thousands of members of the American Academy of Anti-Aging Medicine (A4M; Web site: www.worldhealth.net) without whom our pursuit of innovative medical science would be impossible. Through its nine-year history, A4M has led the preventive health movement as a not-for-profit medical society dedicated to advancing technology to prevent, detect, and treat aging-related disease and to promote research into methods to retard and optimize the human aging process. A4M is also dedicated to educating physicians, scientists, and members of the public on anti-aging issues. A4M believes that the disabilities associated with normal aging are caused by physiological dysfunctions that in many cases can be ameliorated by medical treatment, such that the human life span can be increased and the quality of life improved as one grows chronologically older. A4M seeks to disseminate information concerning innovative science and research as well as treatment modalities designed to prolong the human life span. Although A4M seeks to disseminate information on many types of medical treatments, it does not promote or endorse any specific treatment, nor does it sell or endorse any commercial product.

In our affiliation with A4M as president and chairman, respectively, A4M has given us the opportunity to forge professional relationships with the brightest minds in medicine today. We wish to acknowledge the following individuals for their involvement in *Infection Protection*:

Chief Researcher and Executive Editor
Catherine Cebula
Contributors

Edward Lichten, M.D.	Binyamin Rothstein, D.O.
Carol Osborne, D.V.M.	Ira Shapira, D.D.S.
Anne Vermilye, M.S., C.H.T., C.M.T.	

The following individuals provided research support for the book:

John Abdo, Mark Abrahms, Jerry Fitzpatrick, Alicia Valaquez, Dr. Tom Allen, Dr. Larry Cherry, Joe Partipillo, Stewart Grannen, Stedman Grahm, Oprah Winfrey, Anthony Barone, Goldie and Jerry Klatz, Sid Bobb, Billy Levenson, Richard Furer, Barry Datloff, Ali Berman, Dr. Saroja Bharati, Paul and Sandy Bernstein, Lloyd Blankfein, Bobbie Jandristis, Bob Brahm, Dr. Eric Braverman, Phil Broxham, Perris Calderon, Lorne Caplan, Neil Cauliffe, Simon Chan, Chan Boon Yong, George Chow, Chris Wakeford, Christina Kamm, Paul Chua, Dr. Gerard Chuah, Leslie Cohen, June Colbert, Sam Lamensdorf, Steve Sotiri, Milt Copulos, Mike Crohn, Angie Daniels, Darryll Burleigh, Jo Chua, Dato Harnam, Todd Dawes, Bob Dee, Bob Delmontique, Wayne Demelia, Denie Walters, Dr. Nick DeNubulie, Dr. Eduardo DeRose, Dr. Tom Deters, Dion Friedland, Tom Marinovic, Cory and Allen Dropkin, Dr. Ken Dychwald, Adam Eilenberg, Dr. Wade Exum, Fara Lazzara, Alfreda Green, Dr. Perry Gerard, G. K. Goh, Arnold and Alice Goldman, Paul and Carole Grahm, Mark and Paul Goldman, Dr. Brad Grant, Susan Greenbaum, Lynn Gu, Midred Bonner, Pam Cunningham, Guy Jonkman, Byron Klein, Dr. Harold Hakes, Dr. Hanno Soth, Lee Harris, Warren Price, Dr. Arthur Heath, Tom Heidke, Judy Heifitz, Jack Balani, Dr. Vernon Howard, Andy Hydanto, Mike Interator, Irena Yundov, Izabella Firus, Susanne Archer, Jana Berentson, Joni Pitcock, Dr. Fumihiko Umezawa, Dr. M. Watabe, Julian Grech, Peter Julian, Pam Kagan, Eric Weider, Ben and Joe Weider, Chuck Kaplan, Dr. Mike Katz, Georgia and Sumner Katz, Mitch Kaufman, Dr. Michael Klentze, Dr. Arkady Koltun, Tommy Konig, David Kravitz, Dr. Mitch Kurk, Lalita Mannsauuad, Andy and Bill Lane, Larry Emdur, Dr. Ron Lawrence, Dr. Sherrie

Lechner, Dr. Barry Halliwell, Lee Labrada, Lee Felix, Leon Wah Kneong, Dr. Howard Levine, Dr. Marty Levine, Dr. Ed Lichten, Lee Lidhtee, Dr. Sheri Lieberman, Tony Little, Leon Locke, Jim Lorimer, William Louey, Ross Love, Joe Hing Lowe, Dr. Sidney Malet, Jon Mangion, Jim and Debbie Manion, Mark Brun, U Tin Maug Swee, Mauricio Fernandez, Tim McKeon, Dr. Joe Mercola, Rick Merner, Tom Merridith, Gary Mezei, Dr. Maurice Modavi, Edmund Murphy, Dr. Art Nahas, Neil Spruce, Irene Nathan, Dan Neidermyer, Surya Joshi, O. Ben Seng, Ralph Sesso, Richard Ornstein, Dr. Don Owen, Vic Padillino, Giovanna Breu, David Peppin, Dr. Lee Perry, Dr. Peter Kalish, Kevin Philips, Dr. Lynn Pirie, Jeff Plitt, Glen Pollock, Javier Pollock, Ben Posner, Will and Norm Dabish, Tom Purvis, Grahm and Kathryn Putnam, Dr. Rafael Santonja, Sandy Ranilli, Ran Rahmat, Sharon Ringer, Mel Rich, Steve Stern, Jim Rittenberg, Arlene Robbins, Dr. Jerry Rodos, Dr. Tom Rosandich, Dr. Phil Santiago, Larry and Warren Schiffer, Joe and Holly Schultz, Steve Schussler, Arnold Schwarzenegger, Dr. Marshall Segal, Dr. Uri Schaffer, Brian Sherr, John Sandstrom, Sebina Dussy, Abby Silverberg, Simon Reynolds, Marty and Tracy Silverberg, Dr. Steve Sinatra, Donald Teo, Eugene Hong, Dr. Ym Wong, Janifer Yeo, Dr. S. K. Tan, Amy Sklar, Ann Sobel, Steve Sokol, Steven Speigle, Greg Stavich, Jake Steinfeld, Russ Stewart, John Stokack, Gary Strauch, Larry Stickler, Marc Manuel, Larry Lee, Sukuma Sudiarsana, Jack Sutton, Alan and Linda Tamshen, Dr. Thierry Hertoghe, Dr. Robert Tien, Titus and Vicki Marinas, Stephen Tjandra, Drs. Terry and Jan Todd, Mike Tomzak, Dr. Richard Penfil, T. T. Durai, Jay Tuerk, Tim Tyrrell, Victor Vazquez, Vince Caprio, Gary Vogel, Dr. Bob Voy, David Waite, Wanna Aung, Carole Weidman, Sherri Weinstein, Cliff Wertheim, Bettie and Joseph Whittaker, Brenda Winkle, Kenny Wong, Philip Yeo, Dr. Lynette Yong, Dr. Richard Yong, Dr. Claude Chauchard, Dr. Lindsay Rosenwald, Dr. S. Bergman, Peter Kash, Scott Endsley, Irene Michaels, Arthur Wu, Dr. Francis Nettl, Meesun Boice, Dr. Dato Harnam, Guy Jonkman, Rano Izhar Rahmat, Dr. Robert Peterson.

Finally, we also wish to salute the American Academy of Anti-Aging Medicine in its presentation of a hopeful and attainable model for medicine in the new millennium. Founded on the miracle of the biotech revolution, this new design for health care takes advantage of the continued and expanding arena of discovery and advancement in biotechnology to provide a better understanding of ways to mitigate age-related disability and disease. Conceived by A4M, the concept of technodemography is the application of modern biotechnology to the issues of aging diagnosis, prevention, and intervention, such that one may extrapolate future progress in human aging based on the application of innovative medical interventions on aging. This concept may be illustrated by the Longevity Link, a novel representation of the impact of five key biomedical technologies on gains in human longevity:

$$\lambda \propto \sum_{k=1}^{5} T_k^{\frac{\tau}{3.5}}$$

where:

λ = human longevity

$T_k = \{$

stem cells, giving rise to a supply of human cells, tissues, and organs for use in acute emergency care as well as treatment of chronic, debilitating disease

cloning, a technique holding tremendous promise in producing consistent organs, tissues, and proteins for biomedical use and transplant in humans

nanotechnology, enabling scientists to use tiny tools to manipulate human biology at its most basic levels

artificial organs, making plentiful replacement body parts available

nerve impulse continuity (brain/spinal cord), enabling nerve signal transmission to be maintained without interruption despite physical trauma

$\}$

technological knowledge

and τ = year (after A.D. 2000),

where the exponent $\frac{\tau}{3.5}$ represents the doubling time of medical knowledge and technology every 3.5 years

A4M's technodemographers predict that these advancements will receive widespread application and availability by the year 2029. Visit the World Health Network at www.worldhealth.net, the Internet's leading antiaging portal, to review additional materials on this innovative concept for medicine in the third millennium.

The 10,000 members of the American Academy of Anti-Aging Medicine hailing from 60 countries worldwide share an unwavering commitment to a single purpose. We seek to elevate the quality of medical care available to all so that life-enhancing, life-extending diagnostic and treatment procedures eradicate the disability and disease commonly associated with aging. It is to this unique group of medical innovators that we extend our most sincere thanks and our humblest appreciation.

RONALD M. KLATZ, M.D., D.O., PRESIDENT
AMERICAN ACADEMY OF ANTI-AGING MEDICINE

ROBERT M. GOLDMAN, M.D., D.O., PH.D., CHAIRMAN
AMERICAN ACADEMY OF ANTI-AGING MEDICINE

Introduction:
From Immunity to Infinity

Nature [is] that lovely lady to whom we owe polio, leprosy,
smallpox, syphilis, tuberculosis, cancer.

*—Dr. Stanley N. Cohen, geneticist, Stanford University, quoted by David N. Leff
in a letter to the editor,* New York Times, *March 15, 1987*

Do you feel out of sorts most of the time? Do you cling to cleanliness
as if it were a lifeline that keeps disease at bay? Does it seem like no
matter what you do, you can't seem to shake that persistent runny/
stuffy nose, sore throat, fatigue, weakness, joint swelling, chronic
pain, and allergies, among countless other ailments?

You are *not* a hypochondriac. You are *not* crazy, either. While many of
us, including health care professionals, tend to attribute disease to anything from a bad attitude to laziness, from an unhealthy diet to the environment, many of these problems have a more insidious origin: bugs.

Just 40 years ago, infectious diseases such as tuberculosis, smallpox, and dysentery killed millions. In one of the most significant medical advances of the past millennium, science "conquered" these
diseases with vaccines and antibiotics. But now, thanks to environmental pollutants, food additives, and the remarkable adaptability of
microorganisms, new strains of infection are developing that are
highly resistant to our arsenal of pharmaceuticals.

Most doctors are not aware of how pervasive and relentless these infections can be. They routinely misdiagnose parasitic or viral infections because their conservative tactics are powerless against these tenacious and highly adaptable creatures. Even if your doctor does test you for parasites, chances are overwhelming that the results will come back negative. Why? Because only 50 of the 1,000 species of parasites that can live in your body can be detected by current medical diagnostics.

The truth is that we are in the midst of a huge pandemic that is largely ignored by the traditional medical community. As many as 75% of Americans suffer from some form of bacterial, viral, parasitic, or fungal infection, running the gamut from hardly noticeable to devastating. These infections include conditions such as intestinal parasites manifested as ulcers and gastroenteritis, chronic sinus infection, strep throat, yeast (candida) infection, sexually transmitted disease, and urinary tract infection—to name a few. It's even more frightening that today's most virulent killers—heart disease and cancer—can develop from bacterial, viral, fungal, or parasitic infections.

By measuring how long people live in good health—not just how long they live—the Japanese beat Americans by 4½ years, and the French lived 3 more healthy years. Yet, Japan spends just $1,750 per

The Extent of Infectious Disease in the United States (1997)

DISEASE	NUMBER OF CASES
Hepatitis B	10,420
Tuberculosis	19,850
Syphilis	46,540
Chlamydia	526,650
Gonorrhea	324,900
Salmonella	41,900

Sources: Centers for Disease Control; *Health United States,* 1999.

person on health and France spends $2,100, compared to the United States, which in 1999 spent a whopping $3,724 per person on health annually. The United States is good at expensive, acute emergency care, but fails to provide low-cost preventive care that has kept Europeans and those in the Pacific Rim healthy.

Globally, the population is growing older by the passing minute: The fastest-growing population in most countries is the oldest old, at 80 years plus. Older Americans are at greater risk of infections and are at particular risk for morbidity and mortality due to diarrheal diseases that are likely caused by diminished capacity to fend off infectious agents.

The bottom line: We are in a constant state of war with billions of other creatures—bacteria, viruses, fungi, and parasites—on us, around us, and in us. Although some are harmless, others are eating away at us, causing chronic infections and manifesting as fatigue, premature aging, baldness, skin problems, digestive disorders, periodontal disease, and more. We are finding that most, if not all, chronic diseases have an infectious component—diseases from gastritis *(Helicobacter pylori)* to gonorrhea, from acne to Alzheimer's disease, from carbuncles to cardiac arrest. Infectious disease may well be the trigger

Suspicious Germs

KNOWN TO BE CAUSED BY INFECTION	SUSPECTED TO BE CAUSED BY INFECTION	MIGHT BE CAUSED BY INFECTION
Ulcers	Atherosclerosis, heart	Other cancers
Stomach cancer	disease, stroke	Obesity
Liver cancer	Alzheimer's disease	Schizophrenia
Cervical cancer	Multiple sclerosis	Manic depression
Nasopharangeal cancer	Type I diabetes	
Oral cancer	Asthma	
	Nonmelanoma	
	skin cancer	
	Colon cancer	

that accelerates the onset and/or progression of the chronic degenerative diseases of aging.

Every one of us is infested with good and bad microorganisms. Given a chance, the bad ones will ruthlessly destroy us. Although there is no total escape from these attackers, there is much we can do to protect ourselves internally and externally. *Infection Protection* is a compendium of actions you can take to recognize your risks and start healing yourself today, before you are robbed of your health, youth, vitality, and, quite possibly, your life!

[1]

It's a Bug's Life

We need only to look at the death toll from infectious disease
to see the results of this dangerous trend. We need to make
treating infectious disease a priority.

—*Didier Cherpitel, secretary-general,*
International Federation of Red Cross and Red Crescent Societies, 1999

We are never alone. Catch tuberculosis the next time you take an airplane trip; pick up a brain amoeba in your neighbor's hot tub; order
some food-borne parasites at your local restaurant; sleep with the
wrong person and end up with a sexually transmitted disease; play
with your sister's cat and come down with one of more than 200 pet-
borne diseases. For most of you, *Infection Protection* will be an enlight-
enment—perhaps a rude awakening—that will help you recognize
and reduce risky situations that may lead to your contracting infectious disease.

BE AFRAID, BE VERY AFRAID—
GERMS ARE OUT TO GET YOU!

Without microbes, there would be no food to eat or air to breathe.
Through photosynthesis, algae and bacteria produce about half of

Earth's oxygen. Bacteria and fungi break down dead organisms and natural and manmade wastes, thereby recycling sulfur, nitrogen, carbon, and other elements that keep our world alive.

Microbes naturally present in the human body help digest food, produce vitamins, and protect us from disease. They are important catalysts for making foods such as bread and cheese and drinks such as beer and wine. And they are a source of disease-fighting drugs such as penicillin. Some scientists believe that the cellular engines called mitochondria are descended from bacteria. The fact is that we share our world and our bodies with microbes—and sometimes they are stronger and more adaptable than we are.

The idea that microorganisms—or germs as they are often called—are inherently "evil" began during the second half of the nineteenth century as an outgrowth of Darwin's evolutionary theory. Darwin talked about survival of the fittest, but assigned no "moral value" to the struggle. Some of Darwin's contemporaries, however, imbued germs with a sinister quality, referring to them as cunning and murderous. As cities became overcrowded, water supplies tainted, and waste disposal systems overwhelmed, fevers and plagues—typhoid, pneumonia, scarlet fever, influenza, diphtheria, smallpox, and cholera—were common in America and Europe. It was fairly easy to make the leap to thinking of *all* germs as killers. By the end of the nineteenth century, germ consciousness had become deeply ingrained in the American psyche. And it's still there.

There is a school of thought, however, that maintains it is not the microbes—or germs—themselves that cause infection, but rather the failure of our immune system to keep the relationship between body and microbe in balance. According to this theory, common symptoms of an infection—for example, sneezing, coughing, vomiting, diarrhea, fever, pain, and fatigue—are protective. Rather than suppressing these symptoms with drugs, we should be strengthening our immune system so that it can keep the body in homeostasis—that is, in balance, through nutrition, physical activity, stress reduction, risk management, and immune-boosting supplements.

HORROR HEADLINES

Bubonic Plague

You're dead wrong if you thought that bubonic plague was something that just created a path of devastation in the 1400s, never to be heard

Defining Microbes

MICROBES	WHAT THEY ARE
Bacteria	One-celled bodies about 125,000th of an inch long that can make their own food or feed on live hosts or dead matter.
Viruses	Small (about 1 millionth of an inch across) and simple microbes that reproduce by injecting their genes into a cell to produce thousands of new viruses.
Fungi	Decomposers that break down matter into nutrients that can be reused by plants and animals. There are 100,000 known species; in humans, opportunistic fungal infections strike people with impaired immunity. Fungal infections can occur in healthy people via inhalation or wounds.
Parasites	Microscopic organisms—protozoa, amoebas, and worm-type organisms—that can live in the human body for many years by eating ingested food (e.g., sugar) or living off nutrition from the body's cells. More than 1,000 species may exist, though tests are available for only 40 to 50 types.
Mycoplasmas	Primitive, slow-growing bacteria that create symptoms such as fatigue, headaches, soreness, and joint pain.
Nanobes	Microbes that are smaller than the smallest known bacteria (20 to 150 nanometers in length); roughly the same size as viruses, but they do not need a host in which to live.
Extremeophiles	Microbes that thrive in environments once thought uninhabitable, such as boiling water (thermophiles) and frozen lakes beneath Antarctic ice fields (psychrophiles).

from again. During six weeks in 1994, 53 deaths in India were attributed to the plague, with 5,150 additional suspected diagnoses. Caused by *Yersinia pestis,* the plague is associated with a tremendously high potential for transmission, particularly in an era of mass globetrotting made possible by airline travel. Subsequent to the 1994 outbreak in India, the U.S. Centers for Disease Control and Prevention (CDC) issued orders for the U.S. Customs Service and Immigration and Naturalization Service to quarantine all passengers on planes from India who demonstrated clinical signs of the disease. The CDC did not receive reports of any cases of imported plague as a result of the surveillance program.

Black Death Decimating Prairie Dogs

An outbreak of bubonic plague is consuming north-central Montana prairie dogs. The strain of pathogen is the same one—*Yersinia pestis*—that struck people in 1994 in India (see above). Since the presence of the bacterium that causes the plague was confirmed at Fort Belknap Indian Reservation and a surrounding county, about 3,600 acres of healthy prairie dog towns (colonies) have died off. Health officials are advising people to keep themselves and their pets away from plagued areas and to monitor for fleas.

Bubonic plague can infect deer mice, rats, badgers, coyotes, bobcats, and antelope. Montana has had two confirmed cases of human bubonic plague since 1990. One man contracted it while skinning a bobcat. Another man became ill after administering care to an infected antelope in the field, but later recovered.

Mad Cow Disease

Mad cow disease is a fatal neurological disease that began decimating the British cattle industry in 1986. Beef from cattle infected with bovine spongiform encephalopathy (BSE) was suspected as the source of a similar, rare condition, Creutzfeldt-Jakob disease (CJD), in humans. In 1996, the British government acknowledged that a variant of CJD that is very similar to BSE had indeed infected and killed 10 people. So far in Europe, 56 people in Britain, 2 in France, and 1 in Ireland have died from this variant of CJD. Because the incubation period in humans can be as long as 40 years, it is impossible to know how many people will eventually fall victim to the disease.

Both BSE and CJD are transmissible spongiform encephalopathies (TSEs)—degenerative diseases of the central nervous system that cause fatal dementia. There is no cure. TSEs occur in humans, sheep, cattle, cats, mink, and other mammals.

TSEs are not caused by bacteria or a virus, but rather, researchers theorize, by prions—proteins that normally reside in brain tissue, but cause TSE when malformed. Prions associated with the variant of CJD linked to BSE, however, have been found not only in the brain but also in the tonsils, appendix, spleen, and lymph nodes.

Most TSEs are rare, the exception being scrapie, which infects sheep. TSEs occur sporadically for no known reason. They are not contagious and not easily transmissible, especially between species.

Emerging Infectious Diseases

An infectious disease is labeled "emerging" when it has appeared within the last 20 years or threatens to increase in the near future. A "new" infectious disease can result from genetic change in a pathogen and can appear suddenly in a new population. According to the World Health Organization, at least 30 new disease agents have been identified over the past two decades, and new agents are being added all the time. For example, the Nipah and Hendra viruses were recently identified after outbreaks in Malaysia and Singapore. These are lethal to about 40% of humans. They spread to humans via the urine and mucus of infected animals and cause severe encephalitis.

Some emerging infectious diseases are resurgences of microbes that have become resistant to commonly used drugs—for example, malaria and tuberculosis. Check the U.S. Centers for Disease Control and Prevention (CDC) Web site (www.cdc.gov), the National Foundation for Infectious Disease Web site (www.nfid.gov), and the World Health Organization's Outbreak News Index (www.who.int/emc/outbreak_news/n2000/index.html) for more information on emerging infectious diseases.

Emerging Infectious Diseases Identified Since 1973

YEAR	MICROBE	TYPE	DISEASE
1973	Rotavirus	Virus	Infantile diarrhea
1977	Ebola virus	Virus	Acute hemorrhagic fever
1977	*Legionella pneumophila*	Bacterium	Legionnaires' disease
1980	Human T-lymphotropic virus 1 (HTLV 1)	Virus	T-cell lymphoma/ leukemia
1981	Toxin-producing *Staphylococcus aureus*	Bacterium	Toxic shock syndrome
1982	*Escherichia coli* 0157:H7	Bacterium	Hemorrhagic colitis; hemolytic uremic syndrome
1982	*Borrelia burgdorferi*	Bacterium	Lyme disease
1983	Human immunodeficiency virus (HIV)	Virus	Acquired immunodeficiency syndrome (AIDS)
1983	*Helicobacter pylori*	Bacterium	Peptic ulcer disease
1989	Hepatitis C	Virus	Parenterally transmitted non-A, non-B liver infection
1992	*Vibrio cholerae* 0139	Bacterium	New strain associated with epidemic cholera
1993	Hantavirus	Virus	Adult respiratory distress syndrome
1994	Cryptosporidium	Protozoan	Enteric disease
1995	Ehrlichiosis	Bacterium	Severe arthritis(?)
1996	nvCJD	Prion	New variant Creutzfeldt-Jakob disease
1997	HVN1	Virus	Influenza
1999	Nipah, Hendra	Virus	Severe encephalitis

Sources: U.S. Institute of Medicine, 1997; WHO, 1999.

They can, however, be transmitted readily within a species via cannibalism.

The outbreak of BSE in Britain has been traced to the practice of feeding cattle a protein supplement made from rendered animal wastes from slaughterhouses. It began when cattle were fed scrapie-containing sheep parts. Rendered parts from these cattle were then fed to calves. The practice of using rendered animal parts as feed began as a cost-saving measure, especially for dairy cows whose protein requirements are higher after they are injected with bovine growth hormone. "Cannibalism for profit," as the feeding mode has been called, was stopped in Britain in 1988.

Mad cow disease has not been detected in U.S. cattle, and this country has long banned imported cattle, beef, and beef products from Britain. Many public health advocates believe this precaution is not enough. Consider the following:

- Tainted protein feed made from carcasses of sick animals spread BSE in Europe, and the same feed was sold all over the world even after Britain banned it in 1988.
- The United States continued to import potentially contaminated European meat products well into the 1990s.
- The U.S. Food and Drug Administration has not effectively enforced its 1997 ban against giving feed made from rendered cows to cattle. Approximately 75% of the beef cattle in the United States are fed a diet of animal parts.
- "Downer cattle"—cows that fall down and can't get back up—are a high-risk group for BSE. But they can be slaughtered at FDA-supervised rendering facilities, avoiding inspection and testing by the U.S. Department of Agriculture.

Research by St. Mary's Hospital in London that was published in August 2000 indicates that BSE may be much more widespread than previously believed. Pigs, poultry, and sheep that show no symptoms can be carriers. There is no way to detect TSEs until symptoms develop. Even then, diagnosis cannot be confirmed without a brain autopsy to reveal the disease's characteristic spongelike lesions.

Why Some Diseases Are Making a Comeback

SOURCE	SPECIFIC REASON(S)	REEMERGING DISEASE
Changing lifestyle	• Changes in food processing and handling	*Escherichia coli* 0157:H7 Hepatitis A Listeriosis Salmonellosis
	• Increased use of child care facilities	Cryptosporidiosis Giardiasis Hepatitis A Meningitis Shigellosis
	• Substance abuse and unsafe sexual practices	Chlamydia Hepatitis B Human Immunodeficiency virus (HIV)
	• Increased air travel	All infectious diseases
Growing global population and movement	• Changes in land use	Hantavirus pulmonary syndrome Lyme disease Rabies
	• Increased urbanization in the tropics	Dengue hemorrhagic fever Yellow fever
Changing public policies	• Breakdowns in public health prevention programs	Cryptosporidiosis Dengue hemorrhagic fever Measles Rabies Tuberculosis

Because the incubation period for TSEs is uncertain, infected animals can be slaughtered and enter the food supply before any symptoms of disease have developed.

CJD and other TSEs in humans begin with loss of memory and fatigue, and eventually cause physical as well as mental degeneration, leading to death in about nine months. CJD randomly strikes about 300 Americans each year, mostly older people. These cases, called sporadic CJD, are closely monitored by the CDC for possible BSE involvement. The CJD variant associated with BSE, however, strikes younger people. (The British victims were aged 13 to 43.)

Currently, the only way to ensure that beef is safe is for cattle ranchers to refrain from feeding cattle-rendered parts, and for consumers to select beef that is certified as organic. Although the U.S. Department of Agriculture and other agencies state that U.S. livestock raised for human consumption is safe, for now, from TSEs, a prion disease called chronic wasting disease has infected deer and elk in the western states. Although hunters and their families probably have been exposed to the prions from eating infected meat, it is not known if the disease actually can be transmitted to humans. Scientists, however, have simulated transmission in a test tube and believe it is indeed possible in "real life."

The newest, perhaps most alarming, discovery of a mode of transmission of CJD was brought to broad public attention in October 2000. Tulane University officials reported that a series of surgical transactions may have exposed at least eight hospital patients to the human form of mad cow disease. In March 2000, a Louisiana woman checked into Tulane to undergo brain surgery, and died. In the ensuing weeks, the surgical instruments were washed, sterilized, and reused a multitude of times. After autopsying the woman in May and finding evidence of CJD, Tulane realized that in reusing the surgical instruments on eight subsequent patients, the hospital may have exposed them to this fatal neurological disease. The hospital states it contacted all eight potentially exposed patients and took the instruments out of service. For the unwitting patients, however, an excruciating wait begins: CJD can incubate without symptoms for years, depending on the quantity of exposure to infected material, so most won't know they have it until they begin to experience the early symptoms (typically, depression, personality changes, lack of muscle coordination).

According to the U.S. Centers for Disease Control, 9 out of 10 cases of CJD are caused by tainted medical components, such as corneal implants or transplanted brain tissue. In the 1980s, several people in Switzerland contracted CJD through inadequately cleaned brain imaging electrodes that were used on a patient with the disease.

A Bloody Mistake

The only way to eliminate accidental spread of mad cow disease through tainted hospital and surgical devices is to destroy them after a single use. An obvious reluctance, in which public health is forfeited, is expressed by hospitals, which may spend tens of thousands of dollars on each device.

Ebola

Ebola is a member of the virus family known as Filoviridae. The first known filovirus was Marburg, which appeared in 1967 in Germany. Its source was traced to monkeys imported from Africa for research and vaccine production. There were 31 cases and one generation of secondary transmission (passed by an infected person to another).

Ebola transmission has similarly occurred by handling infected chimpanzees. It is also transmitted by direct contact with the blood, secretions, organs, or semen of infected persons. There are four subtypes of Ebola: Zaire, Sudan, Ivory Coast, and Reston. All but the Reston strain have caused disease in humans.

The Ebola virus was first identified in Sudan and Zaire in 1976, with a second outbreak in Sudan in 1979. In 1989 and 1990, an Ebola-like virus was identified in monkeys imported from the Philippines being held in quarantine in laboratories in Reston, Virginia. A number of the monkeys died. Several workers became infected with the virus but did not become ill. Ebola also occurred in imported monkeys in other research facilities through 1992. Before the fall of 2000, 1,100 human cases with 793 deaths have been attributed to Ebola since it was first identified. Sensational in its aggressive and rapid transmission, a 1995 outbreak of Ebola in Kikwit, the Democratic Republic of the Congo, inspired the best-selling book *The Hot Zone.*

The spread of Ebola across Uganda is current headline news. After first being identified in the capital city of Kampala, Uganda, in mid-October 2000, as of early November, the death toll stood at 92. After infecting a total of 283 people, health officials felt that the epidemic was stabilizing. The strain of the virus involved was identified as Ebola Sudan, which was last detected in neighboring Sudan in 1979.

The exact origin of the Ebola virus is still unknown. Nor do we know where the virus lives between outbreaks, which are often years and hundreds of miles apart. Researchers believe the virus is animal-borne: After the first human is infected from the animal host, the virus can be spread to other people via contact with the infected person's blood and/or secretions, or through contact with contaminated objects such as needles. All the Ebola subtypes have shown an ability to spread through airborne particles under research conditions, although this mode of transmission has never been documented in a real-world setting.

Fatal Course

Ebola is characterized by the sudden onset of fever, weakness, muscle pain, headache, and sore throat. It progresses to vomiting, diarrhea, rash, limited kidney and liver function, and internal and external bleeding. The classic symptom is severe hemorrhagic fever, which is often fatal. There is no vaccine or standard treatment for Ebola. Supportive therapy includes keeping fluids and electrolytes in balance and maintaining oxygen and blood pressure.

Hantavirus

Hantavirus pulmonary syndrome (HPS) is potentially deadly, and immediate intensive care is essential once symptoms appear. Hantaviruses that cause HPS are carried by rodents, especially the deer mouse. Hantavirus was first diagnosed in the southwestern United States in 1993 and has since appeared in other areas of the country. In the first half of 1999, the virus infected 217 people in 30 states. Almost 100 of these people have died.

Rodents shed the hantavirus in their urine, droppings, and saliva. The virus is mainly transmitted to people when they breathe in air contaminated with the virus, as occurs when fresh rodent urine, droppings, or nesting materials are stirred up. The first signs of sickness, especially fever and muscle aches, appear 1 to 5 weeks later, followed by shortness of breath and coughing. Once this phase begins, the disease progresses rapidly, necessitating hospitalization and often ventilation within 24 hours. (See Chapter 11 for tips on how you can minimize your risk of infection.)

Diseases of Luxury

Mycobacteria avium and *fortuitum* multiply in the warm, moist environment provided by indoor hot tubs, and become airborne in the mist produced. People inhale this mist, including bacteria suspended in the water droplets. The lung disease, nontuberculous mycobacteria (NTM), may ensue—particularly in those who are immunocompromised.

Itchy skin lesions caused by bacteria also can result from a dip in hot tubs. *Pseudomonas aeruginosa* flourishes in toasty temperatures and wetness, can readily infect people, and within two days of exposure can create pustules and sores.

New Food-Borne Disease Outbreaks

The U.S. Food and Drug Administration and the CDC are responding to a new strain of bacteria that can infect humans who eat raw or undercooked shellfish. *Vibrio parahaemolyticus* naturally occurs in certain bodies of water. It is credited with triggering a 1998 outbreak of 416 cases of diarrhea, vomiting, and fever in Galveston Bay, Texas, diners who ingested raw oysters. The CDC has received reports of 30 to 40 cases in Alabama, Florida, Louisiana, and Texas. The CDC now urges all coastal states, not just those in the Southeast, to monitor for *V. parahaemolyticus*. Recently, Washington state has seen a flurry of incidents.

On-the-Job Hazards

In October 2000, the CDC reported the first documented case of *Mycobacterium tuberculosis* transmitted from contaminated medical waste to at least one worker at a Washington state medical waste treatment facility. Two other workers became infected with tuberculosis despite no known previous or nonoccupational exposure to the disease. Infectious disease experts urge public health officials to heed this early warning signal that occupationally acquired infections, left undiagnosed, may spread widely and wildly among the general population.

Nanobacteria

Short for *Nanobacterium sanguineum*, a Latin term for "blood bacterium," Nanobacteria (NB) are the smallest known self-replicating bacteria. At just 20 to 200 nanometers (a nanometer is one-billionth of a meter) in size, NB is $1/1,000$ the size of "regular" bacteria, allowing it to move around easily into other cells and invade them.

When exposed to other cells or bacteria, NB causes cell death (known by the medical term *apoptosis*) by altering the gene-expression pattern. NB grows very slowly, reproducing only every three days ("regular" bacteria reproduce in minutes or hours).

Nanobacteria only grow in mammalian blood or serum. Since its discovery in the early 1990s, no benefit for NB to humans has been found. Quite the contrary:

- Chronic inflammatory responses are usually seen in areas where nanobacteria are found.
- Because nanobacteria can infect any tissue or cell, they have been observed killing lymphocytes (see Chapter 2).
- In one of its phases of development during the life cycle, a nanobacterium secretes a calcium biofilm "slime" around itself that both disguises the NB from being detected as foreign to our bodies and allows for multiple NB to connect to function together as a unit. This calcification has been shown by multiple scientific researchers to be the source of diseases including atherosclerotic plaque, coronary artery plaque, heart disease, kidney stones, psoriasis, eczema, liver cysts, breast calcification, dental plaque and periodontal disease, rheumatoid arthritis, fibromyalgia, multiple sclerosis, and Alzheimer's disease.

In May 2001 at the annual meeting of the American Society of Microbiology, NB was reported to be found as a contaminant in medical products previously presumed sterile, specifically IPV polio vaccine. Most human biological vaccines are made in fetal bovine serum—a medium that is now known to be contaminated with NB. It is suspected that production cell lines of viral vaccines are contaminated with NB that can grow in the culture media. Presently, the only way to avoid this contamination is for vaccine manufacturers to pass culture media through filters 20 nanometers in size and irradiate them with 150 megarads to kill any nanobacteria present.

Currently, there are no known natural substances that kill nanobacteria. In order to treat NB infections, doctors must first remove the protective calcium shells and then kill the bacteria with an agent specifically effective as an anti-nanobacterial.

BIOLOGICAL TERRORISM

Biological terrorism involves the release of a biological agent, announced or without warning, with or without a mechanical dispersal mechanism such as a bomb. It raises horrifying concerns of mass casualties, civil unrest, and widespread disabilities and death.

Bioterrorist agents can cause large numbers of casualties with minimal logistical requirements. Those responsible often go undetected. Biological weapons are easy and cheap to produce and can be used to selectively target humans, animals, or plants. The costs of conventional weapons ($2,000), nuclear armaments ($800), and chemical agents ($600) would far outstrip the bargain-basement price of biological weapons ($1) to produce 50% casualties per square kilometer (1969 dollars; source: Internet Dermatology Society at www.telemedicine.org/BioWar/biologic.htm).

Infectious agents are very appealing to bioterrorists because their destructive force is silent. Each year, the United States ships thousands of samples of infectious agents without incident. In general, record keeping on the sale and transfer of such agents is good, and the Centers for Disease Control and Prevention in 1997 made effective an expanded mandate to crack down on the transfer and receipt of 40 select agents that might be used for bioterrorism.

Many experts agree that the United States is more vulnerable to bioterrorist attack than to a war waged with guns, tanks, and naval and air strikes. Preparedness of physicians and health care personnel is paramount, for these people serve as the frontline alert system monitoring the nation's public health.

Life After September 11, 2001

The four September 11, 2001, terrorist hijackings of domestic United States airline flights, and subsequent tragedies at the World Trade Center and the Pentagon and in rural southern Pennsylvania, have forever changed Americans' daily way of life. In the aftermath of that day, clear bioterrorist risks now threaten everything from mail service, to public utilities (including drinking water), to travel on public transportation, airplanes, and trains. We present some tips to help you minimize your risk of contracting a biological agent.

General Advice

DO

The U.S. Postal Service advises all Americans to monitor their mail carefully and to be suspicious of:

- Envelopes or parcels without return addresses
- Envelopes or parcels with stains or odors or containing powdery substances
- Envelopes or parcels with too much postage—a hint that the sender does not want the package returned to him/her

If you receive a suspicious envelope or parcel, the Federal Bureau of Investigation (FBI) recommends:

- Handle with care; don't shake or bump.
- Isolate and look for indicators:

  - Misspelled words
  - Poorly typed or handwritten
  - Incorrect addressee
  - Restrictive markings like "Personal" or "Confidential"
  - Parcels with protruding wires; that are lopsided, rigid, or bulky; or that are packaged with excessive tape or string

- Don't open, smell or taste.
- Place into a plastic bag or container to prevent leakage of contents. OR cover the envelope or package with a trash can. Leave the room, close the door or section off the area.
- Wash your hands with soap and water to prevent spreading to your face (inhalation risk) or any open wounds or abrasions (cutaneous risk).
- CALL THE LOCAL POLICE.

(continued)

(continued)

DO NOT

Do not panic. Identified early, many bioterrost threats may be treated with antibiotics.

Do not waste money purchasing gas masks and environmental suits: The U.S. Centers for Disease Control and Prevention does not recommend these purchases, as they lead to a misguided sense of confidence should a biological or chemical attack occur.

Do not stockpile antibiotics "just in case." Overusing any antibiotic is a sure way to breed pathogens that can resist it. Misusing by self-prescribing the wrong antibiotic may worsen the situation. Unless you are a well-educated and trained medical professional, self-treatment with prescription antibiotics is not a good idea.

Be Prepared

If you become exposed to a biological agent dispersed in the air, first, escape upwind. If you cannot do so, or are at home or in an office, take these measures to reduce the total exposure load:

- Cover your mouth and nose with a makeshift gas mask—a bandanna, shirt, or scarf folded over several times and wetted down with water.
- Close all windows.
- Turn off all fans, heating, and air-conditioning systems.
- Close the fireplace damper.
- Move to the interior of the building with no (or the fewest) windows and doors, taking your Family Disaster Supplies Kit (see below) with you.
- Wet some towels and jam them in the crack under the doors.
- Tape around doors, windows, and exhaust fans or vents. Use the plastic garbage bags from your kit to cover windows, outlets, and heat registers.
- Stay in the room and listen to your radio until you are told all is safe or you are told to evacuate.
- Get medical care—immediately!

The American Red Cross recommends you pack your Family Disaster Supplies Kit with:

- A first-aid kit
- A battery-operated radio, flashlight, and extra batteries
- Bath-size towels
- Plastic garbage bags

(continued)

(continued)

- Wide tape
- A county map
- Bottled water (at least three gallons of water per person)
- Nonperishable snack food
- Medications, and extra eyeglasses and hearing aids

Replace water and medications every three months and food every six months. Batteries should also be replaced on a regular basis.

Leading Bioterrorist Agents

Based on ease of production, stability until delivered, and simplicity of delivery mechanism, the seven most probable biological agents to be selected for twenty-first-century bioterrorist activity are

- anthrax
- plague
- botulinum
- cholera
- smallpox
- tularemia
- viral hemorrhagic fevers

Anthrax Anthrax is caused by the organism *Bacillus anthracis.* In South and Central America, southern and eastern Europe, Asia, Africa, the Caribbean, and the Middle East, the microbe can be found in cattle or other hoofed mammals that graze in fields in which anthrax spores are present. Anthrax in wild livestock has occurred in the United States. Anthrax spores are dormant forms of the bacteria, and germinate when given suitable conditions.

When anthrax affects humans (other than in a case of bioterrorism, see below), it is usually due to occupational exposure to infected animals or their products.

There are three types of anthrax occurring in humans, depending on where the infectious spore has made its entry into the body:

- Cutaneous—least serious. Produces a skin lesion; left untreated, the infection can spread and poison the blood.
- Inhalation (respiratory)—potentially fatal. Occurs when spores are breathed in and lodged into the lung.
- Intestinal—rarely occurs in the United States. Caused by consumption of contaminated meat.

As the most common form of anthrax, cutaneous anthrax enters via a wound on the skin. The infection begins as a raised itchy bump similar to an insect bite and develops into a fluid-filled sac within a day or two. Then it becomes an ulcer with a dark area in the center. Cutaneous anthrax is rarely lethal, killing in 20% of cases when the microbes are carried via the bloodstream to lymph nodes. On the matter of identifying cutaneous anthrax sent in the mail, New York mayor Rudolph Giuliani's recommendation in an October 2001 interview with NBC is: "Let's say you have an envelope and you think there is powder inside, or you happen to open it and you see powder; leave it where it is, get up, leave that room, go to another room, and call 911. Explain what it is and then the police and haz-mat people [hazardous materials specialists] will take over. They'll test it and the vast majority of times it's going to turn out to be talcum powder or something like that." Given the enormous risk of uncertainty, it is best to call for help—better safe than sorry.

Ken Alibek, a top former Soviet germ warfare scientist who is now a U.S.-based author and researcher trying to develop defenses against bioterror, told a surprised congressional briefing held in October 2001 that a hot, moist steam iron and moist fabric could kill anthrax spores. Thus, his suggestion for handling suspicious mail is to "iron your letters," adding that a microwave oven is not as good as an iron and that including moisture is essential because spores can survive dry heat. He suggests that for large amounts of mail handled in postal distribution centers, portable gamma radiation units could be used to sterilize letters.

Being exposed to anthrax spores does not necessarily mean you will develop an infection. Many spores remain dormant and pose no threat. In addition, infection will result only if sufficient numbers of the spores germinate and release harmful bacteria in sufficient quantities. Small amounts of the bacteria can be killed off by the body's immune system. It is estimated that 10,000 spores (each smaller than the size of a period on this page) are needed to trigger infection.

As we have witnessed beginning in the fall of 2001, anthrax is a viable agent of bioterrorism. Culturing large quantities of anthrax spores is a complicated task, but is within the capacity of many nations. During the 1990s, it was suggested that at least 17 nations had some capacity to manufacture anthrax. Presently, the United States, Russia, and Iraq are known to be countries capable of manufacturing anthrax, with many other rogue nations suspected of being able to do so as well.

Plague   Plague is caused by the bacterium *Yersinia pestis*. People get plague from being bitten by a rodent or flea that is carrying the plague bacterium or by handling an infected animal. The two most common forms of plague are bubonic and pneumonic.

In the United States, the last urban plague epidemic occurred in Los Angeles in 1924–1925. Since then, human plague in the United States has occurred as mostly scattered cases in rural areas (an average of 10 to 15 persons each year). Globally, the World Health Organization reports 1,000 to 3,000 cases of plague every year.

When utilized as a bioterrorist agent, plague may be spread by:

- Fleas, acting as contaminated vectors—channels for transmission, spreading the bubonic type.
- Aerosol, causing pneumonic type. This is anticipated to be more common a scenario than fleas spreading bubonic plague.

An aerosolized plague weapon could go misdiagnosed as a flu outbreak. Within two to four days, people would start dying of septic shock. Early treatment and prevention with antibiotics would decrease the number of deaths in those exposed to the agent.

By the 1970s, Soviet scientists were able to manufacture large quantities of *Yersinia pestis* suitable for placing into biological weapons. More than 10 institutes and thousands of scientists were reported to have worked with the plague in the former Soviet Union. In contrast, few scientists in the United States have studied this disease in the detail necessary to be of assistance in the event of a bioterrorist attack using *Yersinia pestis*.

Botulinum (botulism) Botulinum toxin (botox) is the most poisonous substance known. A single gram of crystalline toxin, evenly dispersed and inhaled, would kill more than 1 million people (though technical aspects of dispersal make this difficult to achieve). The basis of the phenomenal potency of botulinum toxin is enzymatic; the toxin operates by disrupting neuromuscular function.

Recently, scientists have been able to understand and put to beneficial use the effects that botulinum has on the neuromuscular system. As such, botulinum has become the first biological toxin to become licensed for treatment of human disease. In the United States, physicians are using botulinum toxin to treat neuromuscular disorders including cervical torticollis, strabismus, and blepharospasm associated with dystonia. It is also used "off label" for a variety of more prevalent conditions that include migraine headache, chronic low back pain, stroke, traumatic brain injury, cerebral palsy, achalasia, and various dystonias.

Terrorists have already attempted to use botulinum toxin as a bioweapon. Aerosols were dispersed at multiple sites in downtown Tokyo, Japan, and at U.S. military installations in Japan on at least three occasions between 1990 and 1995 by the Japanese cult Aum Shinrikyo. These attacks failed, likely as a result of faulty microbiological technique or deficiencies in generating the aerosolized bacterium. The perpetrators obtained their *C. botulinum* from soil that they had collected in northern Japan.

Development and use of botulinum toxin as a possible bioweapon began at least 60 years ago. The head of the Japanese biological warfare group (Unit 731) admitted to feeding cultures of *C. botulinum* to prisoners, with lethal effect, during that country's occupation of Manchuria, which began in the 1930s. The U.S. biological weapons program first produced botulinum toxin during World War II. Because of concerns that Germany had weaponized botulinum toxin, more than 1 million doses of botulinum toxoid vaccine were made for Allied troops preparing to invade Normandy on D day. The U.S. biological weapons program was ended in 1969–1970 by executive orders of Richard M. Nixon, then president. Research pertaining to biowarfare use of botulinum toxin took place in other countries as well.

Beginning in the 1970s, Iraq and the Soviet Union produced botulinum toxin for use as a weapon. Botulinum toxin was one of several agents tested at the Soviet site Aralsk-7 on Vozrozhdeniye Island in the Aral Sea. A former senior scientist of the Russian civilian bioweapons program reported that the Soviets had attempted splicing the botulinum toxin gene from *C. botulinum* into other bacteria. With the economic difficulties in Russia after the demise of the Soviet Union, some of the thousands of scientists formerly employed by its bioweapons program have been recruited by nations attempting to develop biological weapons. Four of the countries listed by the U.S. government as "state sponsors of terrorism" (Iran, Iraq, North Korea, and Syria) have developed, or are believed to be developing, botulinum toxin as a weapon.

After the 1991 Persian Gulf War, Iraq admitted to the United Nations inspection team to having produced 19,000 liters of concentrated botulinum toxin, of which approximately 10,000 liters were loaded into military weapons. These 19,000 liters of concentrated toxin are not fully accounted for and constitute approximately three times the amount needed to kill the entire current total global human population by inhalation—if it could be effectively delivered.

In 1990, Iraq deployed specially designed missiles with a 600-kilometer range; 13 of these were filled with botulinum toxin, 10 with aflatoxin, and 2 with anthrax spores. Iraq also deployed special 400-pound (180-kilogram) bombs for immediate use; 100 bombs contained botulinum toxin and 50 contained anthrax spores.

The potential of botulinum toxin as a bioweapon is constrained due to issues relating to concentrating and stabilizing the toxin for aerosol dissemination. However, these analyses pertain to military uses of botulinum toxin to immobilize an opponent. In contrast, deliberate release of botulinum toxin in a civilian population would be able to cause substantial disruption and distress. For example, it is estimated that a point-source aerosol release of botulinum toxin could incapacitate or kill 10% of persons within half a kilometer. In addition, terrorist use of botulinum toxin might be masked as a deliberate contamination of food. Misuse of toxin in this manner could produce either a large botulism outbreak from a single meal or episodic, widely separated outbreaks.

Cholera Cholera is an acute, diarrheal illness caused by infection of the intestine with the bacterium *Vibrio cholerae*. The infection is often mild or without symptoms, but sometimes it can be severe. Approximately 1 in 20 infected persons has severe disease characterized by profuse watery diarrhea, vomiting, and leg cramps. In these persons, rapid loss of body fluids leads to dehydration and shock. Without treatment, death can occur within hours.

In the U.S., cholera was prevalent in the 1800s, but it has almost been eliminated by modern sewage and water-treatment systems. However, international travel makes Americans traveling to parts of Latin America, Africa, or Asia—where epidemic cholera is occurring—susceptible.

Foodborne outbreaks have been caused by contaminated seafood brought into this country by travelers.

Cholera poses a bioterrorist threat because of the potential to spread it via drinking water. Public water sources—particularly reservoirs—may be attractive targets at which bioterrorists may deposit *Vibrio cholerae*. As many of America's water sources go unprotected or have marginal security measures, it would be fairly easy for a bioterrorist to simply drive or walk up to the shores of a public water reservoir and deposit a dose of the bacterium. If the water-treatment system for that supply does not add chlorine during water processing, the cholera bacteria may pass directly through to harm thousands of people who are served by that water source.

Smallpox   Smallpox is caused by the variola virus and has a very high mortality rate. In the majority of cases, smallpox is spread from one person to another by infected saliva droplets that expose the recipient having face-to-face contact with the infected person. People with smallpox are most infectious during the first week of illness because that is when the largest amount of virus is present in saliva. Contaminated clothing or bed linen can also spread the virus. Disinfectants such as bleach and ammonia can be used for decontamination and cleaning purposes.

A worldwide vaccination program eliminated smallpox in the 1970s. However, approximately half the U.S. population today has never received the vaccination. Additionally, the CDC reports that it does not know how long immunity in those vaccinated lasts. This leaves a startling proportion of Americans at risk for contracting smallpox. In a now highly susceptible, mobile population, smallpox would be able to spread widely and rapidly throughout this country and the world.

Both the United States and the former Soviet Union officially maintained small quantities of the virus at two labs. However, there is the suspicion that it may have been or is still researched and developed at other labs either within Russia or in other countries, thus increasing the concern of smallpox being used as a biological weapon. Recent allegations from Ken Alibek, former Soviet germ warfare scientist turned U.S. anti-bioterrorism expert, have heightened concern that smallpox might be used as a bioweapon. Alibek reported that beginning in 1980, the Soviet government embarked on a successful program to produce the smallpox virus in large quantities and adapt it for use in bombs and intercontinental ballistic missiles; the program had an industrial capacity capable of producing many tons of smallpox virus annually. Furthermore, Alibek reports that Russia even now has a research program that seeks to produce more virulent and contagious recombinant strains. Because financial support for laboratories in Russia has sharply declined in recent years, there are increasing concerns that existing expertise and equipment might fall into non-Russian hands.

The deliberate reintroduction of smallpox as an epidemic disease would have an adverse effect of unprecedented proportions. Potentially, tens of millions of people could die in the most lethal epidemic seen by mankind. An aerosol release of variola virus would disseminate widely: it can be stabilized for widespread dissemination, and the required dose for infection is very small. No antibiotics have yet been proven effective against this viral pathogen.

Tularemia   Tularemia is caused by the bacterium *Francisella tularensis*. It is a zoonotic disease—as a virus that typically infects animals or vectors (such as insects), tularemia can infect humans. It reaches us by exposure via skin, mucous membranes, the gastrointestinal tract, or the lungs. Humans contract tularemia primarily from infected wild rabbits (handling or eating undercooked, infected wild rabbit meat, or handling skins of infected rabbits). Outbreaks have occurred during rabbit-hunting season and during the summer months, when ticks and the deerfly are abundant. Additionally, we can contract tularemia via the bites of certain insects or by drinking contaminated water or breathing contaminated air. Humans do not transmit infection to others.

Tularemia is one of the most infectious pathogenic bacteria known, requiring inoculation or inhalation of as few as 10 organisms to cause disease. Aerosol release would have the greatest adverse medical and public health consequences. Release in a densely populated area would be expected to result in an abrupt onset of large numbers of cases of acute, nonspecific illness beginning 3 to 5 days later (incubation range, 1–14 days), with pneumonia-like symptoms developing in a significant proportion of cases during the ensuing days and weeks. This may be difficult for public health officials to distinguish from an epidemic of influenza or pneumonia.

Viral hemorrhagic fevers   The term "viral hemorrhagic fever" (VHF) refers to a group of illnesses that are caused by several distinct families of viruses. VHFs are caused by viruses of four distinct families:

- Arenaviruses, including Argentine hemorrhagic fever, Bolivian hemorrhagic fever, Sabia-associated hemorrhagic fever, Lassa fever, lymphocytic choriomeningitis, and Venezuelan hemorrhagic fever

- Bunyaviruses, including Crimean-Congo hemorrhagic fever, Rift Valley fever, hantavirus pulmonary syndrome, and hemorrhagic fever with renal syndrome
- Filoviruses, including Ebola hemorrhagic fever and Marburg hemorrhagic fever
- Flaviviruses, including tick-borne encephalitis, Kyassanur Forest disease, and Ornsk hemorrhagic fever

All of these families share a number of features:

- They are all RNA viruses, and all are covered, or enveloped, in a fatty (lipid) coating.
- Their survival is dependent on an animal or insect host, called the natural reservoir.
- The viruses are geographically restricted to the areas where their host species live.
- Humans are not the natural reservoir for any of these viruses. Humans are infected when they come into contact with infected hosts. However, with some viruses, after the accidental transmission from the host, humans can transmit the virus to one another.
- Human cases or outbreaks of hemorrhagic fevers caused by these viruses occur sporadically and irregularly. The occurrence of outbreaks cannot easily be predicted.
- With a few noteworthy exceptions, there is no cure or established drug treatment for VHFs.

In rare cases, other viral and bacterial infections can cause a hemorrhagic fever; scrub typhus is a good example.

VHFs manifest as a severe multisystem syndrome—many organ systems become involved as the disease progresses. Characteristically, VHFs cause overall vascular system damage, thus interrupting the body's ability to regulate itself. This is typically apparent as symptoms of hemorrhage (bleeding). Death occurs in as many as 50% of infections, depending upon virus. VHFs may also result in prolonged convalescence or cause chronic hypertension and renal disease.

Viruses associated with most VHFs are zoonotic. Rats, mice, ticks, and mosquitoes serve as the main channel ("vector") by which most VHFs spread from animals to humans. However, the hosts of some viruses—including Ebola and Marburg viruses—remain unknown.

Taken together, the viruses that cause VHFs are distributed over much of the globe. However, because each virus is associated with one or more particular host species, the virus and the disease it causes are usually seen only where the host species live(s). Some hosts, such as the rodent species carrying several of the New World arenaviruses, live in geographically restricted areas. Therefore, the risk of getting VHFs caused by these viruses is restricted to those areas.

Other hosts range over continents, such as the rodents that carry viruses which cause various forms of hantavirus pulmonary syndrome in North and South America, or the different set of rodents that carry viruses which cause hemorrhagic fever with renal syndrome in Europe and Asia.

A few hosts are distributed nearly worldwide, such as the common rat. It can carry Seoul virus, a cause of hemorrhagic fever with renal syndrome. Therefore, humans can get hemorrhagic fever with renal syndrome anywhere the common rat is found.

While people usually become infected only in areas where the host lives, occasionally people become infected by a host that has been exported from its native habitat. For example, the first outbreaks of Marburg hemorrhagic fever, in Marburg and Frankfurt, Germany, and in Yugoslavia, occurred when laboratory workers handled imported monkeys infected with Marburg virus. Occasionally, a person becomes infected in an area where the virus occurs naturally and then travels elsewhere. If the virus is a type that can be transmitted further by person-to-person contact, the traveler could infect other people. For instance, in 1996, a medical professional treating patients with Ebola hemorrhagic fever in Gabon unknowingly became infected. When he later traveled to South Africa and was treated for Ebola hemorrhagic fever in a hospital, the virus was transmitted to a nurse. She became ill and died. Because more and more people travel each year, outbreaks of these diseases are becoming an increasing threat in places where they have rarely, if ever, been seen before.

Viruses causing hemorrhagic fever are initially transmitted to humans when the activities of infected reservoir hosts or vectors and humans overlap. The viruses carried in rodent reservoirs are transmitted when humans have contact with urine, fecal matter, saliva, or other body excretions from infected rodents. The viruses associated with insect vectors are spread most often when the vector mosquito or tick bites a human, or when a human crushes a tick. However, some of these vectors may spread the virus to animals such as livestock. Humans then become infected when they care for or slaughter the animals.

Some viruses that cause hemorrhagic fever can spread from one person to another, once an initial person has become infected. Ebola, Marburg, Lassa, and Crimean-Congo hemorrhagic fever viruses are examples. This type of secondary transmission of the virus can occur directly, through close contact with infected people or their body fluids. It can also occur indirectly, through contact with objects contaminated with infected body fluids. For example, contaminated syringes and needles have played an important role in spreading infection in outbreaks of Ebola hemorrhagic fever and Lassa fever.

With the exception of yellow fever and Argentine hemorrhagic fever, for which vaccines have been developed, no vaccines exist that can protect against these diseases. Therefore, prevention efforts must concentrate on avoiding contact with host species. If prevention methods fail and a case of VHF does occur, efforts should focus on preventing further transmission from person to person, if the virus can be transmitted in this way.

Because many of the hosts that carry hemorrhagic fever viruses are rodents, disease-prevention efforts include

- controlling rodent populations
- discouraging rodents from entering or living in homes or workplaces
- encouraging safe cleanup of rodent nests and droppings

Additionally:

* For hemorrhagic fever viruses spread by arthropod vectors, prevention efforts often focus on community-wide insect and arthropod control.
* In addition, people are encouraged to use insect repellent, proper clothing, bed nets, window screens, and other insect barriers to avoid being bitten.
* For those hemorrhagic fever viruses that can be transmitted from one person to another, avoiding close physical contact with infected people and their body fluids is the most important way of controlling the spread of disease.
* Barrier nursing or infection-control techniques include isolating infected individuals and wearing protective clothing.
* Other infection-control recommendations include proper use, disinfection, and disposal of instruments and equipment used in treating or caring for patients with VHF, such as needles and thermometers.

The virulence and obscurity of viral hemorrhagic fevers may make them attractive for use by bioterrorists. Preparedness of the United States regarding VHFs is dependent on the work of the CDC's Special Pathogens Branch. They conduct work with Biosafety Level 4 viruses, of which VHFs are a category. As they are the most highly pathogenic of all viruses, the U.S. has designed special facilities to contain them while our scientists conduct their research and investigation.

Profiles of Possible Bioterrorist Agents

ANTHRAX—INHALATION

Contagious?
- No

Lethal?
- Death within 5–9 days of initial exposure if left untreated. 80% of victims die from hemorrhaging in lungs and from meningitis.

Vaccine Available?
- Yes

Possible Method(s) of Delivery as Bioterrorist Weapon:
- Aerosol

Signs and Symptoms:
- Incubation 1–6 days. Stage 1 (first hours to first few days): nonspecific "flulike" symptoms appear: fatigue, malaise, fever/chills, intense thirst, nonproductive cough, mild chest discomfort. Stage 2: sudden fever, difficulty breathing, profuse sweating, delirium, lung hemorrhaging, massive swelling of neck and chest, blue tinge to skin. Prolonged incubation of a period of weeks has been reported.

Treatment:
- Antibiotics effective: penicillin, ethromycin, or tetracycline. FDA has approved ciprofloxacin for preventive treatment in exposed population.

ANTHRAX—CUTANEOUS (SKIN)

Contagious?
- No

Lethal?
- Death in 1 out of 5 cases, occurring when microbes migrate into lymph nodes to cause blood poisoning.

Vaccine Available?
- No

Possible Method(s) of Delivery as Bioterrorist Weapon:
- Cutaneous—anthrax spores enter the skin through minor cuts and abrasions, where they grow into toxin-producing bacteria.

Signs and Symptoms:
- Rash—starting as a welt or swelling; progresses from fluid-filled blister to a black, ulcerous lesion lasting up to two weeks.

Treatment:

• The antibiotic ciprofloxacin is effective if disease caught early; delay lessens chances for survival.

PLAGUE (*YERSINIA PESTIS*)

Contagious?

• Yes—especially via infectious particles from nose and mouth of infected persons.

Lethal?

• Bubonic type—death from collapse of blood vessels, hemorrhage, and blood clots in 50% of untreated patients. Pneumonic type—death rate is 100% in untreated patients, caused by respiratory failure and blood vessel collapse.

Vaccine Available?

• Yes for bubonic type, but efficacy against aerosolized plague unknown.

Possible Method(s) of Delivery as Bioterrorist Weapon:

• For bubonic type—contaminated vectors (such as rodents and their fleas); for pneumonic type—aerosol.

Signs and Symptoms:

• Bubonic type: incubation period 2–10 days; intense, rapid onset marked by malaise, high fever, and tender lymph nodes; may progress spontaneously to bloodstream, thereby infecting nervous system and lungs (producing secondary pneumonic disease). Primary pneumonic: incubation period 2–3 days; onset is intense and rapid, marked by malaise, high fever, chills, headache, aches/pains, cough with bloody sputum, and toxic bacterial overgrowth through body; progresses to result in difficulty breathing and blue tinge to body.

Treatment:

• Antibiotics effective if begun within first 24 hours after first symptom: streptomycin, tetracycline, or chloramphenicol.

BOTULINUM

Contagious?

• No

Lethal?

• Death occurs from respiratory failure due to lung muscles rendered nonfunctional by bacteria. Cases reported in U.S. prior to 1960 had mortality of 60%.

(continued)

(continued)

Vaccine Available?

- Vaccine that is 90% protective after one year for *Clostridium botulinum* types A, B, E is available from CDC but has not been tested in the field. No vaccine for toxin types C, D, F, and G.

Possible Method(s) of Delivery as Bioterrorist Weapon:

- Aerosol

Signs and Symptoms:

- Paralysis, starting with eyes and moving downward to throat, voice, and respiration.

Treatment:

- Antibiotics ineffective. Tracheotomy to assist breathing.

CHOLERA

Contagious?

- Yes

Lethal?

- People with severe disease can die within a few hours after onset, caused by dehydration through profuse diarrhea.

Vaccine Available?

- Current vaccine provides 50% protection lasting for less than 6 months.

Possible Method(s) of Delivery as Bioterrorist Weapon:

- Public water supply

Signs and Symptoms:

- Most infected persons experience no symptoms. Some will experience vomiting and diarrhea. Left untreated, will progress to dehydration and shock.

Treatment:

- Replenish lost fluids and electrolytes.
- Antibiotics effective: tetracycline, ethromycin, chloramphenicol.
- Water department will chlorinate water supply. Affected residents should boil water in dilute bleach solution (½ teaspoon chlorine bleach per 5 gallons water) prior to drinking, cooking, or washing dishes.

SMALLPOX

Contagious?

- Yes

Lethal?

- Death results from overwhelming infection or hemorrhages. 30% mortality among nonimmunized; 3% among immunized. However, immunization lasts only 10 years, so rates for immunized may be much higher.

Vaccine Available?

- In 1965, the World Health Organization (WHO) began a worldwide effort to eradicate smallpox, after commercial production techniques were able to produce a stable freeze-dried vaccine in 1954. Routine vaccination against smallpox ended in 1972. In just 23 years after the first mass smallpox immunization program, public health officials in 1977 declared that smallpox infection was eliminated from the world. Supplies of smallpox vaccine exist today, but are very limited.

Possible Method(s) of Delivery as Bioterrorist Weapon:

- Spray to infect a single group of people.

Signs and Symptoms:

- Incubation period of 12 days. Begins with 2–3 days of flulike symptoms including fever, malaise, achiness, and headache. Over next 7–10 days, lesions appearing as red rash will become bumps, blisters, pustules, then crust to leave scars. Untreated, progresses to systemic infection and hemorrhaging.

Treatment:

- No specific treatment for smallpox.
- Antibiotics used to fight secondary bacterial infection rather than to treat smallpox virus.

TULAREMIA

Contagious?

- No (from human to human)

Lethal?

- Humans with inhalational exposures may develop hemorrhagic inflammation of the airways early in the course of illness, which may progress to bronchopneumonia and lead to death.

Vaccine Available?

- No

Possible Method(s) of Delivery as Bioterrorist Weapon:

- Aerosol

Signs and Symptoms:

- Symptoms usually start 3 days after infection with the bacteria, but the onset may vary from 2 to 10 days. *(continued)*

(continued)

* Symptoms depend on how the infection is acquired: When tularemia infection is transmitted by way of the skin (through a scratch or bite), a sore usually appears at the site where the bacteria entered the body. This is usually accompanied by swelling of the lymph nodes closest to the site of sore. Swallowing the bacteria directly may cause throat infection, stomach pain, diarrhea, and vomiting. Inhaling the infectious material can produce fever and a pneumonia-like illness.

Treatment:

* Antibiotics are effective if prescribed early.

VIRL HEMORRHAGIC FEVER

Contagious?

* For some, yes (human to human)

Lethal?

* Death in as many as 50% of infections, depending upon virus

Vaccine Available?

* With the exception of yellow fever and Argentine hemorrhagic fever, for which vaccines have been developed, no vaccines exist.

Possible Method(s) of Delivery as Bioterrorist Weapon:

* Infected blood or tissue

Signs and Symptoms:

* Specific signs and symptoms vary by the type of VHF, but initial signs and symptoms often include marked fever, fatigue, dizziness, muscle aches, loss of strength, and exhaustion. Patients with severe cases of VHF often show signs of bleeding under the skin, in internal organs, or from body orifices like the mouth, eyes, or ears. However, although they may bleed from many sites around the body, patients rarely die because of blood loss. Severely ill patients may also show shock, nervous system malfunction, coma, delirium, and seizures. Some types of VHF are associated with renal (kidney) failure.

Treatment:

* Patients receive supportive therapy, but generally speaking, there is no other treatment or established cure for VHFs. Ribavirin, an antiviral drug, has been effective in treating some individuals with Lassa fever or hemorrhagic fever with renal syndrome. Treatment with convalescent-phase plasma has been used with success in some patients with Argentine hemorrhagic fever.

FEARFUL FORECASTS

Recent advances in genetic testing—most notably the polymerase chain reaction (PCR) test that became a household term during the O. J. Simpson proceedings—have enabled scientists to cast new light on the fingerprints of viruses and bacteria and how they instigate a

Are You Bugged Out?

DISEASE	POSSIBLE INFECTIOUS DISEASE ORIGIN
Heart disease	*Chlamydia pneumoniae*
	Helicobacter pylori
	Cytomegalovirus
	Pneumonococcal aerogenes
	Enterococci endocarditis
	Staphylococcus aureus
	Enterococci faecalis
	Candida albicans
	Streptococcus
	Herpes virus
Juvenile diabetes	Coxsackie B virus
Obsessive-compulsive disorder (OCD)	Coxsackie B virus
Alzheimer's disease	*Chlamydia pneumoniae*
Schizophrenia	Brona virus
	Influenza virus
Gallstones	Clostridia
	Eubacteria
Crohn's disease	*Mycobacterium pneumoniae*
Breast cancer	Human version of mouse mammary tumor virus

variety of chronic and sometimes debilitating diseases in humans. The genetic component of infectious disease makes some of us the unwitting victims of ominous and predisposing factors over which science currently has no control.

HEART DISEASE

Heart disease is the leading cause of death in the United States and is projected to be the leading cause of disability in the world by 2020. According to the American Heart Association, heart disease caused 459,841 deaths in the United States in 1998—1 of every 5 deaths. It is responsible for 600,000 of the more than 2 million deaths from all causes.

Researchers from Johns Hopkins University studied 900 heart disease patients and found that the more infectious agents that patients tested positive for, the more likely they were to die of a heart attack. Researchers are not sure how infection causes heart disease but hypothesize that it may have something to do with direct infection and inflammation of an artery wall. The healing of the infection results in plaque formation. Although not an established medical fact, it is highly likely that chronic infections contribute to heart disease. The following infectious pathogens are most closely linked to heart disease:

- *Chlamydia pneumoniae* is present in respiratory infections such as pneumonia, sinusitis, and bronchitis. By age 30, 50% of people have been infected with *Chlamydia pneumoniae;* by age 70, that number rises to 80%. Some researchers suggest that an uneventful *Chlamydia pneumoniae* infection during childhood could start a chronic infection of the coronary arteries that goes unnoticed until a heart attack occurs 50 years after the fact.
- In the gastrointestinal tract, the presence of *Helicobacter pylori* has been associated with a chronic low-grade infection. Researchers are now linking the bacteria to heart disease as well. In one British study, heart attacks were twice as common among people infected with *H. pylori* than people not infected with the bacterium.

◆ Gum disease—both gingivitis and periodontal disease—is caused by several types of bacteria. In severe cases, bacteria can escape into the bloodstream and wreak havoc elsewhere in the body. In addition, free radicals generated by the inflammation of periodontal disease may promote the oxidation of low-density lipoproteins (LDLs), enhancing the development of atherosclerosis.

Don't Break Your Heart

People with congenital heart disease (which affects more than 1 million Americans) are at greater risk for developing life-threatening endocarditis, an infection of the heart valve, when they have body parts pierced or tattoos done. Performed improperly, piercing and tattooing open up the skin to potentially deadly bacteria. People at risk for this infection should take preventive antibiotics before undergoing any piercing procedures or tattooing.

Though relatively rare, endocarditis can also occur as a result of periodontal infection, urinary tract infection, pneumonia, and certain dental procedures. Among high-risk people, endocarditis prevention via antibiotics is recommended for dental procedures including the following:

◆ Extractions
◆ Periodontal procedures including surgery and scaling
◆ Dental implants
◆ Root canals
◆ Placement of orthodontic bands
◆ Cleaning of teeth when bleeding is expected

STROKE

Research suggests that frequent and chronic bronchitis is associated with acute cerebrovascular ischemia—otherwise known as stroke. Research has also shown that poor dental health can double the risk of stroke.

CANCER

The first strong link between cancer and infectious disease was uncovered with the discovery that human papilloma virus (HPV) types 16 and 18 are implicated in cervical cancer, the second most frequent malignant tumor in women worldwide. In the 1830s, scientists noticed that celibate women almost never contracted cervical cancer. (This was before Louis Pasteur had introduced the germ theory of disease.) More than 150 years later, German researchers demonstrated that HPV could cause cervical cancer. We now know that HPV is responsible for virtually all cases of cancer of the cervix, which can develop decades after a woman is exposed to the virus. In men, HPV has been implicated in prostate cancer. Preliminary research suggests that an HPV vaccine could be used to protect all women from HPV and to treat existing tumors caused by the virus.

In 1999, German researchers observed that the treatment of fungal infections led to the remission of leukemia in three patients. Up to 30% of leukemia patients develop fungal infections; of those, 50 to 90% will die as a result of high fevers and weakness caused by the infections. The team suspects that cytokines, produced by the body to fight the fungal infections, also fight off leukemia. The findings offer hope for the development of a more targeted way to kill cancer cells without killing healthy cells at the same time.

The most common form of liver cancer—hepatocellular carcinoma, which is almost always fatal—is on the rise in the United States: up more than 70% from the mid-1970s to the mid-1990s. Public health officials expect this rise to continue until chronic hepatitis B and C are reined in. The hepatitis viruses, especially C, cause liver scarring, which leads to cirrhosis and then, often, to cancer.

ALZHEIMER'S DISEASE

Alzheimer's disease is a slow, degenerative condition that affects speech, movement, and mental ability. The brains of people with Alzheimer's are littered with abnormal plaque-like deposits of proteins called amyloid beta peptides. These proteins interfere with the brain's nerve cells. As Americans live longer, the rate of Alzheimer's disease is on the rise. More than 5 million Americans have Alzheimer's disease. Almost 70% are women. By the year 2050, as many as 14.5 million people could be afflicted.

Studies show that *Chlamydia pneumoniae* may be linked to late-onset Alzheimer's disease. Researchers believe that the organism enters brain cells and causes inflammation. Although *Chlamydia pneumoniae* is related to the bacterium that causes the sexually transmitted disease known as chlamydia, it is not sexually transmitted. Rather, it is a common pathogen that is present in respiratory infections such as pneumonia, sinusitis, and bronchitis.

Bugs and the 'Burbs

Scientists at the University of Washington believe they have found a link between Alzheimer's disease and the condition of one's childhood home. In their study, people who grew up in the suburbs were less likely to develop Alzheimer's than people who grew up in poorer farm areas or in more crowded cities, where children are more likely to be exposed to infectious disease.

In August 2000, scientists from Nankai University in Tianjin, China, reported an important discovery about the makeup of both Alzheimer's disease and the human form of mad cow disease, Creutzfeldt-Jakob disease (CJD). Both of the disorders are marked by a gradual and ultimately fatal deterioration of the brain, and both are associated with proteins of very similar structure, known as prions. The protein implicated in Alzheimer's was made up of extra-component reductive amino acids (protein building blocks), which are more prone to attack by free radicals. When enough free radicals accumulate to damage a protein molecule, it can malfunction.

BUG-BUSTING BLOCKBUSTERS

* Wash your hands often throughout the day, especially during cold and flu season. Ten to twenty times per day may not be obsessive-compulsive if in fact you come in contact with many people.
* Keep hot foods hot and cold foods cold.
* Wash kitchen counters and utensils frequently with soap and hot water, especially after preparing poultry and other meat.
* Wash fresh fruits and vegetables before eating.
* Cook poultry, meat, and fish thoroughly.
* Keep immunizations up to date for children, adults, and household pets.
* Use antibiotics exactly as prescribed. Don't self-medicate with antibiotics or lend your medicine to anyone.
* Tell your doctor if an infection does not improve after you have taken a full course of antibiotics.
* Avoid unsafe sex and intravenous (IV) drug use.
* Stay alert to disease threats when you travel. Get all the recommended vaccinations.
* Allow yourself the time necessary to recuperate from an illness.
* Exercise caution around wild animals and domestic animals that are not known to you. If you are bitten, seek medical care immediately.
* Avoid areas of insect infestation. Use insect repellents on skin and clothing when you are in areas where mosquitoes or ticks are common.
* Don't ever drink untreated water while hiking or camping.

[2]

Sworn to
Defend, Protect, and Serve

There is at bottom only one genuinely scientific treatment for
all disease and that is to stimulate the phagocytes.

—*George Bernard Shaw,* The Doctor's Dilemma, *1911*

Optimal health is a state in which our body systems, organs, and cellular processes all function perfectly and in a state of total balance.
This enables us to ward off the very first attempts from foreign substances that try to invade and contaminate this delicate equilibrium.
Tip the scale so that our bodies wind up light on the defense mechanisms, however slightly, and we risk succumbing to infectious disease.

The body's ability to ward off infectious disease depends on the
interplay between and within four major body systems:

1. Endocrine system
2. Immune system
3. Lymphatic system
4. Nervous system

Let's salute these systems and their mechanisms that guard our
good health.

THE ENDOCRINE SYSTEM:
COMMAND AND CONTROL CENTRAL

In this era of increasingly sophisticated communications technology, it's easy to lose sight of one of the most amazingly complex yet efficient communications networks of all. And it's right under your nose (so to speak). It's hormone HQ—that is, your endocrine system.

The endocrine system is made up of a number of glands, including the adrenals, ovaries, testes, thyroid, parathyroid, and pituitary. These glands secrete hormones—or chemical messengers that influence the function of organs throughout the body. Too much or too little of any hormone will cause an imbalance that can have serious consequences.

The health of your endocrine system is also intimately tied to your biological age. When your endocrine system is in peak performance condition, you are likely to feel good, look good, and successfully defend yourself against almost all infection and chronic disease.

Lots of internal signals and external factors, called modulators or disrupters, can impact or even short-circuit the endocrine communications system—for example, excessive exercise, disordered sleep, pregnancy, malnutrition, pharmaceuticals, phytochemicals (bioactive substances in plants), seasonal changes in light and temperature, and environmental toxins.

The Adrenal Glands

The adrenal glands, which sit atop the kidneys, act like shock absorbers in a 3,000-mile all-terrain endurance race, continually modulating their production of hormones in response to stress. The outer area of the adrenal gland, called the cortex, secretes the steroid hormones cortisol and dehydroepiandrosterone (DHEA), which it synthesizes from cholesterol.

Cortisol Cortisol is secreted by the adrenal glands according to a circadian (24-hour) rhythm established during infancy. A normal daily cycle begins with a peak level in the morning that gradually tapers off as the day progresses. Throughout the day, healthy cortisol levels help your body to effectively use nutrients, maintain muscle, and promote heart health.

Cortisol levels are regulated by hormones produced by the pituitary gland and the hypothalamus. These hormones and cortisol counterregulate each other, forming a feedback loop that keeps cortisol at an optimal level. This checks-and-balances system can be interrupted by lack of sleep, stress, and certain physical conditions.

Large amounts of cortisol are released in response to physical stress such as exercise; physiological stress such as severe illnesses, surgery, or burns; and psychological stress such as a lost job, bad relationship, or demanding lifestyle. As long as the stress—real or imagined—remains, so also does the high level of cortisol. Prolonged stress damages the feedback loop that regulates cortisol levels. Stress-related disruptions in cortisol levels have been associated with premature aging and depression. Long-term oversecretion of cortisol due to chronic prolonged stress can lead to Addison's disease, hypertension, and hypoglycemia, each of which can be deadly.

Unrestrained cortisol secretion exhausts the body. It can inhibit immunity, slow protein synthesis (necessary for tissue repair), and lead to neuronal loss, brain damage, bone loss, muscle wasting, increased abdominal fat, psychosis, premature aging, and death.

DHEA Dehydroepiandrosterone, better known as DHEA, has been dubbed the "mother of all steroids." The most abundant steroid in the human body, it is involved in the manufacture of testosterone, estrogen, progesterone, and corticosterone. DHEA levels begin to rise at about age 7, keep rising for the next 20 years or so, and then decline gradually until very little remains in circulation by age 75.

DHEA appears to be a potent immune system booster. Dr. Raymond Daynes, head of the division of cell biology and immunology at the University of Utah at Salt Lake City, found that it rejuvenated many measurements of immune function in mice, including the production of T cells and other immune factors, which decline with age. Older people do not respond as well to vaccines as younger people. But when Daynes gave old mice vaccines laced with DHEA, their ability to mount defenses to such diseases as hepatitis B, influenza, diphtheria, and tetanus equaled that of a young animal.

DHEA may also be beneficial in fighting autoimmune disease, in which the body's immune system attacks its own tissue as though it were a foreign invader. In a clinical trial of 57 women with the autoimmune disease systemic lupus erythematosus, researchers at Stanford University Hospital found that DHEA relieved symptoms such as skin rashes, joint pain, headaches, and fatigue. Many also reported a higher tolerance for exercise and better concentration.

Although DHEA can reverse the immune suppression caused by excess cortisol, when stress becomes chronic, the adrenals can no longer maintain production of the extra DHEA needed to do the job. An elevated cortisol-to-DHEA ratio signals the initial stage of adrenal exhaustion, resulting in impaired immunity.

DHEA's Quad Play

- Maintains immune resistance against infection
- Necessary for stable blood sugar levels
- Converts fat to lean muscle
- Decline correlated to onset of age-related diseases, including cancer, coronary artery disease, and osteoporosis

The Thyroid

The thyroid is a small butterfly-shaped gland located behind the hollow of the throat. It synthesizes two hormones, thyroxine (T4) and triiodothyronine (T3), which directly affect virtually all of the body's metabolic processes, steadying everything from body temperature to heartbeat. Hypothyroidism, in which levels of either, or both, thyroid

Symptoms of a Sluggish Thyroid

+ Labored breathing
+ Muscle cramps
+ Persistent lower-back pain
+ Bruising easily
+ Mental sluggishness
+ Emotional instability with crying jags
+ Mood swings
+ Temper tantrums
+ Getting cold easily (particularly in the hands and feet)
+ Dry, coarse, leathery, or pale skin
+ Coarse hair and/or loss of hair
+ Loss of appetite
+ Stiff joints
+ Atherosclerosis (hardening of the arteries)

Home Detection of Hypothyroidism
(Barnes Basal Temperature Test)

1. Shake down an oral thermometer and place it next to your bed before going to sleep.
2. As soon as you awake, place the thermometer under your armpit and leave it there for 10 minutes before getting up.
3. Record the temperature. If it is below normal rising temperature (97.8° to 98.2°F) for two consecutive days, you are very likely to be hypothyroid. (Menstruating women should wait until after the first day of their period before taking this test.)

If you are low according to the Barnes test, have your doctor conduct a thyroid-stimulating hormone (TSH) blood test.

hormones are low, can create a host of vague symptoms such as lack of energy, weakness, and mental sluggishness. Hypothyroidism also disrupts the body's equilibrium, and colds, viruses, and respiratory ailments may take hold more easily. An estimated 15 to 40% of the population suffers from an underactive thyroid.

In the summer of 2000, researchers at the Morehouse School of Medicine in Atlanta announced proof positive that stress hormones do indeed help infections take hold. Culturing two species of pneumonia bacteria with and without the stress hormones adrenaline and noradrenaline, Tesfay Belay and colleagues found that both strains grew faster in the presence of hormone. In one, concentrations of the bacteria were measured to be 4,000 times that in the control (nonhormone-treated) culture. Given that people release large quantities of stress hormones in times of physical injury, Dr. Belay's study shows a clear interconnection between the endocrine and immune systems that can quite literally "bug us."

THE IMMUNE SYSTEM: THE DEFENSE DEPARTMENT

A clear concept of an immune system emerged only in the mid-1970s. Today, the development of techniques for measuring immune system response has become one of the hottest topics in medical research. We are learning how keenly sensitive the immune system is to fluctuations in environment, diet, exercise, sleep, and stress.

We can't see the immune system; its complex network is spread all over the body. Without an immune system, anything could attach itself to you—inside or out—and grow unchecked.

Who Am I?

Immunocompetence, which is the body's biological sense of what is self and what is not, develops in the womb and in the first few months after birth. In the fetus, stem cells produced by bone marrow are called to "boot camp" in the thymus gland, where they develop into T cells. The T cells graduate if they learn how to recognize "self" by reading a unique molecular code that appears on the surface of all the cells in the body; if not, they are eliminated. This activity is part of a process called histocompatibility—a term you are likely to hear more frequently as organ transplant technology evolves.

A healthy immune system captures and destroys things in the body that shouldn't be there—bacteria, viruses, parasites, chemicals, even splinters. Invaders that stay outside the cells are easier to conquer than those that enter the cells. White blood cells are a key component of the immune system. A cubic millimeter (cc mm) of blood normally contains 4,000 to 10,000 white blood cells. The ideal white count is about 6,000 to 7,000 per cc mm of blood. Too few white blood cells means your immune response is low; too many means that your immune system is working inefficiently. Knowing the type of white blood cell that is elevated signals what kind of infection you have—bacterial, viral, or parasitic.

Battle Strategy

A nonspecific reaction is the immune system's most basic tactical move. When you cut yourself and the area swells and turns hot and pink, you're experiencing the symptoms of a nonspecific reaction. The more researchers study this initial reaction, the more they appreciate its complexity and importance.

Neutrophils, a type of white blood cell that patrols the body at all times, are the first to arrive at the trouble site. Neutrophils send distress signals and block the area so that the infectious agent can't spread.

Macrophages, cells stationed at strategic points all over the body, are next on the scene. They start chewing up the invader and send out chemical messengers called cytokines that activate still more immune cells. Macrophages also prepare a rap sheet on the invader, packaging little pieces of the culprit as evidence for the helper T cells that arrive later to assess the threat and plan a larger attack.

When a foreign element enters a cell, the cell itself has the ability to summon T cells to the site. If the invader doesn't match the unique molecular code on the outside of the cell—that indicator of "self" discussed earlier—the T cells will destroy it and will make new T cells programmed to always remember that particular invader. This immunological memory is the power behind vaccines.

The immune system's special forces, white blood cells called *lymphocytes,* or *T cells* and *B cells,* are part of the learned or combinatorial immune system. They can slice and dice, shuffle and combine, a limited number of genes to make tens of millions of antibodies and killer T cells in response to specific invaders. While even the most primitive creatures have an immune system, it appears that only jawed vertebrates have the more advanced combinatorial system as well, and scientists still don't know why.

Like neutrophils, lymphocytes originate from stem cells in the bone marrow. Some mature in the bone marrow and become B cells, which produce and secrete antibodies. B cells remain on alert in the lymphatic system until they are called into action.

Other lymphocytes become T cells during a stay in the thymus gland. They circulate through the lymphatic system—a network of vessels, ducts, and nodes that includes organs such as the tonsils, adenoids, spleen, and appendix. The lymphatic system removes bacteria, viruses, antigens, and other biowaste from circulation. The lymphatic system connects to every organ in the body except the brain. It goes into high gear during infection, and the lymph nodes nearest the infection become swollen with the filtered "nonself" microbes and biowaste from the infection itself.

There are several different kinds of T cells, each with a specific duty. *Helper T cells* dispatch and coordinate other T cells and direct B cells to make antibodies. Helper T cells can live a long time and remember the invaders they've encountered. They can help the immune system to react even faster in a repeat attack.

Some helper T cells (TH1) deal with the immune response to bacteria, viruses, and parasites; others (TH2) focus on allergic reactions and antibody responses. Research indicates that poor diet, high stress, and exposure to environmental toxins can suppress TH1 activity. It's the nature of the system that when TH1 activity decreases, TH2 activity is increased. When this happens, TH2 cells secrete chronically high amounts of compounds that stimulate inflammation and fever. This reaction, when stimulated inappropriately or chronically, leads to inflammatory diseases such as arthritis and autoimmune conditions such as asthma, lupus, multiple sclerosis, and chronic fatigue.

Killer T cells (also called natural killer (NK) cells) have special receptors on their surface that recognize certain antigens, or invaders. When a cell is infected with a virus, for example, the cell presents a fragment of the virus on its surface. The killer T cell latches on to this fragment, recognizes it as "nonself," and injects a chemical called a cytokine into the cell to destroy the virus. Killer T cells are the kamikazes of the lymphocyte army. All NK cells demonstrate an ability to inject a lethal substance to cause the cell to explode.

Suppressor T cells are the immune system's "cease-fire" switch, keeping B cells and helper T cells under control. Like killer T cells, *B cells* focus on only one antigen, bind with the antigen, and morph into large plasma cells that produce antibodies called immunoglobulins. These immunoglobulins patrol the body like smart bombs looking for their targets. Antibodies that respond to the first exposure to an antigen are very different from antibodies that cause an immediate allergic reaction.

The Thymus Gland: Commanding the T-Cell Brigade

The thymus gland, located in the chest, is a primary organ of the immune system. It activates T cells and produces hormones key to the immune system. At puberty, our immune system reaches its zenith, and our thymus gland is at its largest. The thymus begins to shrink until it is a shriveled shadow of its former self by age 40. By age 70, more than 95% of it has turned to fat or fibrous tissue. The shrinking thymus correlates with a rise in the diseases associated with aging, including cancer, autoimmune diseases, and infectious diseases. There is also a decline in T cells and immune factors such as interleukin-2. As such, scientists believe that restoring thymus gland function can rejuvenate the immune system.

Key Thymus Functions The thymus produces T lymphocytes, which are essential for resistance to infection from moldlike bacteria, yeast (including *Candida albicans*), fungi, parasites, and viruses, and for protection against development of cancer and autoimmune disorders, including allergies and rheumatoid arthritis.

The thymus gland also releases hormones (thymosin, thymopoietin, and serum thymic factor), low levels of which are associated with depressed immunity and increased susceptibility to infection. Typically, thymic hormone levels will be very low in the elderly, individuals prone to infection, cancer and AIDS (acquired immunodeficiency syndrome) patients, and when an individual is exposed to excess stress.

Pumping Up the Thymus Zinc is perhaps the most critical mineral to thymus gland function. When zinc levels are low, the number of T cells is reduced, thymic hormone levels are lower, and many critical white blood cell functions are severely lacking.

Melatonin, a hormone that is produced by the pineal gland in the brain and is responsible for regulating sleep patterns, stimulates the thymus. Melatonin levels are highest around puberty, when the thymus is at its largest size. Starting in the late teen years, melatonin levels decline and the thymus starts to shrink. The thymic-stimulating model of aging suggests that the decline in melatonin levels causes the thymus to shrink and the immune system to falter, leading to disease vulnerability.

When Italian immunologist Walter Pierpaoli, M.D., Ph.D., and his associates put melatonin in the drinking water of older mice, the animals became much more resistant to disease. The weight of their thymus glands increased and their thymus cells became more active, suggesting that they were producing new, active immune cells.

In 1985, Keith Kelley, M.D., a research immunologist at the University of Illinois at Urbana-Champaign, showed that injections of cells that secrete human growth hormone (HGH) could regrow the shriveled thymus gland in old rats so that it was as large and robust as that of young rats. Kelley's work was subsequently confirmed by

Israeli scientists, who used bovine growth hormone to reverse thymus shrinking in mice, and similar results have been shown in dogs.

HGH Improves Immune Activities

- Manufacture of new antibodies
- Increased production of T cells and interleukin-2
- Greater proliferation and activity of disease-fighting white blood cells
- Greater activity of anticancer natural killer cells
- Stimulation of bacteria-fighting macrophages
- Increased maturation of neutrophils
- Increased production of new red blood cells

Albumin: One of the Most Important
Markers of Immune Status

The battle against germs is waged by the immune system by launching protein-based substances such as albumin. Normally found in most animal tissues, sharp declines in albumin levels correlate to an increase in the risk of contracting serious infectious disease.

Albumin is assembled in the liver from more than 500 amino acids—that is, protein building blocks obtained from food or manufactured within the body. It serves the following important functions:

- Protects tissue from free radical attack, which can destroy cells by interrupting their normal processes
- Guards against heart disease by transporting antioxidants, which help keep coronary arteries clear, capture fats that can clog arteries, and stabilize the ratio between HDL (good) and LDL (bad) cholesterols

- Binds waste products, toxins, and drugs that would otherwise cause damage
- Maintains pH balance (see Chapter 16)
- Reduces the propensity for red blood cells to clump together to form plaques that might clog arteries
- Transports a range of nutrients from blood to cells
- Stabilizes red blood cells and growth hormones
- Plays a major role in controlling the amount of water in body tissues
- Transports thyroid hormones
- Maintains the blood-brain barrier
- Maintains mineral levels in the bones
- Binds to cortisol to move it away from vital organs

Albumin levels fall when the immune system is burdened by toxins that we consume, inhale, or touch. The link between albumin levels and cancer was observed as early as the 1700s. Chimney sweeps, who suffered from a high rate of scrotal cancer, were urged to wash thoroughly every day to remove the soot from their bodies. Their risk of developing scrotal cancer dropped to nil. A relationship between albumin and heart disease was established in the late 1980s by a British study. Low levels of albumin are also associated with a range of other diseases.

In 2001, researchers at the University of Ferrara, Italy, studied 344 older men and women living in nursing homes and found that low albumin levels were a strong predictor of mortality risk. Increasing disability was likewise correlated to depressed albumin levels. No one in the study group exhibited indicators of acute illness.

To maintain overall health, a program of regular and fastidious hand-washing (see Chapter 7) will significantly decrease the potential load of infectious agents trying to gain access to your body.

THE LYMPHATIC SYSTEM:
SOLDIERS THAT BATTLE INVADERS

Lymph is a plasmalike substance that drains water, proteins, and electrolytes from body tissues in a system of vessels called lymph vessels, or lymphatics. The lymph flowing through these vessels ultimately empties into the bloodstream via a large vein in the neck. Lymph nodes, which are nodular structures about the size of a pea (or less), are clustered along the lymph vessels. Groups of lymph nodes are found in the neck, behind the ears, in the armpits, below and above the elbows, in the groin area, and in the hollow of each collarbone. Lymph nodes serve three purposes:

1. They trap contaminants so that white blood cells can scavenge them before they cause harm.
2. They filter lymph to prevent foreign particles from entering the bloodstream.
3. They function as sites of storage and proliferation of B and T lymphocytes.

The lymphatic system may be considered as the terrain in which the immune system operates. When the lymph nodes become enlarged and tender, it means they're responding to an infection that you've contracted.

THE NERVOUS SYSTEM:
SENTRIES WATCHING OVER THE IMMUNE
RESPONSE

One of the most threatening endocrine disrupters today is physical, emotional, and psychological stress. High stress and anxiety are killers and are probably the most common cause of premature aging. During World War II, concentration camp survivors frequently developed many age-related disorders, including the very early onset of Alzheimer's-like disorders—as early as age 35.

A two-way flow of information, conducted through hormones or hormone-like proteins, engages the immune and nervous systems in an interlocked function in the presence of stress. This interplay involves the following:

- The adrenal glands, which release cortisol after receiving stress messages sent by the brain
- Hormones and neuropeptides (hormone-like chemicals released by nerve cells), which convey messages to cells of the nervous system, as well as organs throughout the body and throughout the immune system
- Macrophages and T cells, which carry receptors to certain neuropeptides, to which killer cells respond
- Activated lymphocytes, which transmit information to the nervous system
- Thymus hormones, which act on cells in the brain
- The brain, which sends messages along networks of nerve fibers connected to the thymus gland, spleen, lymph nodes, and bone marrow

Autoimmune Disease

In autoimmune disease, the immune system mistakes part of your body for a foreign invader and attacks your own tissue, trying to kill what it considers as hostile. According to the American Autoimmune Related Disease Association (AARDA), approximately 50 million Americans (20% of the population) suffer from autoimmune disease. Of these, the majority—some say as many as 30 million—are women.

Autoimmunity is now established as, or highly suspected to be, the underlying cause of more than 80 chronic diseases, including lupus, Type I diabetes, rheumatoid arthritis, thyroid disease, ulcerative colitis, Crohn's disease, scleroderma, Sjögren's syndrome, endometriosis, and multiple sclerosis. Advocates such as AARDA are encouraging the medical community to consider these disorders as a unique category of diseases that differ anatomically but share a common etiology (cause)—that is, autoimmunity—and to explore effective treatments across medical disciplines addressing the fundamental cause of autoimmune disease rather than the symptoms of various disorders.

Very early in life, the immune system learns to distinguish "self" from "nonself," but some of the immune system's cells (lymphocytes) remain capable of reacting against "self." As long as these cells are suppressed, all is well. Trouble can begin when immune system cells begin to attack your own tissue—either because they are not suppressed or because there is an alteration in your body tissue that they mistakenly identify as "nonself." Virtually everyone experiences some degree of autoimmunity, and for the most part, no harm is done. Autoimmune disease occurs when there is actual damage to the body.

Medical science doesn't have all the answers for why your immune system might turn against you. The genetic susceptibility to autoimmune disease is a tendency toward autoimmunity in general. Thus, people in the same family may have different autoimmune disorders.

Vestigial or Vital?

Often referred to as vestigial organs, implying that they might have served a functional purpose in our ancient ancestors but evolution has outmoded their use, the tonsils, adenoids, appendix, and spleen are also part of the immune system. Scientists are revisiting this demotion, suspecting that surgical removal of these organs may compromise immunity.

Anders Moller and Johannes Erritzoe of Université Pierre et Marie Curie in Paris, France, compared the health of birds killed in accidents to those killed by domestic cats. Examining more than 500 birds from 18 species, Drs. Moller and Erritzoe found that:

- Birds succumbing to repeated infections or infested with parasites had smaller spleens than their healthy counterparts.
- In 16 species, the spleens of birds killed by cats were, on average, 30% smaller than those that died of accidental causes, lending truth to the phrase "survival of the fittest."

Source: The Economist, June 3, 2000.

The other half of the equation is environment. Autoimmune conditions became more prevalent in the last half of the twentieth century. Some scientists think autoimmune diseases are a modern phenomenon triggered by the toxins and pollutants that now regularly bombard our bodies.

Autoimmune processes can slowly destroy cells or tissue, interfere with organ function, or stimulate certain organs to grow excessively. Some people may experience multiple disorders. Autoimmune diseases are generally classified into the following two categories:

1. Organ-specific disorders, in which the autoimmune process is directed mostly against one organ such as the thyroid (Hashimoto's thyroiditis), stomach (pernicious anemia), adrenal glands (Addison's disease), or pancreas (insulin-dependent diabetes)
2. Non-organ-specific disorders, in which autoimmune activity is spread throughout the body as in rheumatoid arthritis, systemic lupus, and dermatomyositis

While the media and popular press are filled with information on how to boost or enhance your immune system, it's equally important

Everyday Encounters That Destroy the Immune System

- Pollution
- Food additives
- Food-processing techniques
- Certain drugs
- Nutritional deficiencies
- Certain bacterial infections (such as salmonella)
- "Foreign" materials such as silicone implants and perhaps mercury alloy dental fillings, as well as plastic and titanium joint replacements
- Mental and emotional stress

to understand that in some people the immune system can make a mistake that leads to autoimmune disease.

BUG-BUSTING BLOCKBUSTERS

Be Good to Your Adrenal Glands

- Eat a whole-foods diet, and minimize (preferably, eliminate) substances that stress the adrenals such as sugar, caffeine, and alcohol.
- Go outside and enjoy nature for an hour a day. Researchers are finding that, in addition to causing seasonal depression, a lack of natural light may hamper the function of the adrenal glands.
- Adopt stress management techniques:
  - List your daily activities and rank them in order of priority. Accomplish what you can, but don't fret if everything doesn't get done.
  - Enjoy leisure activities. This reduces the constant taxing of stress on the adrenals.
  - If you find yourself embroiled with conflicts at work, home, or anywhere else, take the time to resolve the matter with those involved. If necessary, seek professional counsel. If you keep negative emotions bottled up, your adrenals might figuratively explode.
- Siberian ginseng contains a component that the body uses to manufacture pregnenolone, the precursor to DHEA. Supplement 100 milligrams once or twice a day (take only a morning dose if the effects are too stimulating).

Reduce Your Levels of Cortisol, the "Hormone of Death"

Chronic excess cortisol compromises your immune system. To protect yourself, consider the following:

• Make simple lifestyle changes, including:

  • Set aside 30 minutes daily for quiet self-reflection: no television, no radio, no disruptions of any kind (no exceptions, no excuses).
  • Do a moderate exercise workout daily—for example, 15 minutes of aerobic activity.
  • If you are in a high-stress work situation, take a 15- to 20-minute midday nap to prepare you for the climb of cortisol levels in the afternoon.
  • Practice deep breathing for 10 minutes three times per day.

• Take vitamin B complex and vitamin C (500–1,000 mg daily), both of which have been shown to reduce the cellular damage caused by external stress.
• Get a dog—a great stress buster and the best fitness coach on four legs.

Maintain Healthy Levels of DHEA

• For DHEA supplementation, divide a starting dose of 10 to 25 milligrams into three or four administrations across the day, and be sure to have your physician test your blood levels quarterly. Be mindful that taking too much DHEA (more than 100 mg per day) can turn off your own internal production. Take it every other day, or alternate it with a DHEA precursor, such as dioscorea (wild yam) capsules.
Warning: DHEA should not be taken by anyone with a history of prostate or ovarian cancer because it can metabolize to testosterone and estrogen in the blood. Check with your doctor before taking.
• Reduce stress. In a study at the Institute of Heartmath in Boulder Creek, California, people who lowered their stress by relaxation techniques and listening to music had a 100% increase in their DHEA levels and a 23% decrease in cortisol.

Help Your Thyroid Help You

- Eat the following foods in moderation (less than four times a week), as they may suppress thyroid function:

Brussels sprouts	Peaches
Mustard greens	Pears
Spinach	Turnips
Cabbage	Broccoli
Kale	

- Take a kelp supplement, which contains iodine, a basic ingredient of thyroid hormone.
- Use bottled water for drinking and brushing. Fluoride (found in toothpaste and most municipal water sources) and chlorine (in tap water) suppress thyroid function.

Note: While thyroid supplements may be available from health food stores, we advise you not to treat yourself. It is possible to overdose on thyroid hormone. Check with your physician.

Always Seek Qualified, Expert Medical Care

An American Autoimmune Related Disease Association (AARDA) survey showed that more than 65% of patients with autoimmune disease have been labeled hypochondriacs or chronic complainers in the early stages of their illness. Find a physician who is updated on these latest interventions for successful treatment of autoimmune disease:

- First, correcting any deficiencies the autoimmune disease may be causing, such as hormone, thyroid, or insulin deficiencies. In blood-related autoimmune disorders, certain blood components may be replaced via transfusion.
- Next, controlling or balancing the activity of the immune system, a process known as modulating. The goal is to diminish

the damaging autoimmune response while preserving the immune system's ability to fight disease in general. Corticosteroid drugs are usually used to help achieve this balance. In some cases, however, more powerful drugs are needed.

[3]

You Are What You Eat

The gastrointestinal (GI) tract, the largest system in the body, is 28 to 30 feet long with a total surface area of almost 6,000 square feet—about the dimensions of a tennis court! It is where the majority of infectious disease battles are fought. From the time a substance enters your mouth, until its unwanted ingredients or by-products exit the anus, you are at risk for that substance to cause you harm.

As we age, certain physiological changes increase our risk for succumbing to food-borne illnesses. The stomach produces less acid; the immune system slows. A food-borne illness can weaken older folks quickly, complicating any chronic ailment they may have. Declines in mental function also can impair correct food handling and personal hygiene practices.

THE DIGESTIVE PROCESS

Digestion begins in the mouth, where saliva begins to break down food. Once in the stomach, the chyme (mixed food) is broken down further by pancreatic enzymes and hydrochloric acid. The gallbladder releases bile salts, which help break down fat. Ideally, small particles of food enter the small intestine. Nutrients are absorbed by the body and the waste products enter the colon (large intestine), where they are formed into feces that move through the colon propelled by rhythmic muscle contractions called peristaltic action. If food has not been well digested in the small intestine, it can serve as sustenance for unfriendly bacteria living in the colon.

MODERN-DAY DINING TRENDS

Today's food-borne outbreaks are widespread and sporadic, and it is often difficult for public health officials to isolate the ultimate source and alert those at risk in a timely fashion. Due in large part to health promotion campaigns urging Americans to choose more fresh fruits and vegetables, the United States has increased importation of foods, many from countries that lack proper food safety standards. The consumer demand for preservative-free products is a trend that ultimately gives the bugs a clear advantage.

Preservatives, added by food manufacturers to prevent spoilage during the time it takes to transport foods over long distances to stores and our kitchens, function as either antimicrobials or antioxidants, or both. As antimicrobials, they prevent the growth of molds, yeasts, and bacteria. As antioxidants, they keep foods from becoming rancid, browning, or developing black spots. Antioxidants also mini-

Unappetizing Condiments

In May 2000, three teenagers were apprehended and charged with serving hamburgers topped with spit, urine, and cleaning solvents for months at a New York State Thruway Burger King. The teens allegedly sprayed burgers with oven cleaner, caustic stove cleaner, and abrasive cleanser with bleach. Any of the diners could have suffered symptoms ranging from burning or irritation of the lining of the mouth to severe burning of the stomach or esophagus. The Burger King restaurant in which these incidents took place had just passed health inspection two months earlier.

mize the damage to some essential amino acids—the building blocks of proteins—and minimize the loss of some vitamins.

Through the complicated system of growing, processing, importing, distributing, handling, preparing, and serving prepared food, you literally put your health in the dirty hands of strangers. You can, however, make simple changes and smart decisions to reduce the odds that you'll regret going to the grocery store, restaurant, or local fundraising picnic.

FOOD-BORNE DISEASE

Since 1975, scientists have identified 30 new microorganisms implicated in the recent rise in food-borne and water-borne infectious diseases in the United States. The growing epidemic is attributed to three major factors:

1. Changes in the ethnic composition and eating habits of the American population
2. Increasingly complex—and global—system of food distribution

Gambling in Our Schools

School districts across the United States are playing roulette with thousands of school-age children. When the U.S. Department of Agriculture (USDA) recently instituted a zero tolerance standard for salmonella and *Escherichia coli* in beef sold to schools, the new requirements caused a 50% increase in the cost of ground beef sold to schools. Instead of paying the extra cost, many school districts are opting out of the government program and are now buying less rigorously inspected open-market beef—and hoping that the cafeteria workers cook it thoroughly before serving it.

3. Retraction of surveillance for infectious agents at local, state, national, and international levels

Food-borne infectious diseases not only cause acute gastrointestinal (GI) distress (commonly nausea, vomiting, and diarrhea) but notably increase the vulnerability of those with chronic illnesses.

Food Bug Basics

The U.S. food supply has changed greatly since the last generation, when 70% of foodstuffs were produced within 100 miles of home. Now supermarkets carry items from around the world. The General Accounting Office reports that the number of imported food entries into the United States more than doubled between 1992 and 1997, to 2.7 million items. Yet, FDA inspections declined from 8% of total imports to less than 2% during the same period.

In October 2000, Canadian researchers from the University of Manitoba in Winnepeg reported that pesticide sprays encourage bacteria, including salmonella, *Escherichia coli,* and shigella, to flourish on crops. The team warns that these bugs can pose a notable threat to

Leading Food Poisoning Offenders

FOOD	NUMBER OF OUTBREAKS SINCE 1990
Seafood (including finfish and shellfish)	237
Eggs	170, mostly as salmonella
Beef	91, 40 from ground beef
Fruits and vegetables (composite)	82, mostly sprouts and lettuce

An outbreak occurs when two or more people are infected from a single identified food.

Source: Center for Science in the Public Interest (CSPI), August 2000

people eating raw strawberries, raspberries, and lettuce. The bacteria thrived in a third of all pesticides, growing best in four of the most widely used fungicides, weed killers, and insecticides. The researchers determined that the bacteria multiply rampantly in tanks where pesticides are stored and are released during the widespread routine preventive spraying conducted during growing seasons.

What's Bugging You?

The media has confounded the seriousness of food-borne illnesses by flurries of coverage that may not truly serve the public benefit. Contrary to what the public may perceive from exhaustive coverage on television and in the newspapers, *E. coli* is not the second leading cause of food-borne infection (to salmonella). *Campylobacter jejuni,* commonly found in chicken intestines, is food-borne public enemy number 2. Campylobacter is a sporadically occurring illness, which may lead to Guillain-Barré syndrome, a condition marked by increased protein in the cerebrospinal fluid. Symptoms include numbness of the limbs, muscular weakness, and paralysis. *E. coli* grabs headlines because it causes outbreaks among clustered population segments at a time. Indeed, the CDC reports that overall incidence of food-borne disease declined from 1996 to 1998, due to decreases in salmonella and campylobacter infections.

Fast Facts on Food Poisoning

• While it is nearly impossible to obtain a precise count, the Centers for Disease Control and Prevention (CDC) estimates that there are from 6 to 80 million cases of food poisoning a year.

• Medical costs and lost wages due to food-borne salmonellosis, only one of many types of food-borne infections, have been estimated to be more than $1 billion per year.

• Infants, the elderly, and the immunocompromised are at increased risk of serious illness and death from food poisoning.

FOOD SAFETY FOR HOME

What comes to mind when you think of a clean kitchen? Gleaming floors . . . polished countertops . . . neatly arranged cupboards? A truly clean kitchen is one that ensures safe foods. This relies on more than just appearances—it means continual vigilance in following safe food practices in four major areas:

1. Selection of foods
2. Food storage
3. Food handling (before cooking)
4. Cooking and cleanup processes

Better Safe Than Sorry
At the Supermarket
   • Pick up packaged and canned foods first so that perishable
     foods spend minimal time away from refrigeration. Place
     frozen foods and meat, fish, and poultry in separate plastic bags
     so that drippings don't contaminate other foods.

Port-of-Entry Food Inspection Deficits

Because only a tiny fraction of food poisoning is reported to officials, actual attributable cases of outbreaks may be as much as 10 to 100 times higher than documented:

   • 1987: Salmonella from Mexican cantaloupes caused more than 25,000 illnesses in the United States.
   • 1997: An outbreak of hepatitis A in the United States was caused by frozen strawberries from Mexico.
   • 1997–1998: Guatemalan raspberries sickened 2,500 people in 20 American states and Canada.

- Don't buy foods in cans that are dented or bulging or in jars that are cracked or have loose or bulging lids.
- Check expiration dates and never buy outdated foods.
- Check the "use by" or "sell by" date on dairy products and other items that are dated and pick the ones that will stay fresh the longest.
- Choose eggs that are refrigerated. Cook eggs thoroughly. Salmonella will not grow at temperatures below 40°F and is killed at 160°F.
- Buy pasteurized apple juice and cider.
- Purchase fruits and vegetables that are in season. They likely have not been shipped from another country. Due to staffing limitations, the Food and Drug Administration inspects only one or two out of every 100 shipments of imported food.
- Check for cleanliness at the meat counter and salad bar.
- Have a cooler in your car for cold and frozen foods if it will take you more than an hour to get groceries home.

At Home
- Keep it clean—the refrigerator, the counter, the cupboards, the utensils, etc.
- Use an instant-read thermometer to ensure meat and poultry are thoroughly cooked. Ground beef and pork should be cooked to an internal temperature of 160°F; beef, veal, lamb, steaks, and fish to 145°F; chicken and turkey to 180°F.

The world's largest *E. coli* outbreak ever reported (10,000 documented cases) occurred in 1996 in Japan. The source implicated was the ingestion of raw radish (daikon) sprouts.

In an effort to reduce *E. coli* outbreaks, federal agencies, including the Food and Drug Administration and the U.S. Centers for Disease Control and Prevention, have approved irradiation of ground beef. Irradiation uses electric or radioactive beams to kill bacteria at the processing plant.

Bacteria Sources and Symptoms

BACTERIA	SOURCE	SYMPTOMS	HOW SOON IT STRIKES	HOW SOON IT ENDS
Escherichia coli	Ground beef, raw milk, lettuce, sprouts, unpasteurized juices	Severe abdominal pain, watery (then bloody) diarrhea, occasional vomiting	Within 1 to 8 days	Requires immediate treatment
Campylobacter	Raw/undercooked chicken, raw milk	Diarrhea (can be bloody), fever, abdominal pain, nausea, headache, muscle pain	Within 2 to 5 days	7 to 10 days
Salmonella	Poultry, eggs, raw meat, milk, and dairy products, fish, shrimp, sauces and salad dressings, cream-filled desserts and toppings, fresh produce	Nausea, vomiting, abdominal cramps, diarrhea, fever, headache	Within 6 hours to 2 days	1 to 2 days
Listeria	Hot dogs, deli meats, raw milk, soft-ripened cheese, raw and cooked poultry, raw meats, ice cream, raw vegetables, raw and smoked fish	Fever, chills, and other flulike symptoms; diarrhea; infections of the blood (septicemia); inflammation of the brain (encephalitis) or membranes of the brain or spinal cord (meningitis); spontaneous abortion or stillbirth	Within a few days to 3 weeks	Requires immediate treatment
Vibrio haemolyticus	Raw oysters and clams, crabs, shrimp	Diarrhea, abdominal pain, nausea, vomiting, headache, fever, chills	Within 4 hours to 4 days	2½ days

(continued)

(continued)

BACTERIA	SOURCE	SYMPTOMS	HOW SOON IT STRIKES	HOW SOON IT ENDS
Vibrio vulnificus	Raw oysters and clams, crabs	Diarrhea (in healthy people), bloodstream infection (in people with liver disease, diabetes, or weak immune systems)	Within 16 hours (diarrhea)	Requires immediate treatment
Norwalk virus	Shellfish, salads	Nausea, vomiting, diarrhea, abdominal pain, headache, low-grade fever	Within 1 to 2 days	1 to 2½ days
Hepatitis A	Shellfish, salads, cold cuts, sandwiches, fruits, vegetables, fruit juices, milk, milk products	Fever, malaise, nausea, loss of appetite, abdominal pain, jaundice	Within 10 to 50 days	1 to 2 weeks

Source: Center for Science in the Public Interest (CSPI).

- Keep hot foods hot and cold foods cold after they are prepared.
- Refrigerate or freeze perishables right away. The refrigerator temperature should be 40° to 45°F and the freezer should be at 0°F.
- Thaw frozen foods in the refrigerator or the microwave rather than letting them sit at room temperature.
- Marinate foods in the refrigerator. Don't use marinade from raw meat, poultry, or seafood on cooked food unless you boil it first to kill bacteria.
- Always check labels to determine how foods should be stored initially and after being opened.
- Don't store food near household cleaning products.
- When storing meat, fish, and poultry, be sure juices can't escape and contaminate other foods.

- Store leftovers in airtight, labeled and dated containers and use within three days.
- Store eggs in their carton in the refrigerator, where it is cooler than on the door. Discard cracked eggs.
- Rewash packaged prewashed lettuce before you use it.
- Don't crowd the refrigerator or freezer so much that air can't circulate.

Dr. Klatz's Personal Regimen for the Uneasy Queasies

My personal regimen for ridding food-borne bugs is a low-tech, drug-free approach, and one for which you can keep supplies on hand:

1. Within the first 25 minutes of those uneasy queasies (for me, it's usually an unexpected cramping, gurgling, or sloshing in my stomach), I induce emesis—that is, vomiting. Trigger your gag reflex (stick your finger down into your throat; do not jab) or take a dose of syrup of ipecac (follow label directions) followed by 3 cups of warm tap water with 1/2 teaspoon of salt in each cup.
2. I've found that letting diarrhea run its course is the body's most effective purging system. If, however, diarrhea continues past one hour, you might try the following:

   a. Sip aloe vera juice, 2 ounces every hour.
   b. Sip Pepto-Bismol, 2 ounces every hour.
   c. Consume whey protein (the immunoglobulins deactivate various toxins), 2 to 3 tablespoons, dissolved in 6 ounces of water.
   d. Use ileocecal bowel massage (see Chapter 17) to help open the ileocecal valve (ICV), located between the small and large intestines, which, when not functioning properly, allows waste material to accumulate in the small intestine where it becomes toxic.

Helpful hint: Begin Immodium (follow package directions) to slow bowels if diarrhea is not controlled after one hour of evacuation.

Note: Take care to stay hydrated (page 96).

Important: For diarrhea lasting past 24 hours (in adults) or 8 hours (in children), or if delirium, loss/altered consciousness, or dehydration occurs, seek emergency medical attention immediately.

- Throw out anything that looks or smells suspicious.
- Scrub and rinse raw fruits and vegetables thoroughly.
- Never eat raw sprouts. Seeds for sprouts start with a high number of microorganisms hitching a ride after they leave the farm, and germination and sprouting (with its high moisture and warm temperature) produces high numbers of pathogenic bacteria ready for you to ingest.
- Move older canned goods to the front of the cupboard, to be used first.
- Wash and sanitize cutting boards after use. Either put them in the dishwasher or wash and rinse in a solution of 1 teaspoon of chlorine bleach to 1 quart of water. Consider two cutting boards: one for raw foods and one for cooked foods.
- Wash lids of canned foods before opening them. Wipe down jars and bottles before returning them to the refrigerator.
- Wash the blades of can openers after every use.
- Thoroughly clean food processors and meat grinders after use.
- Wash hands regularly while handling all food. Wash with warm water and liberal amounts of soap for at least 20 seconds. Be sure to clean under nails (and close to the nail beds), where 90% of all bacteria hide. Use a clean, dry paper towel to dry your hands (never a sponge or kitchen towel that has already been used).
- Anyone experiencing diarrhea, a cold, or the flu should not prepare food for themselves or others until the illness subsides.

Sickening Liquids

Generic liquid dishwashing soap is up to 100 times more effective than antibacterial soaps in killing respiratory synctial virus, which can cause life-threatening infant respiratory diseases. The simple fact is that frequent and thorough handwashing is the number 1 proven way to prevent getting and spreading infectious diseases.

- Wash your hands after handling raw chicken or meat. The government's "sniff and poke" inspection system does not detect microbial contamination. For example, as much as 60% of the raw poultry sold at retail probably carries some disease-causing bacteria.
- Either clean dishes with an automatic dishwasher and then air-dry, or wash them by hand right away with hot water and soap and then air-dry. Leaving dishes to soak in water creates a soup in which bacteria receive the nutrients they need to multiply. When washing dishes by hand, do so within two hours. Air-drying reduces the chances for human contact to transfer bacteria to the clean dishes.

Leftovers Can Be a Land Mine

Refrigerate hot foods as soon as possible after cooking, within two hours maximum. Never keep any food that has been standing out for more than two hours. Date leftovers so they can be used within three days of refrigeration.

Punch Up the Flavor, Punch Out the Bugs

A taste for spicy foods may have evolved in hot climates because spices help cleanse foods of pathogens. Some spices are so powerful that they can kill or stop the growth of dozens of types of bacteria. The following spices have been shown to inhibit at least 30 bacteria species:

Garlic	Caraway
Onion	Mint
Allspice	Sage
Oregano	Fennel
Thyme	Coriander
Cinnamon	Dill
Tarragon	Nutmeg
Cumin	Basil

Cloves

Parsley

Lemongrass

Cardamom

Bay leaf

Pepper

Chili/cayenne

Ginger

Rosemary

Anise seed

Marjoram

Celery seed

Mustard

Lemon

Lime

How Long Will It Keep?

PRODUCT	STORAGE PERIOD	
	REFRIGERATOR	FREEZER
Ground beef	1–2 days	3–4 months
Steaks and roasts	3–5 days	6–12 months
Pork chops	3–5 days	3–4 months
Ground pork	1–2 days	1–2 months
Pork roast	3–5 days	4–8 months
Lunch meat	3–5 days	1–2 months
Sausage	1–2 days	1–2 months
Lean fish	1–2 days	Up to 6 months
Fatty fish	1–2 days	2–3 months
Whole chicken	1–2 days	12 months
Chicken parts	1–2 days	9 months
Swiss, brick, processed cheese	3–4 weeks	Freezing will affect texture and taste.
Milk	5 days	1 month
Fresh eggs in shell	3–5 days	Not applicable
Hard-boiled eggs	1 week	Not applicable

Sources: Food Marketing Institute; U.S. Department of Agriculture.

Use vinegar-based dressings liberally. Vinegar markedly reduces the number of colonies of *E. coli* on vegetables, particularly those standing at room temperature. Additionally, salt, which is found in nearly all commercially prepared dressings, enhances the bactericidal activity of vinegar.

Raw honey (sold at bee farms, not commercial products commonly sold in supermarkets) can be a sweet way to boost your immunity. In a lab study of 345 unpasteurized honey samples, the majority exhibited antibacterial action against the food-poisoning bacteria *Staphylococcus aureus*. Researchers found that the raw honey contains an enzyme that, in the presence of a little water, produces hydrogen peroxide—a mild antiseptic. In general, stronger, darker honeys (such as buckwheat, sagebrush, and tupelo) have greater antimicrobial activity—enough, actually, to act as food preservatives.

Cinnamon to the Rescue

Kansas State University researchers report that just 1 teaspoon of cinnamon powder killed 99.5% of *E. coli* (populated to 100 times typical contamination levels for the experiment) within three days. The same researchers suggest that cinnamon would also have antimicrobial effects on other food-borne illnesses.

Commercial Counterparts to Homemade Recipes

Commercial products such as cookie dough, ice cream, mayonnaise, Caesar salad dressing, and eggnog are, by law, made with pasteurized eggs—that is, eggs that have been heated sufficiently to kill bacteria—and also may contain an acidifying agent that kills bacteria.

At Risk with "Farm Fresh"

We owe a great debt of gratitude to Louis Pasteur, whose experiment of heat treating and rapid cooling of milk gave rise to the bacteria-killing food preparation process that bears his name. Yet, in seeking foods that are "natural" or "farm fresh," we have unwittingly departed from the primary infectious disease prevention tactic invented over 150 years ago.

Raw juices (such as fresh pressed apple cider) are a particular risk. While just 2% of the nation's juice supply is estimated to be "raw," these beverages make us vulnerable to infectious disease in four ways:

1. Raw juices are not subjected to pasteurization.
2. Pathogens on just one or a few pieces of fruit can spread throughout an entire batch of juice.
3. Low-level contamination can cause severe illness, especially in young children, the elderly, and those with chronic disease.
4. Certain pathogens can survive acidic conditions in juice at refrigerator temperatures.

If you insist on drinking unpasteurized juices, follow these five steps to minimize exposure to *E. coli* and other bacteria that may be harbored by these drinks:

1. Consume before the "use by" date.
2. Do not buy raw juices that are unrefrigerated.
3. Keep raw juices refrigerated at home, and do not leave out after pouring.
4. Heat the raw juice to a boil (or 180°F minimum) for one second; consume immediately while piping hot or refrigerate promptly to avoid recontamination.
5. Be very careful about serving raw juices to children, seniors, the immune-impaired, and pregnant women.

Who Cares?

Men may be less safe about food practices than women. When asked if they believed that cooked food left at room temperature overnight is safe to eat without reheating (the correct answer is no), 12% of men responded yes (only 5% of women did). Nearly 40% of those under age 40 indicated they did not adequately wash cutting boards, while only 25% of those age 60 and over indicated the same.

FOOD SAFETY FOR DINING OUT

Today, the average person consumes four restaurant meals a week, supporting an industry making $376 billion. Coincident with this trend, according to the U.S. Centers for Disease Control and Prevention, about 60% of food-borne disease occurred outside the home in 1970, but the number skyrocketed to as high as 80% by the 1990s.

The booming food service industry has placed a largely unmanageable burden on local health officials to inspect dining establishments on a frequent and intensive basis. The Center for Science in the Public Interest's (Washington, D.C.) study of 45 municipalities in "Dine at Your Own Risk" reports the following:

- Only half were able to inspect restaurants at least twice a year.
- None enforced all 12 key FDA food safety guidelines.
- Only 13% enforced the FDA's Food Code on cooking temperatures for meats, poultry, fish, and eggs.
- Only 64% required that hamburgers be cooked at high temperatures for the sufficient time to kill *E. coli*.

Dining Out Defense: A Checklist

[ ] *Does the dining establishment display its most recent inspection report?* While there is no national requirement to do so, restaurants that post the report in a location visible to patrons are likely to have

less to hide than facilities that don't post it at all. Look for a sparkling record, the equivalent of an A+, on this report card.

[ ] *What does the bathroom look like?* A poorly maintained bathroom may reflect deficits in other areas of the establishment. Is there soap in the bathroom? If not, odds are the employees don't wash properly before returning to their posts.

[ ] *How are tables cleaned?* Do bus personnel use the same cloth or sponge on all tables? Do they use any disinfectant solution? Do they clean their hands before setting the table for the next patrons?

[ ] *If it's an open kitchen (where you can see the food being prepared and cooked), does everyone use gloves?* Even if so, verify that the handler doesn't use the same gloves to perform a nonfood prep function (such as tending the register or answering the phone), then return to food preparation duty wearing the same gloves.

[ ] *Keep your order simple.* At a sit-down restaurant, don't choose anything elaborate—the more steps involved in creating a dish, the greater the chances are for mishandling and contamination.

[ ] *Speak up.* If your food is supposed to be served hot, it should be piping hot; if it's supposed to be served cold, it should be chilly. If a poultry dish is bloody or pink, send it back.

[ ] *Get out . . . or get sick.* If the wait staff gives you a difficult time when you alert them to potential infectious disease land mines in the establishment, leave.

Advocacy for Proper Hygiene and Sanitation at Dining Establishments

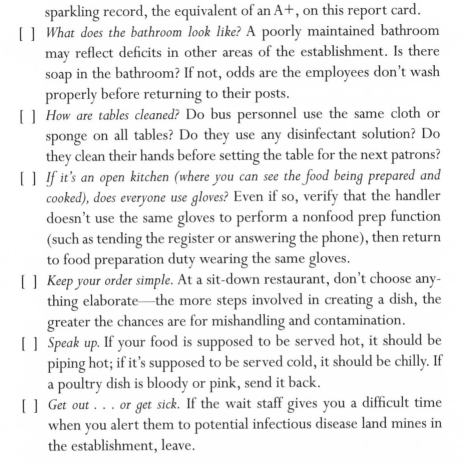

C onsumers for
E ducation,
A wareness, and
S afety of
E ateries

Established in 2000 by the American Academy of Anti-Aging Medicine (A4M, Chicago, IL), the Consumers for Education, Awareness, and Safety of Eateries (CEASE) encourages restaurant patrons to alert establishment owners and managers of flagrant hygiene and sanitation violations that, left uncorrected, may result in anything from discomfort to death. CEASE encourages all restaurant patrons to carry two copies of the CEASE Violation Notice (Appendix G) whenever dining out. If you

Wise Diners . . .

+ Do not eat at a salad bar unless a plastic or glass covering (a sneeze guard) is installed over the area, reducing the chances that bodily fluids, hair, and skin of fellow patrons become items you tote away from the bar. Get your servings from as far back in the containers as you can reach.
+ Do not order "salad" sandwiches (chicken salad, turkey salad, etc.). Typically made with leftovers, the environment is a bacteria haven.
+ At fast-food outlets, special order the main selection. This will increase the chances that you will not be served an item sitting under a warmer and thus harboring bacteria.

observe violations that put your own health and those dining with you at risk, complete the notice. Hand-deliver one copy to the owner or manager on duty. When you get home, log on to the Better Business Bureau's Internet Web site at www.bbbonline.com. Follow the instructions to file an on-line complaint, being sure to list the offenses that you observed and marked on the CEASE form.

Dirty Money

Dr. Love of the University of California has reported that at least 10% of the dollar bills she has cultured contain potentially pathogenic bacteria capable of causing disease, namely *E. coli* and *Staphylococcus*—common food-poisoning offenders.

This finding confirms the earlier work of Dr. Theodore Pope and his colleagues at Wright-Patterson Air Force Base Medical Center. The team found that more than 75% of the dollar bills they examined contained bacteria that can cause significant infections in the immunocompromised. Says Pope, "Paper currency is widely exchanged for goods and services. . . . If some of these bills are contaminated with bacteria, there is potential to spread these organisms from person to person. Our results suggest that paper currency . . . may play a role in the transmission of potentially harmful organisms."

Source: MedServe Medical News, May 24, 2001.

STOMACH HEALTH IN THE AGE OF RISING
FOOD-BORNE DISEASE

Peptic Ulcers

You won't get them from too much stress, a night of bar hopping, your daily dose of lattes or cappuccinos, or your penchant for spicy or fried foods. Rather, as many as 90% of peptic ulcers are caused by the bacteria *Helicobacter pylori* infection (the other 10% result from chronic/ overuse of aspirin and other nonsteroidal anti-inflammatory drugs [NSAIDs]). Peptic ulcers (an ulcer is an erosion of body tissue) occur in either the stomach (gastric ulcer) or in the first portion of the small intestine (duodenal ulcer). Duodenal ulcers occur in an estimated 6 to 12% of the U.S. population, affect four times as many men as women, and are four to five times more common than gastric ulcers.

Gastric acid helps us digest the food we eat. It is highly corrosive: If it were placed on the skin, it would eat straight through to the bone. Ulcers form when gastric acid comes into contact with the stomach or small intestine tissue, which is normally protected by a layer of mucin, a slippery layer of mucus. *H. pylori,* aspirin, and other NSAIDs are the three primary culprits that break down the protective layer to create a situation where gastric ulcers can readily form.

Helicobacter Pylori Most people acquire *H. pylori* bacteria in childhood, and it is estimated that one-third to one-half of the world's population is infected. For most, the bacteria remain dormant, but for others a peptic ulcer results. Ninety to one hundred percent of patients with duodenal ulcers, seventy percent with gastric ulcers, and fifty percent of people over the age of 50 test positive for this bacterium.

Peptic ulcers may lead to serious medical complications if untreated, including hemorrhage, perforation (erosion of the ulcer through GI tissue), and obstruction. For some people, *H. pylori* infection can lead to stomach cancer. In fact, in 1994, the World Health Organization declared the bacterium a carcinogen. It is not yet known

Signs and Symptoms of a Peptic Ulcer

You may experience abdominal discomfort:

- 45 to 60 minutes after meals or during the night, described as gnawing, burning, cramplike, or aching, or as "heartburn"—present when the stomach is empty, such as between meals or in the early morning. Pain may last several hours.
- Discomfort is relieved by food, antacids, or vomiting.
- Abdominal tenderness.

Your physician may use the following diagnostics to confirm the presence of a peptic ulcer:

- X ray or fiber optics (endoscopic exam).
- Positive test for blood in the stool.
- Food allergy testing: Food allergens are triggers for recurrent ulcers.

whether it is a good idea to eradicate *H. pylori* in people who test positive for the bacterium but have no negative symptoms.

Low gastric acid output and low antioxidant content in the GI lining are the primary factors that make people vulnerable to peptic ulcers. *H. pylori* infection increases gastric pH, which leads to ulcer formation, which leads to more *H. pylori* infection.

H. pylori is diagnosed either by measuring antibodies to *H. pylori* present in blood or saliva, or by culturing material during endoscopy (a visual inspection of the intestinal tract). If testing confirms you have *H. pylori,* your doctor may prescribe one or more of the following:

- Antibiotics for the bacterial infection
- H-2 blockers, drugs that reduce stomach acid and are commonly prescribed for ulcer treatment
- Medications to coat the ulcer area
- Antacids to neutralize excess stomach acid

Be sure to follow dosing instructions exactly, and tell your physician right away if your stools become bloody, dark, or tarry-looking.

Bismuth, a naturally occurring mineral, acts as an antacid that wipes out *H. pylori*. Whereas bacteria may develop resistance to antibiotic strains, they are unlikely to do so with bismuth. The best-known and most widely used bismuth preparation is bismuth subsalicylate (Pepto-Bismol).

When to See the Doctor

- Vomiting, beginning as bloody or having the appearance of containing coffee grounds
- Stool that is bloody, black, or tarry-looking
- Diarrhea as a result of antacid use
- Severe abdominal pain
- Weakness, paleness

Dietary Enzymes

Our bodies make enzymes and also obtain them from food, particularly raw food. So far, about 3,000 enzymes have been identified. Some enzymes break down large nutrient molecules such as proteins,

Fizzling Relief

With as many as 70 million Americans affected by some type of digestive malady, total costs of treatment are upwards of $107 billion per year. A substantial portion of this bill is for over-the-counter GI remedies, including antacids. While antacids lower the likelihood of a person developing a peptic ulcer by reducing the acidity of the stomach lining, they also raise the risk of contracting a food-borne infection, since pathogens may survive in a less acidic environment.

carbohydrates, and fats. Others govern the storage and release of energy from nutrients, while still others oversee the circulatory, respiratory, and other systems. Together, enzymes act in a chain reaction of biochemical activity known as metabolic reactions.

With age, enzyme quality and quantity deteriorate, and, therefore, so does the digestive process. But the speed at which this happens can depend a great deal upon lifestyle factors such as diet. For example, enzymes need vitamins, known as coenzymes, and minerals, known as cofactors, to help them do their work.

Enzymes can be influenced negatively by trauma, chemotherapy, surgery, chronic pain, depression, stress, and chronic illness; and by environmental triggers such as exposure to pesticides and heavy metals (e.g., lead and mercury). It's important to maintain an internal equilibrium that's friendly to digestive enzymes, as their mutiny can be a primary cause of abdominal aches and pains.

H. Pylori Vaccine Under Development

In July 2000, researchers at the University of Padua in Italy announced that a vaccine to flush H. pylori out of its hiding place deep in the crevices of the GI lining is readying for clinical trials. Dr. Cesare Montecucco discovered that H. pylori injects a toxin called VacA into cells that line the gut, causing them to swell and expel their enzymes. These enzymes help to degrade the protective mucous layer, making food for the bacterium directly available—and enabling ulcers to form when the gastric acid comes into contact with the gut tissue.

BUG-BUSTING BLOCKBUSTERS

Be Compulsive About Safe Food Practices

- Make sure your fridge is running at 40°F (5°C) or less, freezer at 0°F (−18°C) or less.
- Don't open the fridge or freezer needlessly. Doing so raises the temperature. Make a mental list of everything you need to grab

from the fridge to make dinner, then haul it all out at once.
Teach children to do the same.

* Thaw foods in the fridge or microwave, or submerge in cold
  water that's freshened on the half hour.

* Wipe the tops of cans before opening, to prevent foreign
  agents from entering the food.

* Wash hands before, between, during, and after preparing
  meals.

* Wash all vegetables, including the precut kind. These veggies,
  sometimes sold as ready-to-eat salad or salad mix-ins, may be
  advertised as "no rinsing necessary," but during the misting
  process common in supermarket produce sections, they
  become moist, even within sealed packaging, and hence can
  harbor bacteria. The washing procedure before packaging is
  also questionable.

* Refrigerate hot foods as soon as possible—no more than two
  hours after cooking.

* Date all leftovers to use within three days. Throw out all
  leftovers once they've passed that time frame. If in doubt,
  throw it out. Never taste-test leftovers (a single bug-blooming
  bite is all you need to contract food-borne illness).

Sanitize to Keep Bacteria at Bay

* The FDA's Center for Food Safety and Applied Nutrition
  reports that the kitchen sink drain, disposal pipe, and
  connecting pipe are breeding grounds for bug growth. Pour a
  solution of 1 teaspoon (5 ml) of chlorine bleach in 1 quart (1
  L) of water down the sink, at least once a week.

* Use a solution of 1 teaspoon (5 ml) of chlorine bleach in 1
  quart (1 L) of water to clean the cutting board between
  handling raw meats, poultry, and fish, and other foods (such as
  vegetables, fruits, and breads).

* Use a solution of 1 teaspoon (5 ml) of chlorine bleach in 1
  quart (1 L) of water to clean kitchen countertops and other
  surfaces in contact with food.

• Sanitize countertop sponges by microwaving (for 60 to 90 seconds, but take care not to melt your sponge), or immerse in a solution of 4 teaspoons (20 ml) of hydrogen peroxide in 1 quart (1 L) of water.

Plant and Animal Enzymes with Anti-inflammatory and Antimicrobial Functions

ENZYME	SOURCE	FUNCTION
Pancreatin	Animal	Alleviates disturbed digestion
Lipases	Plant	Break down and digest fat
Amylases	Plant	Break down and digest carbohydrates
Proteases	Plant	Break down and digest proteins
Papain	Unripe papaya	Relieves inflammation; used to treat sports injuries, respiratory ailments, viral diseases, and degenerative diseases; destroys gastritis-causing bacteria; used to treat ulcers; stimulates tumor necrosis factor (TNF), a cancer-killing agent
Bromelain	Pineapple	Assists stomach digestion and small intestine in absorption; relieves inflammation; used to treat sports injuries, respiratory ailments, viral diseases, degenerative diseases, burns, skin infections, and dental inflammations; stimulates tumor necrosis factor (TNF), a cancer-killing agent
Rutin	Plant	Antiviral and antibacterial
Lactase	Plant	Breaks down and digests lactose (sugar in milk)
Cellulase	Plant	Breaks down and digests fiber

General Peptic Ulcer Treatment Options

- Tell your physician if you are taking more than 50 milligrams of aspirin per day on a regular (three to four times a week) basis.
- Stop smoking. Smoking increases the backflow of bile salts (highly irritating agents) toward the stomach, decreases the secretion of bicarbonate (which neutralizes gastric acid) by the pancreas, and accelerates passage of food to the duodenum.
- Check your stool daily for bleeding and tell your doctor if you see blood.
- Reduce stress. Although it is not a causative factor in ulcers, stress is certainly a contributory one.
- Consume a diet rich in fiber. Diets rich in plant fibers are used to reduce the recurrence rate of duodenal ulcers.
- Consume raw cabbage juice. A quart a day (divided doses) has been shown to heal ulcers in an average of 10 days.
- Glutamine, 500 milligrams three times a day, can be taken instead of raw cabbage juice. It's the effective antiulcer ingredient in raw cabbage juice.
- Aloe vera juice soothes gut mucosa and is believed to possess antibiotic and cellular-healing properties. Consume 1 quart per day if active bleeding of an ulcer is present.
- Always talk with your doctor before starting a self-treatment program.

[4]

Digestion, Immunity, and Parasites

The intestines—the lower part of the gastrointestinal (GI) tract—conduct the final digestive processes from which the body harvests nutrients from food before it becomes waste. Our intestines remove toxins created by the digestive and cellular processes. The intestines are home sweet home for bacteria (called intestinal flora). Representing 400 different species, these microorganisms typically comprise 2 to 3½ pounds of body weight. In all, the intestines may be home to as many as 100 trillion organisms—more than the number of cells in the entire body!

We all have armies of "good" and "bad" bacteria in our intestines. The good bacteria perform functions necessary to sustain life—from vitamin and enzyme production to enhancing digestion and absorption of proteins. Good bacteria also suppress potentially threatening microorganisms from multiplying and spreading. For example, *Candida albicans,* normally a quiet resident in our bowels, spreads aggressively to cause disease if there is an insufficient quantity of good bacteria to prevent it from overgrowing.

Friend or Foe?

Mark Konlee, editor at the nonprofit organization Keep Hope Alive Limited (www.keephope.net) and publisher of a nationally distributed newsletter on immunity and advances in nontoxic HIV treatments, suggests this simple self-check to determine if your gut is home to friendly flora:

• Are your stools large in diameter, brown, and float on water?
• Is your urine yellow at least once or twice daily? (It will get lighter if you consume lots of water, yellow after taking a B-complex vitamin.)

Answering yes to both these questions is indicative of intestinal health. Stools that measure 1 to 1½ inches in diameter indicate there is no inflammation in the colon. Stools float when your bifido (natural flora bacteria) are producing a healthy quantity of fatty products. Stools that are often yellow or light in color, or urine that is consistently brown, may indicate that you have a hepatitis infection.

The Good Guys

Of the 400 or so known species of bacteria that colonize the upper and lower gastrointestinal tract, lactobacilli and bifidobacteria are the most important and beneficial.

Lactobacilli, found in the lower portion of the small intestine, produce the enzyme lactase, which is necessary for the digestion of milk-based foods. They also produce lactic acid, which helps maintain an optimum acidic environment in the gastrointestinal tract, thus preventing the growth of harmful alkaline-loving microorganisms. Most important among the lactobacilli is *L. acidophilus,* which helps to control the overgrowth of opportunistic organisms such as yeasts. Lactobacilli perform the following functions:

• Through the production of lactic acid, acidify the colon to inhibit the growth of undesirable bacteria such as salmonella, *Escherichia coli,* and *Helicobacter pylori.*
• Produce a fatty acid that makes it difficult for fungi and yeast *(Candida albicans)* to grow.

- Decrease the time it takes for waste products to move through the digestive system (transit time).
- Aid the synthesis of vitamins B and K.
- Aid the synthesis of butyric acid, which helps prevent colon cancer.
- Help convert more cholesterol to bile acid, thus allowing less cholesterol to accumulate in the bloodstream.
- Help metabolize toxic environmental chemicals.
- Help regulate hormones. Estrogen is reactivated from bile acid by lactobacilli and reabsorbed.
- Eliminate bad breath caused by waste products and gas produced by unfriendly bacteria.

Yogurt is a familiar source of *Lactobacillus acidophilus,* but not all commercially produced yogurts contain living bacteria. Tufts University reports that most often store-bought yogurt contains as few as 100,000 cells of *L. acidophilus* bacteria or less per gram, which means you'd have to consume upwards of ten 6-ounce servings of yogurt to approach the recommended therapeutic dose.

Bifidobacteria, found primarily in the large intestine, produce acetic and lactic acid, along with B vitamins. Bifidobacteria also inhibit the bacteria that convert nitrates into potentially cancer-causing nitrites, thereby lowering the risk of gastrointestinal cancer. The growth of bifidobacteria in the lower intestine is largely dependent on the fiber and complex sugars (fructooligosaccharides, or FOSs) in your diet.

Acidophilus in Your Diet

The best way to add acidophilus to your diet is to make your own yogurt or take a supplement that has been tested by an independent laboratory and lists the concentrations of live bacteria on its label. Choose a well-known name brand with the highest count of live bacteria.

If you were delivered vaginally and were breast-fed, you received a double dose of healthful intestinal flora from your mother. Breast milk helps infants maintain the acidic pH in the intestines conducive to the growth of healthy bacteria. Formula-fed babies typically have a neutral or slightly alkaline intestinal pH.

Bacteria coexist in the intestine with colonies of yeast. In fact, bacteria keep yeast growth in check. Frequent or prolonged use of antibiotics can kill enough bacteria to destroy this balance and cause an overgrowth of yeast, which leads to infections such as vaginitis and chronic diarrhea. Out-of-control intestinal yeast is also thought to precipitate allergic symptoms or to aggravate existing allergies.

Certain strains of friendly bacteria produce powerful antibiotics, all produce acids, and some produce hydrogen peroxide (H_2O_2)—a powerful free radical scavenger. These products all effectively inhibit harmful bacteria, but none of them actually destroys bad microorganisms.

Unlike synthetic drugs produced in laboratories, natural antibi-

Good Bacteria

BACTERIA	SOURCE	PRODUCES ANTIBIOTIC(S)
Bifidobacterium bifidum	Supplements, bifido-enriched milk	Bifidin
Lactobacillus acidophilus	Supplements, acidophilus-enriched milk	Acidolin, Acidophilin, Lactobacillin, Lactocidin
Lactobacillus brevis	Milk, kefir, cheese, sauerkraut	Lactobrevin
Lactobacillus bulgaricus	Supplements, yogurt, cheese	Bulgarican
Streptococcus lactis	Cheese, cottage cheese, cultured buttermilk, raw milk products	Nisin

otics (and the other products of friendly flora) wield their bad bug–chasing powers without causing uncomfortable or dangerous side effects. Acidolin, produced by *L. acidophilus,* creates a highly acidic environment in the intestine that disintegrates cells cultured with both the polio and cowpox viruses. People with bowel disorders, even just bloating, may benefit from consuming probiotic supplements such as acidophilus after a meal.

The Bad Guys

Most people also have another type of resident in their intestines: parasites. Contrary to popular belief, parasitic infection is not just a third-world phenomenon. Parasites—worms and protozoa—do not seem to serve any useful function in the intestine and may contribute to allergic reactions. Infection with the protozoa *Giardia lamblia,* which contaminate streams and lakes and have been found in drinking water, is common among people with chronic gastrointestinal problems such as irritable bowel syndrome. The digestive disruption and nutrient absorption problems created by *Giardia* can cause diarrhea and fatigue.

The Good Worm

Generally, parasites such as roundworms and tapeworms are not good things. But a certain type of intestinal worm, a species of the helminth, may be an exception. University of Iowa researchers have suggested that the helminth worm can be used to trigger an immune modulation that dampens the immune response sometimes raised by the body against normal intestinal bacteria that can lead to inflammatory bowel diseases such as Crohn's disease and ulcerative colitis. Research is still in its early stages, but one day this helminth may turn out to be as popular as lactobacillus for intestinal well-being, especially among those with irritable bowel syndrome.

BOWEL FUNCTION

Once in a while, most of us go to the bathroom either too much (diarrhea) or not enough (constipation). Diarrhea is characterized by passing many loose, watery, or unformed bowel movements. Usually, diarrhea is a short-term reaction to a specific irritant such as mildly contaminated food, a minor infection, or stress. Diarrhea is your body's natural way of coping with insults (ingesting pathogenic foods or beverages, toxic exposures, or medication use) that the body considers disagreeable. It is generally safe to let diarrhea run its course, normally taking a day or so to subside. Because diarrhea is a symptom, not a disease, people with recurrent bouts should see their doctor to find the underlying cause and treat it properly.

One of the greatest risks with diarrhea is dehydration, which is characterized by dry mouth, wrinkled skin, excessive thirst, and little or no urination. In the case of diarrhea caused by infection, dehydration contributes to the success of the infectious agent in conquering your immune system. Replace the approximate volume lost in diarrhea by drinking about 8 ounces of water after every visit to the bathroom, plus 2 to 4 more cups per day. Rehydration also replenishes the essential minerals (sodium, potassium, calcium, magnesium) known as electrolytes. Temporary measures to institute immediate rehydration include sipping half-strength tea with lemon and sugar, or taking commercial Pedialyte.

When to See the Doctor

- Severe, continuous diarrhea with cramping and/or vomiting lasting 12 hours or more
- Moderate diarrhea lasts more than 5 to 7 days continuously
- Mucus, blood, or worms appear in your stool
- Diarrhea is accompanied by fever above 101°F (38.3°C), or by acute abdominal pain

If diarrhea continues past two hours, it is best to prepare and sip a homemade rehydration solution until the diarrhea subsides.

Into 1 quart of bottled water, add the following:

½ teaspoon of table salt
¼ teaspoon of salt substitute
½ teaspoon of baking soda
2 tablespoons of sugar

Adults should sip at least 3 quarts of this mixture during each day that diarrhea is present. Children (6 months and older) should drink at least 1 quart each day affected.

Other natural ways to help recover from a bout of diarrhea include the following:

- Eat a bland carbohydrate diet. Sweet, sour, and spicy foods tend to promote the wavelike contractions that aid digestion, which may hasten diarrhea. Limit your diet to bananas, rice, applesauce, and toast.
- Avoid carbonated beverages. They only add gas to an already delicate situation.
- Consume a mixture of 1 tablespoon of carob powder in applesauce or honey, one to three times a day.

Constipation is defined as infrequent or difficult bowel movements. It affects more than 4 million people in the United States on a regular basis. Common causes include the following:

- Failing to consume fiber
- Not drinking enough water
- Not exercising enough (exercise stimulates the bowels)

If an underlying disease is ruled out as the cause, simple lifestyle and dietary changes are effective. Many Americans are too reliant on laxatives. Laxative dependency has created an annual business of $500 million.

Irritable Bowel Syndrome

Irritable bowel syndrome (IBS) is characterized by alternating bouts of diarrhea and constipation as well as abdominal pain, flatulence, heartburn, and possibly nausea. IBS accounts for about 50% of all visits to gastroenterologists. Symptoms vary widely from person to person, which makes IBS difficult to define precisely. We do know, however, that emotional stress appears to play a key role.

A Minty Treat

Researchers in Taiwan confirm that peppermint (*Mentha piperita*) contains volatile oils that contribute to the herb's ability to quiet the churning and gurgling sometimes associated with IBS. Sip a few cups of peppermint tea a day. If symptoms don't improve within a week, you should see a physician.

Leaky Gut Syndrome

When the intestinal wall breaks down—due to an overaccumulation of waste material, food allergies, alcohol abuse, or the overuse of antacids, antibiotics, and nonsteroidal anti-inflammatory pain relievers (aspirin and ibuprofen)—the intestine is prone to inflammation. The body then absorbs damaging debris. This condition is known as leaky gut syndrome or intestinal permeability. Excessive absorption of toxins into the bloodstream can overstimulate the immune system, resulting in allergies and autoimmune diseases, including rheumatoid arthritis, lupus, fibromyalgia, and chronic fatigue syndrome.

The following natural substances may lower intestinal permeability and heal the gut:

- Glutamine: an amino acid that prevents and reverses intestinal mucosal damage while decreasing bacterial colonization.
- Bentonite clay (aluminum silicate): A well-known intestinal adsorbent, its large surface area soaks up many times its weight in toxins and bacteria.
- Quercetin: a natural bioflavonoid, similar in molecular structure to the prescription medication cromolyn sodium that is administered to suppress the allergenic reaction of the gut in response to foods.
- Aloe vera juice: for its gut-soothing and cell-healing properties.
- Fast of fruit or vegetable juice: Fasting for one to three days each month allows the gut to rest from its round-the-clock nutrient delivery functions.

USING NATURAL PRODUCTS

Fiber

The intestinal lining has the fastest growth rate of any tissue of the body; a new lining is generated approximately every three to six days. Daily consumption of 20 to 30 grams of fiber promotes lining regeneration, and 35 grams or more reduces the risk of chronic diseases. Sadly, the American Dietetic Association reports that most Americans consume only 11 grams daily. Fiber is composed of complex carbohydrates, and the only source is plant foods. It is sometimes referred to as a prebiotic, as it promotes growth of friendly flora while suppressing overpopulation of bad bacteria.

Fiber is categorized as either soluble or insoluble. Soluble fiber (which forms a glue-like paste in water) in whole grains, seeds, nuts, vegetables, and fruits promotes the production of short-chain fatty acids (SCFAs), which nourish the cells of the intestines, stimulate healing, and reduce the risk of cancer. SCFAs also inhibit the growth of yeasts, promote the growth of healthful bacteria, and reduce the liver's production of cholesterol. Inadequate consumption of soluble fiber can lead to intestinal permeability, and consuming too much (in the form of vegetable-based stimulant powders) can cause you to go to the bathroom excessively. Over time, you could become dependent on laxatives for bowel function.

Insoluble fiber, so named because it does not dissolve in water, helps prevent parasites and unhealthful bacteria from clinging to intestinal walls. Studies show that it lowers the risk for colon cancer.

Fructooligosaccharides

Fructooligosaccharides (FOSs) are indigestible carbohydrates that, like fiber, act as prebiotics by feeding both *L. acidophilus* and *L. bifidus*. FOS is present in a variety of fruits, vegetables, and grains, and is most plentiful in Jerusalem artichokes. It is resistant to digestive enzymes, and,

Fiber Sources

SOURCES OF SOLUBLE FIBER

Apples, bananas, citrus fruits, prunes, carrots, barley, oats and oat bran, lima beans, psyllium husks

SOURCES OF INSOLUBLE FIBER

Whole wheat, wheat bran, brown rice, rice bran, rye, cooked lentils, asparagus, brussels sprouts, flaxseed

SOURCES OF BOTH SOLUBLE AND INSOLUBLE FIBER

Kidney beans, navy beans, green beans, green peas, winter squash, corn

DOUBLE-DUTY PERFORMERS

Carrots, blueberries, and raspberries are sources of insoluble fiber that contain FOS contrary to what you might think based on the *saccharide* in the name, FOS does not raise blood sugar levels. As a therapy for diarrhea, constipation, foul-smelling stools, and gas, FOS is taken at up to 8 grams daily (1 teaspoon twice a day). As a general preventive measure, FOS may be taken at a dose of 1 gram per day. Too much FOS will cause diarrhea.

Cook Smarts

A number of culinary herbs and spices are natural antibiotics that can contribute to intestinal health.

Spices and Their Benefits

SPICE	BENEFIT
Garlic	Albert Schweitzer used garlic to treat amoebic dysentery at his clinic in Africa. Recommended dose: 3 small cloves daily.*
Onion	Although not as potent an antimicrobial as garlic, onion is easier to consume in large quantities. Recommended dose: 1 medium onion daily.*
Turmeric	A major ingredient in curry, turmeric lowers the number of gas-forming bacteria in the intestine. It is also an anti-fungal. Recommended dose: ¼ teaspoon daily.*
Ginger	Long used to relieve digestive upsets, ginger protects the intestinal lining and is thought to be effective against parasites. Recommended dose: ½ teaspoon twice daily.*
Sage	Sage contains an essential oil that kills yeast, bacteria, and worms. Recommended dose: ½ teaspoon daily.*
Rosemary	Rosemary contains an essential oil that kills yeast, bacteria, and worms. Recommended dose: 1 teaspoon twice daily.*
Oregano	Oregano contains an abundance of antibiotic, antiviral, antiparasitic, and antifungal substances. Recommended dose: 1 teaspoon twice daily.*
Thyme	Thyme is known for its antiparasitic abilities. Recommended dose: ¼ teaspoon twice daily.*

*Recommended doses listed here are amounts that should be added to food.

Probiotics

The term *probiotic* may not be a household word—yet. But probiotics are likely to become as common as antibiotics in your everyday health vocabulary. *Biotic* means "life." Whereas *antibiotics* inhibit life, *probiotics* promote life.

Probiotic therapy—the use of supplements of beneficial bacteria—has a long history. Farmers use probiotics to promote growth and health in livestock. Chickens are given a multibacterial probiotic to prevent deadly salmonella from growing in their intestinal tract.

Beneficial bacteria fend off harmful bacteria, viruses, and fungi, and also lower cholesterol, fight cancer and stomach ulcers, protect against food poisoning, and keep potentially harmful microorganisms in check. They are important in boosting immune function, preventing and treating a whole range of bowel problems from constipation to ulcerative colitis, manufacturing B vitamins, and aiding in digestion (especially of milk-based foods).

Antibiotics have many uses, but they do not distinguish between good and bad bacteria—they kill everything. Because many bad bacteria have developed strains that are resistant to antibiotics, it's the beneficial bacteria that often suffer the most casualties from antibiotic treatment. If you lose too many good bacteria, your body's natural defenses against infection and disease become seriously impaired.

Probiotics may be helpful in treating the following conditions:

- Anxiety, depression, stress
- Yeast infections
- Dental problems
- Diabetes
- Food poisoning
- Gastrointestinal conditions, including colitis, constipation, Crohn's disease, diarrhea (helpful if taken as soon as symptoms appear), irritable bowel syndrome, and toxic bowel syndrome

- Headache
- Osteoporosis
- Rheumatoid arthritis
- Skin problems such as acne and aging skin
- Urinary tract infection
- Vaginitis

Proper nutrition and maintaining a probiotic-friendly level of acidity (pH) in the gut are important to maximize your benefit from probiotic supplementation. For example, fruits, vegetables, and grains, which are high in fiber, promote the growth of bifidobacteria in the large intestine. Similarly, maintaining a neutral pH in the stomach supports the growth of friendly bacteria. Overuse of antacids can upset this ideal pH.

You can take a probiotic supplement daily to promote the growth of beneficial bacteria. Select it carefully, as quality, ingredients, and processing techniques vary widely. Keep the following considerations in mind:

- Among *L. acidophilus* strains, experts recommend *L. acidophilus* DDS-1 superstrain and *L. acidophilus* NAS superadhesion strain.
- Among bifidobacteria strains, experts recommend *Bifidobacteria bifidum* Malyoth superstrain.
- Read the label. The ideal probiotic supplement will guarantee a count of at least 2 billion bacteria of a specific superstrain. Look for products made with the full-culture production method (rather than centrifuging or ultrafiltration). This method preserves the bacteria's supernatant or growth base, which is rich in beneficial metabolic by-products.
- Freeze-dried powders, capsules, and wafers are preferred rather than liquid supplements, which are highly perishable.
- Glass bottles are preferable. Acidophilus packed in plastic bottles tend to lose potency and quality.
- Mind the expiration date. Bacteria counts drop as the product ages. Don't bother buying or taking supplements past the expiration date.

Generally, health experts recommend that people who simply wish to maintain healthy levels of friendly flora take one to two capsules of acidophilus containing 1 to 2 billion (that's *billion,* sometimes noted on labels as $\times 10^9$, not *million*) colony-forming units per dose. Some also suggest that acidophilus be taken before a meal (on an empty stomach), since stomach acid is lowest at that time, thus increasing the chances for the supplement to take residence in the intestine. When taking antibiotics, supplement with probiotics two hours after each dose, at bedtime, and for two to three weeks after finishing the course of antibiotics.

If you are taking probiotics to combat abnormal bowel function, be mindful that you may experience a temporary and transient set of mildly uncomfortable reactions. Dubbed Herxheimer's reaction (for the German physician who discovered it), the death of large numbers of harmful bacteria or fungi caused by the introduction of friendly flora sometimes causes bloating, gas, and/or headaches. These symptoms indicate the supplement is taking effect, deactivating and displacing the bad bugs. Depending on the severity of your GI imbalance at the time you initiate probiotic therapy, you may consider taking the minimum recommended dose and gradually increasing the amount and frequency.

Colostrum

Colostrum is the breast fluid produced by mothers just after delivering their babies. It is known as "first food." Colostrum is packed with the following:

- Immunoglobulins, to promote immune response
- Leukocytes that slow the multiplication of viruses
- Lactoferrin, an iron-binding protein with anti-inflammatory, antiviral, and antibacterial properties
- Lysozyme, an enzyme that destroys bacteria and viruses
- Proline-rich polypeptides, to boost T-cell production
- Cytokines and lymphokines, with antiviral and anticancer proteins

• Growth factors that promote wound healing and tissue repair, and stimulate growth and regeneration of muscles, bone, nerves, and cartilage
• An assortment of vitamins and minerals

Cow colostrum is the basis of all commercially available colostrum preparations. Unlike humans, who receive about 80% of their immune system gifts via the placenta, newborn calves are delivered with a blank immune slate and receive immunity solely from mother's milk. Bovine colostrum contains a high concentration of immune and growth factors. Humans can receive these nutrients by dietary supplementation.

Broad-spectrum antibodies in bovine (cow) colostrum have been shown in many studies to destroy *Escherichia coli,* cryptosporidia, rotavirus, streptococcus, salmonella, and shigella. *Helicobacter pylori* can only be killed by antibiotics and bovine colostrum. For those with leaky gut, colostrum has been likened to a dietary source for the "glue" that allows the cells of the gut to strengthen and support themselves once again. Those with milk (lactose) intolerance should be cautious, as colostrum is, after all, the first milk.

Not all bovine colostrum products are equally effective, nor do they contain the same amount of bioactive factors. Select a product in which the ingredients were not heat treated and contain no less than 15% immunoglobulins, as well as high concentrations of immune and growth factors. Colostrum is available in tablets, capsules, lozenges, bulk powders, meal replacement bars, and drink mixes. Choose the form that's most convenient for you.

A standard daily dosage of colostrum for maintaining good intestinal health is one to two tablets (providing about 15% immunoglobulin G [IgG]) or 1 to 5 grams of bulk powder. In illness (such as diarrhea, food poisoning, or other infection), take up to 10 grams per day. Always follow the label for brand-specific instructions.

BUG-BUSTING BLOCKBUSTERS

Banish parasites from your GI system. The following suggestions are from Keep Hope Alive's Mark Konlee:

- Slice a clove of raw garlic and serve on rye crisp. Consume with meals three times daily.
- Drink 4 ounces of sauerkraut juice before meals two to three times daily, or take 2 tablespoons of apple cider vinegar in water three times daily with meals for two to three weeks to help detoxify the gut. Reduce to once or twice daily thereafter.
- Take 10 drops of grapefruit seed extract in a glass of water four times a day, for three to five days (ending after five days). This extract kills most intestinal infections.

One of the best things you can do for your immune function is to maintain a healthy colon. It is your body's last bastion against aging and infectious disease. Follow these suggestions:

- Eat plenty of fiber. High-fiber foods help keep the colon clean.
- Start your meal with a salad. The digestive enzymes in raw vegetables and fruits will boost your digestive enzymes.
- Consider taking an enzyme supplement (check with your physician to review potential adverse effects). Select a combination of enzymes that resists stomach acid. Start with a small dose, and take 30 minutes before or after meals. Too much can cause diarrhea, nausea, and headache.
- Drink lots of water. The only way to replenish the water your body loses through breathing, urinating, and perspiring is to consume it. Choose bottled water from a reliable source.
- Slow down! Many of us are dashboard diners—eating on the go or eating too fast strains the digestive system.

- Avoid stress. Food doesn't move through the digestive tract when you are in a stressful situation, which is a common cause of constipation. Try meditation, yoga, tai chi, hypnotherapy, biofeedback, or flotation to relax.
- Exercise. Physical activity is a stress reliever and bowel stimulator.
- Wash your hands regularly. This protects against intestinal pathogens, and, as a bonus, reduces your chances of contracting a respiratory ailment (see Chapter 6).
- Avoid antibiotic overuse. Antibiotics destroy good intestinal flora, particularly lactobacilli.
- Use aspirin and other nonsteroidal anti-inflammatory drugs (NSAIDs) sparingly. They can cause intestinal permeability.
- Use antacids and laxatives sparingly. Your body can become dependent on both. Additionally, the constant suppression of stomach acid by antacids increases the risk of intestinal infection. If you have frequent heartburn, eat smaller low-fat meals, chew a calcium tablet after each meal, and do not eat within four hours of bedtime. Avoid coffee, chocolate, alcohol, and spicy foods until the heartburn stops.
- Engage in ileocecal massage (see Chapter 17) to relieve pressure associated with intestinal gas and to promote GI transit.
- Ask your physician to test you for food allergies. About 25% of people of European descent and about 75% of Asian, African, or Native American heritage are lactose intolerant: They cannot properly digest milk products. Other common allergies include nuts, wheat, eggs, meat, chocolate, and plants from the nightshade family (tomatoes, eggplant, zucchini, and peppers). Once diagnosed, the removal of offending foods from your diet often improves digestion.
- Don't smoke. It contributes to ulcers and heartburn, compromises the liver's ability to filter toxins, and interferes with food absorption.
- Spice your foods liberally with garlic, onion, turmeric, ginger,

sage, and rosemary—all of which are known as intestinal health–boosting condiments.

- Drink alcohol in moderation. In damaging the lining of the small intestine, alcohol amplifies digestive problems. An irritated small intestine also interferes with your ability to absorb nutrients and may lead to ulcers.
- Reduce dietary fat. Excess dietary fat contributes to colon cancer. The more fat you eat, the more bile your liver sends to your colon. At elevated levels, bile is thought to be a carcinogen.
- Watch the sugar. Too much refined sugar causes constipation.
- Keep caffeine in check. It can overstimulate the intestine and cause diarrhea (or worsen it).
- Deworm your pets regularly to reduce your chances of catching a bug from them (see Chapter 11). Also, always wash your hands after handling a pet, and keep your pets out of the bedroom (especially off the bed).
- Follow established guidelines for the handling of food (see Chapter 3).
- Make sure the source of your drinking water follows established regulatory guidelines.
- Explore the following herbal and other natural remedies:

  - Psyllium, buckthorn, and aloe are helpful in treating constipation.
  - Goldenseal can prevent or treat traveler's diarrhea.
  - Ginger and peppermint oil (enteric coated) can help relieve irritable bowel syndrome.
  - Lemon juice and lemon water are excellent cleansing agents for the colon.
  - Flaxseed and slippery elm teas are good bowel lubricants. Slippery elm also soothes the inflammation of ulcers, gastritis, and colitis.
  - Fresh or reconstituted dried figs improve constipation without the strong laxative effect of prunes.

• When you've gotta go, go! When you repeatedly ignore your
  body's signals that it's time to defecate, you may weaken the
  signal and force your body to do something drastic to get your
  attention. Two defecations of well-formed stools per day,
  approximately 20 to 30 minutes after a meal, are signs of
  colonic health.

[5]

Bladder, Kidneys, and Genitourinary Complaints

The sexual revolution is over and the microbes have won.

—*P. J. O'Rourke,* Give War a Chance, *1992*

URINARY TRACT INFECTIONS

Americans make 8 million doctor visits a year for urinary tract infections (UTIs), also known as bladder infections or cystitis. Half of American women have at least one UTI in their lifetimes. Far fewer men have UTIs than women. Recurrent UTIs may be caused by frequent reinfection or unresolved infection: 2 to 4% of apparently healthy women have elevated levels of bacteria in their urine. Recurrent UTIs can cause progressive damage and scarring of the kidneys, which may lead to kidney failure.

Signs of a urinary tract infection include the following:

• Burning and stinging upon urination
• Frequent urination, especially at night (although urine output may be a small amount)
• Increased urge to urinate
• Pain in the pubic area

- Lower back pain
- Blood in the urine, or bad-smelling urine
- Low-grade fever
- Painful sexual intercourse
- In some, lack of urinary control
- In men, penile discharge
- In children, bedwetting; in infants, irritability

While many women self-diagnose and self-treat UTI, the condition shares symptoms with vaginitis and some sexually transmitted diseases, so it's important to inform your physician when you suspect UTI. Your physician may test for UTI by measuring for high levels of bacteria (the cause) and white blood cells (the body's response) in urine. Unfortunately, these tests are rather imprecise and generally do not correlate well to symptoms. In fact, only 60% of women with UTI symptoms actually have significant levels of bacteria in their urine.

The universal cause of UTI is bacterial contamination of the urinary tract. *Escherichia coli* is responsible for 90% of all bladder infections when bacteria can be identified as the source. Urine, secreted by the kidneys, is sterile until it reaches the urethra, the canal through which urine passes from the bladder to exit the body. Bacteria can reach the urinary tract by making their way up the urethra (or, on rare occasions, through the bloodstream). Women are more vulnerable to UTIs because they have shorter urethras, and the proximity of the anus and urethra to the vagina promotes bacterial migration.

The healthy person normally mounts the following multifront preemptive defense mechanism that minimizes bacterial growth in the urinary tract:

- Urine flow washes away most bacteria.
- Urine pH inhibits growth of many bacteria.
- The surface of the bladder is antimicrobial.
- In men, the prostatic fluid is antimicrobial.
- White cells are secreted into the urine to fight infection in the event that bacteria invade the urethra.

Nevertheless, a variety of risk factors sometimes weaken the genitourinary (GU) defense mechanism and allow an environment in which UTI bacteria flourish:

- Sexual activity, which drives bacteria into the urethra—the cause of 75% of UTIs
- Change in the vaginal flora (such as that caused by use of spermicides and diaphragms)
- Urinary or fecal incontinence
- Menopause without hormone replacement therapy
- Diabetes or another immunocompromised state
- Incomplete bladder emptying
- Anatomic changes caused by pregnancy and childbirth
- Age 65 years and older
- Frequent bubble baths or salt baths
- In men, obstruction of urine flow in the urinary tract (usually caused by enlarged prostate)

UTIs are treated with an analgesic to relieve pain plus short-term therapy with an antimicrobial that targets the bacteria causing the infection. Antibiotic resistance is particularly problematic for UTI patients. In February 1999, researchers from the University of Washington School of Medicine announced that bladder infections are starting to fail to respond to the common antibiotics of choice. Instead, individuals with recurrent UTIs should first receive a culture and sensitivity test to specifically determine a second-tier targeted antibiotic—rather than the old standard general spectrum antibiotic.

Women with recurrent UTIs are advised to drink anywhere from eight glasses of water per day to one glass of water per waking hour. To soothe UTI discomfort, take one or two warm baths a day. Women might pour a cup of warm water over the genital area while urinating to relieve burning and stinging. Refrain from sexual intercourse until symptom-free for two weeks. The use of lubricant cream or oil during sex can help limit irritation to the urethra and even inhibit the egress of bacteria into the urethra, making for safer sex. Be sure to clean away the lubricant with soap and water immediately after intercourse, as some bacteria may be held suspended within the lubricant.

For postmenopausal women with recurrent UTIs, vaginal estrogen may be helpful—even if they are already taking hormone replacement therapy. Lack of estrogen can lead to structural and pH changes in the vagina that affect the urethra and promote bacterial growth.

Cranberry juice contains bacterial inhibitors that make it difficult for bacteria to cling to the linings of the bladder and urethra. To be effective, 100% cranberry juice (not "cocktail") is needed. Blueberry juice contains the same bacterial inhibitor.

- As a treatment, drink four to six 4-ounce glasses of unsweetened cranberry juice, mixed with 2 ounces of unsweetened apple juice and 2 ounces of water.
- As a preventive measure, 10 ounces of cranberry juice a day can reduce the risk of developing UTI and can speed up the clearing of an existing infection.
- In women diagnosed with recurrent UTI, cranberry extract in capsule form (400 milligrams per day) significantly reduces new infections.

Women may also follow these preventive measures:

- Wear loose underclothing that allows body fluids to evaporate.
- Take showers instead of tub baths.

When to See the Doctor

- Pain, stinging, burning, itching with urination.
- Fever is above 100°F.
- Blood appears in urine.
- Discomfort and other symptoms do not improve within a week.

- Wipe from front to back with toilet tissue to avoid introducing fecal bacteria to the urethra.
- Follow these procedures for sexual intercourse:
  - Urinate and wash the genital area immediately after sexual intercourse.
  - Drink a glass of water before sexual intercourse to get the kidneys to produce urine and move it along the urinary system.
  - Have sex in the lateral position or with the woman on top, to reduce the chances of injuring or transmitting bacteria to the urethra (since a woman's is of a shorter length and more prone to invasion by bacteria that may be mobilized upward during sex).

YEAST OVERGROWTH AND INFECTION

Candida albicans are common yeast cells found in relatively small numbers in the gastrointestinal and genital tracts, and in the mouth, throat, and esophagus. Normally, candida lives in harmony with other flora. When the body's internal environment is disturbed, the bacteria that control candida are killed and yeast overgrowth results.

Candida displays a Dr. Jekyll/Mr. Hyde persona: In its balanced state, candida is a spore and is somewhat round in shape. When yeast overgrowth occurs, candida turns into a fungus with roots that can plant themselves in the intestine wall or any other mucous membrane. Candida often spreads first in the GI tract, causing gas, bloating, indigestion, heartburn, nausea, constipation, and diarrhea. As you succumb to the associated major cravings for sugar, starches, and alcohol, candida proliferates, releasing toxins and interfering with digestion, making you feel worse. The yeast can enter the bloodstream and spread through the body, overwhelming the immune system. As the candida spreads, symptoms grow more diffuse and may include depression, lethargy, mental confusion/fog, mood swings, premenstrual syndrome (PMS), confused thyroid function, susceptibility to infections (sinus, respiratory, bladder, gums, etc.), sensitivity to pollutants and fumes (which can become full-blown environmental illness), achy muscles and/or joints, and skin fungus, among others.

Candida is much more common in women than men. Predisposing factors include the following:

- Bowel flora environment less hospitable to good bacteria, permitting bad bacteria to flourish (see Chapter 4)
- Decrease in digestive enzyme secretions, allowing food to pass to intestine in a less digested state
- Use of medications, particularly cortisone and birth-control pills
- Prolonged antibiotic use
- Impaired immunity
- Impaired liver function
- Chemotherapy and radiation treatment, surgery

Symptoms of Chronic Candidiasis

General symptoms: chronic fatigue, loss of energy, generalized malaise, decreased sex drive

Gastrointestinal symptoms: bloating, gas, intestinal cramps, rectal itching, altered bowel function

Genitourinary symptoms: vaginal yeast infection, frequent bladder infections

Endocrine system manifestations: menstrual symptoms, including premenstrual tension, cramps, bloating, headache, moodiness

Nervous system manifestations: depression, irritability, difficulty concentrating

Immune system manifestations: allergies, chemical sensitivities, low immune function

Dermatological manifestations: eczema, psoriasis

Related conditions: Leaky gut, food allergies

An overgrowth of yeast causes a very common form of vaginitis. The vaginal "ecosystem" is very delicate and can be disturbed easily by diet, medication, and even the type of undergarments worn. Vaginal yeast infections cause intense itching and burning, which may be accompanied by a thick, white, cottage cheese–like vaginal discharge. If experiencing yeast overgrowth, avoid these substances:

- Foods containing refined sugar, which promote yeast growth
- Meat and dairy products that have been treated with antibiotics
- Birth-control pills, antibiotics, and cortisone-like medications
- Moldy conditions in the home
- Certain chemicals such as perfume, smoke, and insecticides

Your physician will approach a case of yeast overgrowth based on how extensive it is and the extent to which the immune system has been compromised. Possible treatments include the following:

- Prescription antifungal drugs
- Diet modification
- Nutritional supplements that support immunity
- *Lactobacillus acidophilus* to restore the balance of flora in the gastrointestinal tract (plain unflavored yogurt; acidophilus milk, powders, and tablets)
- Fructooligosaccharides (FOSs), which feed *Lactobacillus acidophilus* and encourage its growth
- Identifying and addressing allergies to yeast and mold
- Stress reduction and adequate sleep to boost the immune system
- Various commercial herbal blends as well as garlic, berberines (goldenseal and barberry), tea tree oil (topical)
- Hydrogen peroxide (food grade and intravenous)
- Ozone (oral and intravenous)

Douching with 2 tablespoons of vinegar, the juice of half a lemon, and 1 quart of water can help restore the vagina's naturally acidic pH.

Eating plain unflavored yogurt regularly for several weeks may also help. If yeast toxins have spread throughout the body, a complicated six-month course of antiyeast drugs accompanied by a comprehensive year-long program of dietary and lifestyle modification to reestablish balance may be necessary.

VAGINAL INFECTIONS

Vaginal infections account for more than 10 million visits to the doctor a year, making them the most frequent reason women visit their gynecologic health care provider. There are three types of vaginal infections. Although the vast majority of women have heard of yeast infections, far fewer know about trichomoniasis, which is caused by a protozoan, or BV (bacterial vaginosis). Untreated BV can lead to pelvic inflammatory disease (PID) and may increase risk for human immunodeficiency virus (HIV) infection. In pregnant women, vaginosis and trichomoniasis have been linked to premature birth and low

Symptoms of Vaginal Infections

BACTERIAL VAGINOSIS	TRICHOMONIASIS VAGINITIS	CANDIDA VAGINITIS (YEAST)*
• Unpleasant fishy- or musty-smelling vaginal discharge/odor	• Severe internal and external itching	• White cottage cheese-like discharge
• Increased vaginal discharge	• Yellow-green frothy discharge	• No odor
• Vaginal itching and irritation	• Foul, fishy vaginal odor	
	• Abdominal pain	

*Yeast infections are not sexually transmitted diseases (STDs). This information is presented for comparison only.

birth weight. Women who smoke are at least three and a half times more likely to develop BV than women who don't.

Expert Insights on Vaginal Infections
by Edward M. Lichten, M.D.

Dr. Lichten is a board-certified ob/gyn specialist in private practice in Southfield, Michigan, specializing in gynecology and antiaging, and alternative medicine. He became interested in natural approaches for GU disorders while a resident at Ohio State University's College of Medicine in 1975, when the chairman of gynecology used alternative medical treatments. His wife had developed a vaginal infection postoperatively, and she was experiencing pain coupled with an odorous discharge. Rather than allowing the use of standard prescribed antibiotics, he instructed that she be given vitamins A, E, and C along with a vinegar douche. Within two days of this recommendation, the woman left the hospital symptom-free.

What is your perspective on when and why natural treatments for vaginal infections are superior to the conventional drug-based approach?

My nearly 30 years of experience in managing female infections has brought me to the realization that natural therapies should often be the initial approach to treatment. Only when these alternatives fail should prescription drugs be recommended. I have come to this conclusion for a number of reasons. Foremost is that systemic antibiotics are commonly used as the first treatment of women's vaginal maladies. Nonetheless, frequent use of antibiotics leads to an imbalance in the body of both helpful and harmful bacteria. Therefore, the use of antibiotics may create an obstacle for the body's natural ability to fight infections.

Once diagnosed, what is your integrative program for treating vaginal yeast infections?

The foundation for natural treatment is topical gentian violet and oral vitamins. Dilute gentian violet is a dye that has been used by gynecologists for more than 80 years. To this, we add oral vitamin A

(10,000 IU per day) or beta-carotene (50,000 IU per day) to enhance the integrity of the vaginal lining, aiding in both the prevention and the recurrence of BV infections. (*Important:* Sexually active women of childbearing age should not use vitamin A without effective birth control.) Zinc (30 mg per day) and vitamin E (400 to 800 IU per day) are indispensable in supporting immune function, thus helping to prevent vaginal infections such as BV. It is when immunity is suppressed that one is likely to get these outbreaks. Additionally, oral vitamin C (1,000 mg three to four times per day) augments immunity and helps reestablish the integrity of the vaginal lining. (*Important:* High-dose vitamin C supplementation (at 3 to 4 grams total daily intake) should only be administered under a physician's supervision and should not be continued for an extended period of time [discontinue after two weeks of continuous use].)

Changes in dietary habits are equally important. Reduce alcohol, simple sugars, and refined foods. When vaginal yeasts persist, some physicians may recommend an avoidance of fruits. When yeast is the diagnosis, the patient may be placed on essential fatty acid (EFA) supplementation, which helps to reduce inflammation. A mix of omega-3 (found in evening primrose) and omega-6 (found in flaxseed) fatty acids, 2 tablespoons of oil a day, or 1,000 to 1,500 mg in capsule form twice a day, is the appropriate dosage. Reducing the consumption of animal fats while increasing the intake of fish and nuts is another way to increase the intake of essential fatty acids.

Antifungal herbs and spices such as garlic, oregano, cinnamon, sage, and cloves should also be added to the diet. There is scientific proof that growth of *Candida albicans* is actually inhibited by garlic. Some physicians who practice alternative medicine recommend that women experiencing vaginal yeast infections should supplement their diets with garlic capsules. Alternatively, eating one clove of uncooked garlic per day or taking an oral supplement containing 5,000 mcg of allicin is a means by which to enhance the effectiveness of the intravaginal garlic and other natural formulations. Oral lactobacillus capsules or powder reduce the GI concentration of yeast while vaginal capsules increase the normal bacteria lactobacillus and decrease local yeast.

Of course, standard medications may be prescribed in conjunction with alternative remedies and should not be overlooked. To date, *after a proper diagnosis is made,* there are numerous standard medicines with which to treat vaginal yeast infections. *Note that natural and alternative therapies in the treatment of vaginal yeast infections may be offered not only as additions to these standard treatment modalities, but, at times, in place of them.*

What do you recommend to alleviate the discomfort of vaginal infections?

Chamomile *(Matricaria recutita)* and licorice *(Glycyrrhiza glabra)* can be made into teas and consumed three times daily for six weeks. They are both natural antifungal agents. Tea tree oil *(Melaleuca alternifolia)* or lavender essential oil *(Lavandula* species) can be applied topically two to three times a day for relief of symptoms of some types of vaginal infections. Some nutritionally oriented health care providers suggest using one-third part tea tree oil to two-thirds part vitamin E oil. Saturate a tampon with this mixture or put the mixture in a capsule and insert it in the vagina daily for a maximum of two weeks. This treatment has been especially successful in the treatment of recurrent vaginal yeast infections. Another herbal preparation, fireweed *(Epilobium parviflorum),* can be taken as a tea to treat oral, vaginal, and intestinal candidiasis. Finally, in regard to herbal preparations, marigold *(Calendula officinalis)* can be mixed into a salve and applied three to five times a day for relief of external vaginal discomfort.

Is vaginal yeast infection contagious?

Currently, there is no evidence for sexual transmission of vaginal yeast infections. It's unnecessary to treat the male sexual partner of the person affected.

BACTERIAL PROSTATITIS

The prostate, a donut-shaped male sex gland, is the most common site of disorders in the male genitourinary system. Encircling the urethra, contraction of the prostate muscle squeezes fluids in the organ (the ingredients in semen) into the urethral tract during ejaculation. Prostatitis, an inflammation of the prostate, can affect men of all ages, and may be acute or chronic.

Most often, prostatitis is caused by a bacterial infection usually from either *Escherichia coli* or *Proteus mirabilis,* which find their way to the prostate via the urethra, the bloodstream, or the lymphatic system. Prostatitis can partially or totally block the flow of urine from the bladder, weakening the bladder and making it susceptible to infection from bacteria in the retained urine, which can transmit the infection further, up into the kidneys.

If you suspect prostatitis, your doctor will conduct cultures of urine and also a digital rectal and prostate examination. To treat the condition, your doctor may prescribe the following:

* Antibiotics to fight the infection (usually taken for a month)
* Stool softeners to avoid constipation
* Medications to lower fever if you have one
* Bed rest until pain and fever subside

Signs of Prostatitis

* Urgency to urinate
* Burning with urination
* Frequent urination; waking to urinate at night
* Difficulty starting urination and emptying the bladder completely
* Fever
* Chills
* Pain between scrotum and anus
* Joint and muscle aches
* Lower back pain
* Sometimes, blood in urine

Natural remedies that can ease symptoms and may help prevent recurrent attacks include the following:

- Saw palmetto (extract and flower pollens)
- Hydrotherapy: sitting in 6 to 8 inches of warm to hot water for about 15 minutes at least three times a day
- Avoiding alcohol, coffee, spicy foods, chocolate, and tomato products to prevent further irritation of the urethra
- Drinking at least eight glasses of water a day to promote adequate urine production and flow

Bee-neficial

A review conducted by Drs. MacDonald, Ishani, and colleagues, published in the May 2000 issue of the *British Journal of Urology,* reports that ryegrass pollen (Ceranilton) can modestly improve symptoms of benign prostate hyperplasia. This finding supports the work of Drs. Jabib and Ross and colleagues from the University Department of Surgery at Western General Hospital (Edinburgh, Scotland) that isolated the active ingredient as FV-7, which was demonstrated to have a strong inhibitory effect on the growth of prostate cancer cells.

BUG-BUSTING BLOCKBUSTERS

Harmonize Your Urinary Tract

Men and women can take these simple measures to decrease the odds of getting a bladder infection:

- Drink at least 2 quarts of fluids daily (best is distilled bottled water), including 10 to 16 ounces of unsweetened cranberry juice.
- After sexual intercourse, urinate and wash around genitalia with soap and water promptly, and dry thoroughly.
- Avoid simple sugars and refined carbohydrates, which act as food for bad bugs in the GU tract.

Women, Take Heed: Recommendations to
Keep Candida at Bay

- Keep the genital area clean and free from sweat (wearing cotton undergarments instead of other fibers will help).
- Don't lounge around in wet clothing, especially a wet bathing suit.
- Use unscented soap and take showers rather than tub baths.

Men, Hear This: Make Sure Your Diet Is Rich in Zinc

Zinc deficiency has been associated with reduced immune system activity and a range of prostate-related ailments, including prostatitis. Significant sources of zinc are egg yolks, lamb chops, lima beans, pecans, pumpkin seeds, soybeans, and sunflower seeds. Take a zinc supplement (50 milligrams daily) if you are not getting enough of this trace element through food sources.

[6]

The Breath of Life:
The Respiratory System

A bunch of germs were whooping it up
In the bronchial saloon
The bacillus handling the larynx
Was jazzing a gag-time tune
While back of the tongue in a solo game
Sat dangerous An Kerchoo
And watching his luck was his light of love
The malady known as flu.

—Cal Beacock, the Pundit, *published by the International Save the Pun Foundation,*
quoted in Reader's Digest, *January 1986*

The respiratory system delivers oxygen to cells throughout the body and removes carbon dioxide, a by-product of cellular processes. Starting with inhalation at our nose and mouth, air enters the lungs through the trachea and bronchus into the two major passageways: the right and left main bronchi. It travels through the highly branched structure of the lung (formed by several hundred million bronchioles and alveolar ducts), to arrive at air sacs called alveoli. At the alveoli, which are covered with tiny blood vessels, blood drops off carbon dioxide picked up from cells at which it has deposited oxygen and refreshes itself with more oxygen, to repeat its delivery cycle over and over again with each breath you take.

On average, we breathe about once every five seconds. The

process of taking 20,000 breaths a day puts our bodies at particular risk to airborne pathogens.

SNEEZING

When a piece of dust, dirt, or mucus in the nasal passageway impedes smooth airflow, the nose sends a message to the brain to ask the lungs to send out a big burst of air to blast out the bothersome agent . . . *achooooo!*

Contrary to popular practice, sneezing into your hands is not a wise germ-fighting measure. Our palms provide a warm, moist haven where viruses can breed. If you sneeze into your hands and then touch an object (such as a telephone, a TV remote control, or a computer mouse) with which someone else has contact within 10 minutes, you've just aided and abetted the germ. To receive a sneeze, use a tissue, handkerchief, or (moms out there, take note) your sleeve—these objects will not enable germs to live long enough to be transmitted to someone else. Above all, handwashing is the best tactic, especially during cold and flu season (see Chapter 7).

Frequent sneezing not associated with a cold or flu is likely related to allergies, particularly hay fever. If you have sneezing spells—where you sneeze more than two or three times in a row more than three times a day—see your doctor.

COUGHING

Coughing is a generally healthy reflex that dislodges phlegm, mucus, and foreign agents such as dirt or pollen, preventing them from traveling deep into the air passageways. Physicians categorize coughs as "good" or "bad"—good coughs produce phlegm, whereas bad coughs are dry, hacking episodes that cause irritation to the throat.

If you are suffering from repeated episodes of any type, it is important that your physician identify the underlying source. You may have a cold, flu, or bronchitis if your productive cough is accompanied by a runny or stuffy nose, fever, aches, sneezing, or sore throat. Generally, productive coughs should be allowed to take their course; cough suppressants should be used only if you're losing sleep or if the cough bothers others.

Dr. Robert Stockley and colleagues at the Queen Elizabeth Hospital in England recently reported that sputum (a medical term for phlegm) that isn't clear or milky in color (mucoid), but is instead brown, green, or yellow with a pungent odor (purulent), is more likely to be loaded with bacteria.

A common problem experienced during respiratory tract infections is an inability to clear secretions. Try these simple methods to provide mechanical support during the coughing process or to promote deep breathing:

1. Wrap a bath towel around the chest, holding on to both ends with your arms across your chest.
2. Pull the towel tightly to splint ribs while coughing or inhaling deeply.
3. Additionally, run a hot shower and breathe the steam for 10 to 15 minutes, up to six times a day, to loosen secretions sufficiently to cough them up.

When to See the Doctor

- Cough lasts more than a week without improvement
- Cough is accompanied by fever, chills, or muscle aches
- Cough produces green, brown (blood-tinged), or yellow sputum, possibly indicating a secondary bacterial infection
- Cough can be characterized as deep, gurgly, and feels like it's coming from the lungs (as opposed to the throat area), which may be a sign of bronchitis
- Cough is accompanied by wheezing, shortness of breath, or tightness in the chest, possibly an early indicator of pneumonia

These methods are preferred to using humidifiers and vaporizers, since this equipment can breed large quantities of bacteria and disperse them into the air (see discussion on pneumonia later in this chapter). The combination of deep breathing, a good strong cough, and expectoration in the shower is a very effective way to break up congestion from a cold or flu.

COLDS AND FLU

Colds and flu can strike year-round and are the most frequent medical condition experienced by Americans, totaling 600 million cases each year.

Colds

Any of 200 different strains within five different viral families can cause the common cold. About half of all colds are caused by one of about 100 strains of the rhinovirus. Because succumbing to one strain does not confer immunity from the others, you can continue to catch cold after cold. With age, immunity to the common cold does build, which is why adults have fewer colds than children. The average adult will catch 2 to 4 colds a year; the average school-aged child will have 6 to 10.

Stress can worsen cold symptoms. Research at Carnegie-Mellon University suggests that people under stress have an exaggerated immune system response to the cold virus, resulting in more intense physical symptoms such as coughing and sneezing. Psychological stress stimulates production of a chemical messenger known as interleukin-6 (IL-6). IL-6 attracts immune cells to fight off a virus and creates cold symptoms, but its overproduction intensifies cold symptoms.

Because it is caused by a virus, the common cold cannot be treated with antibiotics. When a cold develops into a sinus infection, bacterial bronchitis, or secondary infection, however, antibiotics are often correctly prescribed.

Flu

Flu symptoms were first described by Hippocrates in 412 B.C. The term *influenza* was coined in 1357 A.D. It derives from the Latin word for "influence"—because the flu was blamed on the influence of the stars. The first recorded flu pandemic (global spread) occurred in 1580, starting in Asia and moving through Africa, Europe, and the Americas. The worst pandemic to date occurred in 1918, killing 20 million—perhaps even 100 million—worldwide, which is far more than the 8.5 million lives lost in World War I. The 1918 pandemic infected more than 25 million Americans and killed half a million, at a time when our population was only 40% of what it is today. If a pandemic similar to the 1918 experience were to strike today, 1.5 million Americans would die. That would be more deaths than the combined effect of heart disease, cancer, stroke, chronic pulmonary disease, AIDS, and Alzheimer's!

Where people went for medical care dramatically influenced whether they died from the flu. Osteopathic (D.O.) physicians, who are fully qualified doctors licensed to perform surgery and prescribe medication in all 50 states and who receive extra training in the musculoskeletal system (the body's interconnected system of nerves, muscles, and bones that makes up two-thirds of its body mass), practice manual healing methods, including osteopathic manipulative treatment (OMT). In the early part of the twentieth century, osteo-

Taking a Flu Shot to Heart

An annual flu shot may do more than protect from influenza. Researchers at the University of Texas suggest that flu can inflame the plaque buildup that clogs arteries; thus, heart patients who are vaccinated against influenza may improve their chances of avoiding a subsequent heart attack.

pathic physicians were much more successful in treating flu than their allopathic (M.D.) counterparts.

In a time when antibiotics were not widely available, osteopathic medical hospitals treated flu and pneumonia victims with therapies including lymphatic pump postural drainage (see Chapter 17) and hydration. The death rate among flu victims in this group was just 0.5%, whereas the rate at allopathic hospitals stood at 6%. Osteopathic treatment of pneumonia resulted in a 10% death rate, while M.D.-administered treatment resulted in a 33% death rate. We don't know why the flu of 1918 was so virulent. Scientists are working hard to stay a step ahead of today's flu viruses.

The flu virus is airborne, triggered when someone with the infection coughs or sneezes, releasing droplets of respiratory fluid into the air. Three types of viruses cause the flu:

1. Influenza A: a potentially severe illness that spreads easily and affects large numbers of people
2. Influenza B: a generally less severe illness that tends to infect fewer people
3. Influenza C: considered clinically irrelevant because its symptoms are so mild

Different strains of each type of flu are named for the place they were first identified—for example, the Hong Kong, Sydney, Beijing, and Russian flus. Scientists are generally able to predict how a flu virus

Lifesaver

Diabetics are three to four times more likely to die as a result of flu complications, and five times more likely to be hospitalized for flu. The Centers for Disease Control and Prevention (CDC) estimates that by raising the number of diabetics receiving the influenza and pneumococcal vaccination from 40 to 60%, 8,000 lives a year could be saved.

will mutate as it spreads throughout a population, but about every decade or so we are surprised with a brand-new unexpected strain.

Each year, infectious disease teams prepare an influenza vaccine they predict will help prevent the spread of the likeliest flu strains. Composed of inactivated organisms from several strains of flu, the vaccine protects only against the flu caused by those strains and typically takes up to two weeks to reach full protective levels in vaccinated individuals. It is about 70 to 90% effective in young, healthy people, and less effective in the elderly and those with certain chronic medical conditions.

Treatment for flu is largely the same as for a bad cold: bed rest, extra fluids, decongestants, and an aspirin substitute to relieve muscle discomfort and inflammation and reduce fever.

Recently, a new category of medication has made a big impact on this malady. The flu is now being treated successfully with one of two M-2 inhibitor drugs (amantadine or rimantadine). However, the efficacy of M-2 inhibitors has been declining because they induce viral resistance. Two new neuraminidase inhibitors (zanamivir and oseltamivir) were made available in 2000. These drugs bind and inactivate the enzyme responsible for the release of the virus from affected cells. If administered within 48 hours of the onset of symptoms, flu symptoms are effectively managed to reduce odds of complications. So far, tolerance has been good and adverse effects have been nominal.

Double Duty

Zanamivir may not just alleviate symptoms of flu, but may prevent it. When Dr. F. G. Hayden at the University of Virginia administered the drug once a day to both the initial flu patient as well as family members in the same household, only 4% of the family members came down with flu, compared to 19% in the control group. This translates to a 79% rate of protection. Additionally, the administration of zanamivir to elderly populations as a prophylactic treatment has prevented up to 92% of flu cases in that group.

Prevention of Colds and Flu

Perhaps the most effective prevention method to employ is to make your body as inhospitable and unattractive a host to cold and flu viruses as possible. Consider the following:

1. Limit your sugar intake. Sugars are the food on which bacteria love to feast, and cold and flu viruses are no exception. Foods that increase mucus formation, such as bananas, oranges (and citrus juices), peanuts, and dairy, should be eaten in moderation. Resist the urge to reach for that cookie or scoop of ice cream, too.
2. If you're taking a multivitamin with iron, check with your physician on whether you really need the iron, since it's a mineral that feeds bacteria.
3. Minimize your exposure to immune-taxing molds and mildews. During the fall months when temperatures drop at night and cause condensation by morning, keep windows and bathrooms dry by weatherproofing and properly ventilating. Don't jump into raked piles of leaves, as doing so will deliver a potent dose of unwanted mold exposure.
4. Keep yourself hydrated. Drinking at least eight glasses of distilled water a day is perhaps the most inexpensive way to keep your body systems in proper balance.

The Love Bug-Buster

Psychologists at Wilkes University (Pennsylvania) found that college students having sex at least once a week (but not more than two times a week) had immune systems that were more resilient to fending off colds and flu. Is this a case of too much of a good thing?

Is It a Cold or the Flu?

Generally, flu is more likely to be associated with high fever, body aches, dry cough, and severe fatigue, whereas a cold is characterized more by sneezing and a runny nose. Both conditions may cause a sore throat and chest discomfort.

Diagnosing Colds or Flu

SYMPTOMS	COLD	FLU
Fever	Rare	High (102–104°F); lasts three to four days
Headache	Rare	Prominent
General aches/pains	Slight	Usual; often severe
Fatigue, weakness	Quite mild	Can last up to two to three weeks
Extreme exhaustion	Never	Early and prominent
Stuffy nose	Common	Sometimes
Sneezing	Usual	Sometimes
Sore throat	Common	Sometimes
Chest discomfort	Mild to moderate	Common; can become severe
Cough	Hacking	
Complications	Sinus congestion or earache	Bronchitis, pneumonia; can be life-threatening

Source: National Institute of Allergy and Infectious Disease.

Populations at Risk for Flu-Related Complications

◆ Anyone over age 50
◆ Residents of nursing homes and other chronic care facilities
◆ Children and adults who have chronic pulmonary or cardiovascular disorders, including asthma
◆ Children and adults who have needed regular medical follow-up or hospitalization during the preceding year because of chronic metabolic diseases (including diabetes), renal dysfunction, hemoglobinopathies, or immunosuppression
◆ Women in the second or third trimester of pregnancy during the flu season

Natural Remedies for Colds and Flu

REMEDY	DESCRIPTION
Vitamins and Minerals (more information in Chapter 17)	
Vitamin A, 10,000 IU daily for up to four days; beta-carotene, 25,000 IU per day (contraindicated in pregnant women/ women of childbearing age not using birth control)	Long established as effective agent to combat infectious disease. Vitamin A deficiency can manifest as increased infection by cold and flu viruses.
Vitamin C, 2,000 mg, divided into four to five doses a day	Antiviral and antibacterial properties reduce duration and severity of colds and flu, enhance white blood cell production, increase interferon, enhance antibody responses, and maintain the integrity of mucous membranes.
Zinc lozenges (15–25 mg elemental zinc each), one under tongue every three hours for first three days, one every four hours for three days thereafter	Deficiencies associated with immune system disorders and susceptibility to infectious disease. Zinc gluconate lozenges prevent onset of colds and decrease their duration.

(continued)

(continued)

REMEDY	DESCRIPTION
Herbs (more information in Chapter 17)	
Astragalus, as extract (70% polysaccharides); as capsule, 250–500 mg daily; or as tincture (1:5), 1½ teaspoons daily	Popular in Chinese herbal medicine, clinical trials demonstrate effectiveness in reducing severity and duration of the common cold.
Cat's claw (2% oxindole alkaloids), 100 mg daily	Enhances the body's immune response to the pneumonia vaccine.
Echinacea, as extract (3.5% echinacosides); as capsule, 150 mg three times a day; or as tincture (1:5), 2–4 ml three times per day	Promotes movement of white blood cells to area of infection, stimulates activity of T cells and natural killer cells, enhances performance of macrophages, blocks virus receptors and inhibits ability of viruses to spread, stimulates production of interferon (inhibits virus reproduction).
Elderberry, as capsule, 350–500 mg four times a day; or as tincture, 30–60 drops four times a day	Accelerates recovery from flu by two to four days.
Garlic capsules (70:1 extract, 5,000 mg), three times daily	Broad antiviral action, activates natural killer cells, macrophages, and B cells.
Goldenseal	Contains ingredients (most notably berberine) that inhibit activity of bacteria and viruses, stimulate the immune system, and maintain healthy mucous membranes (making them less susceptible to irritation from cold and flu infection).
Licorice	Immune stimulant, prevents bacterial and viral infections, lowers the impact of stress on the body.
Peppermint	Menthol is helpful in treating symptoms of colds and flu such as sore throat and irritated lips and nose. Various mints

(continued)

(continued)

REMEDY	DESCRIPTION
Peppermint *(cont.)*	(especially as tea) possess antiviral properties.
Willow bark	The herb from which aspirin is derived, willow bark is an analgesic and anti-inflammatory. Relieves symptoms of infection.

Other

Fever	Fever is one of the body's natural defenses. A higher-than-normal body temperature can inhibit the reproduction of some viruses. Reducing a fever with aspirin or acetaminophen may extend the length of illness. Generally, temperatures below 102°F can be left untreated. Temperatures 103°F and higher in an adult can be dangerous and should be reduced, especially in the elderly and in people with cardiovascular disease.
Teas and soups	Increase mucus flow; hot caffeine-free beverages help purge viruses.
Stress reduction	Stress management helps prevent onset of colds and flu and shortens their duration.
Nasal rinse	A warm saline solution used as a nasal rinse helps prevent colds and shortens their duration. Combine 2 cups of warm water, 1 teaspoon of salt, and a pinch of baking soda in a large saucer. Pinch one nostril and inhale slightly to cleanse nostrils and sinuses.

PNEUMONIA

Pneumococcal disease, a common cause of pneumonia, can be a complication of the flu. *Streptococcus pneumoniae* kills 40,000 people annually in the United States, 90% of whom are elderly. Numerous studies have shown that the pneumococcal vaccination significantly reduces hospitalization and death rates among elderly patients with lung disease, but only 25% of people who are candidates for the vaccine actually receive it.

Those most susceptible to pneumococcal disease are the same group targeted for the flu vaccine. For high-risk people, the CDC urges doctors to augment the flu vaccine with a pneumococcal vaccination every 10 years.

Pneumococcus bacterium, the most common cause of bacterial pneumonia, is spread when an infected person coughs, sneezes, or comes in close contact with someone. Recently, researchers demonstrated that smoking as well as inhaling secondhand smoke is a significant risk factor for pneumococcal disease. Chemicals in tobacco impair the lungs' ability to move mucus, likely trapping harmful microbes that irritate the lungs' lining and make them even more susceptible to the bacteria and viruses that cause the serious lung inflammation known as pneumonia.

Our nervous system connects the lung tissue to the upper thoracic spine. Osteopathic physicians refer to the physical connection between the musculoskeletal system and organs affected by disease as somatic dysfunction. Through osteopathic protocols involving the manipulation of the spine (OMT), D.O.s achieve a faster recovery rate for their pneumonia patients than their allopathic (M.D.) counterparts. In December 2000, a study conducted at Kirksville College of Osteopathic Medicine (Kirksville, Missouri) found that treating elderly patients hospitalized for pneumonia with OMT shortened the duration of their intravenous antibiotic treatment and total hospital stay.

To alleviate the discomfort associated with pneumonia, try the following suggestions:

• Using a cool-mist, ultrasonic humidifier to increase air moisture. Regular addition of a liquid water conditioner solution will help to control odor (resulting from a buildup of fungus and bacteria). Twice a week, run the humidifier outside, filled with a dilute vinegar solution made of 1 part vinegar (acetic acid) to 9 parts water, a strong disinfectant

Signs, Symptoms, and Treatment of Pneumonia

• Symptoms of pneumonia include fever, shortness of breath, chills, cough, chest pain, and increased mucus production. The infection leads to an accumulation of fluid in the lungs, causing congestion.
• Pneumonia caused by pneumococcus or any other bacteria must be treated with antibiotics. It can take four to six weeks to recover from pneumonia. If complications arise, it can take much longer.
• Both chronic bronchitis and asthma can develop after a respiratory infection and last for months, even years. Thus, effective and aggressive treatment of pneumonia is a must. Pneumonia kills 40,000 people each year.

When to See the Doctor

• Fever 101°F or above
• Pain that is not relieved by heat or medication
• Increased shortness of breath
• Difficulty breathing when lying down
• Increased chest pain
• Dark or bluish fingernails, toenails, or skin
• Blood in sputum
• Nausea, vomiting, or diarrhea

that will sanitize your humidifier. Never leave water in the
unit over an extended period of nonuse. Germ-free warm
mist humidifiers use ultraviolet light and vaporization
(boiling), and claim to kill 99.99% of bacteria, molds, and
spores that can breed in tap water.

* If you have a productive cough, do not use cough suppressant,
  as coughing is the body's natural way of ridding lung
  secretions. Tell your doctor if the cough is dry and hacking.
* Using a heating pad or hot compress to relieve chest pain.
* Staying in bed and conserving your energy.
* Avoiding mucus-promoting foods, including all dairy products,
  especially cheese; bananas; oranges (and citrus juices); and
  peanuts.
* Staying hydrated. Consume at least one glass of distilled water
  every hour. Drink ten to fourteen 8-ounce glasses of distilled
  water each day you're sick and for several days afterward.
* Using tissues to capture your sneezes and coughs, and
  disposing of them promptly.
* Taking acidophilus to replace the friendly flora killed by
  prescription antibiotics (see Chapter 4).

SINUSITIS

Sinusitis is an inflammation of the nasal sinuses that accompanies
upper respiratory infection. Acute sinusitis is frequently caused by
colds or bacterial and viral infections of the nose, throat, and upper
respiratory tract. Chronic sinusitis, the most common chronic disease
in the United States, affecting 14% of the population, may be caused
by small growths in the nose, injury to the nasal bones, smoking, and
irritant fumes and smells. Chronic inflammation from allergies or
repeated colds can weaken mucous membranes and thus impair the
immune system, precipitating more colds and allergies, which lead to
more sinus infections. Over 50% of all cases of sinusitis are caused by
bacteria.

In all types of sinusitis, the mucous membranes of the sinuses swell and drainage passageways are blocked for the fluid that cleans and moisturizes the membranes. If drainage is clear after a week, you probably do not have an infection. Greenish or yellowish mucus indicates infection. If the drainage is clear and you do not have a cold, you may have allergies, not sinusitis.

Chronic sinusitis can be very difficult to clear up. Researchers suspect that most people with this condition suffer from a microscopic fungus that naturally resides in the nose, and, for some people, triggers an immune response. In addition, Mayo Clinic researchers have shown that sinusitis patients using steroid medication inhalers (such as Nasacort, Beconase, or Flonase) put themselves at a greater risk of developing a sinus fungus. Many patients with chronic sinusitis often suffer from yeast syndrome (chronic candidiasis; see Chapter 5), whereas others may suffer from *Helicobacter pylori* infection—the bacteria linked to ulcers (see Chapter 3)—for which treatment frequently also resolves sinusitis.

Signs and Symptoms of Sinus Infection

- ◆ Green, yellow, or blood-tinged nasal discharge, signaling an 8 in 10 chance that you've got a bacterial infection requiring antibiotic treatment.
- ◆ Postnasal drip.
- ◆ Sensation of pressure in the head.
- ◆ Headache, worsening in the morning or when bending forward. Headaches in chronic sinusitis may last for weeks at a time.
- ◆ Earache.
- ◆ Cheek pain that resembles a toothache.
- ◆ Facial pain.
- ◆ Loss of sense of smell.
- ◆ Tenderness over forehead and cheekbones.
- ◆ Fatigue, lack of energy.
- ◆ Cough (sometimes nonproductive).
- ◆ Fever (sometimes).

The first line of defense against a sinus infection is antihistamines, which offer short-term relief but can have a rebound effect if used for a long period of time and then discontinued. Antihistamines are also associated with debilitating side effects, including fatigue, dizziness, and anxiety. The next recourse is antibiotics. Some sinus infections respond well to a short course of antibiotics, but others are far more stubborn. Over time, most people who use an antibiotic to treat recurrent sinus infections will become resistant to the drug, and their repetitive use may ultimately weaken the immune system.

The best way to address chronic sinusitis is to institute long-term control measures that minimize the exposure to irritants that precipitate the condition. Studies show that 25 to 75% of people with allergies have sinusitis. This population can be helped by creating a sinus-friendly home environment (see Chapter 15), including the following:

+ Using air-filtering vacuum cleaners
+ Installing a HEPA (high-efficiency particulate air) filter on central forced-air systems
+ Placing a HEPA filtration machine by the head of the bed to condition breathing air while asleep
+ In extreme cases, removing pets, carpeting, and feather bedding
+ Not smoking and not allowing others to smoke inside your residence
+ Identifying and eliminating food allergens

When to See the Doctor

+ Immediately if you experience swelling around the eyes (including forehead and sides of nose and cheeks)
+ If you experience blurred vision

Left untreated, sinusitis can progress to asthma, bronchitis, pneumonia, and other respiratory disorders.

A nutritional supplementation support program for sinusitis can include the following:

- Vitamin C, 500 milligrams every two hours
- Bioflavonoids, 1,000 milligrams per day
- Vitamin A, 5,000 IU per day (contraindicated in pregnant women and women of childbearing age not on birth control)
- Beta-carotene, 15,000 IU per day (contraindicated in pregnant women and women of childbearing age not on birth control)
- Zinc, 20 milligrams per day

To soothe sinusitis, try the following:

- A warm compress to relieve pain in the sinuses and nose.
- Inhaling shower steam or using a vaporizer several times a day to loosen secretions so that you can expel them.
- Blowing your nose gently. Forceful blowing will lodge mucus into the sinus cavities.
- Limiting mucus-forming foods, such as bananas, oranges (and citrus juices), peanuts, and dairy.
- Drinking plenty of distilled water, juices, and hot broths.

Soup Is Really Good Food

In October 2000, Dr. Stephen Rennard, a chest specialist from Nebraska, reported on his lab tests of homemade and commercially available chicken soups. The tests found that both the chicken and the vegetables present in the soup inhibited the movement of neutrophils, cells that stimulate the production of mucus. The soup broth exhibited a mild anti-inflammatory effect, which soothes upper respiratory symptoms.

EAR INFECTIONS

If you have raised children, you know the drill: Your child has some upper respiratory symptoms, spikes a fever, goes to the doctor, and is diagnosed with a middle ear infection (acute otitis media). The question is: When should you expect to receive an antibiotic prescription for the infection?

Nearly 75% of all American children have at least one ear infection by the time they are 2 years old. After colds, ear infections are the second most common infection in children. A propensity toward ear infections can be genetic and is related to the shape of the middle ear. Parents who smoke expose children to contaminants through the air and are much more likely to have children with chronic ear or respiratory infections.

Upper respiratory and ear infections account for the lion's share of overuse of antibiotics in children. Most upper respiratory infections are viral and will not respond to antibiotics, and most ear infections will heal without antibiotic intervention. Some research shows that giving an antibiotic early in an ear infection may actually prolong the infection and precipitate recurrence. Introducing an antibiotic too early in an infection interrupts the immune system's natural defense against the infection and contributes to antibiotic resistance. *Streptococcus pneumoniae,* a common bacterial cause of ear infection, is becoming highly resistant to many antibiotics.

Many clinicians believe that food allergies are the underlying

When to See the Doctor

If an ear infection lasts for more than a week or interferes with a child's ability to eat or drink, or if significant hearing loss is noticed, an antibiotic may be necessary.

cause of ear infections. The most common offenders include milk, eggs, wheat, soy, corn, peanuts, chocolate, and tomatoes.

Consider following these recommendations to avoid childhood ear infections:

* Enhance the immune system with a good vitamin-mineral formula that includes vitamin C and the B vitamins.
* Avoid allergens. Ask your physician to test for both food and inhalant allergies.
* Impart antibodies by breast-feeding your infant.

ASTHMA

Asthma is a complex, multifaceted disease that triggers attacks of wheezing and shortness of breath, known as bronchial hyperreactivity. In a severe attack, airways may shut down completely. Although it manifests itself in an episodic manner, asthma is a chronic disease that

Signs and Symptoms of Asthma

* Repeated attacks of shortness of breath or rapid, shallow breathing.
* Cough, which may expel clear/milky (mucoid) sputum.
* Wheezing.
* Chest tightness.
* Neck stiffness/tightness.
* Laboratory testing shows increased serum immunoglobulin E (IgE), positive food and/or inhalant allergies, or increased levels of eosinophils.
* Reduction in peak flow—the amount of air you can blow out of your chest and how quickly you can do it. Most people can blow all the air out of their chest within three seconds. People with asthma, however, have a much harder time accomplishing this feat. At-home monitoring with a peak flow meter device is a useful advance warning approach.

demands constant vigilance, and thus may be considered an autoimmune disorder affecting the respiratory system.

Incidence of asthma in the United States rose almost 100% between 1982 and 1996. Among children, asthma is one of the most common chronic illnesses and the leading cause of hospitalizations and school absenteeism. Contrary to popular opinion, children do not "outgrow" asthma; however, asthma may cause fewer problems as children grow because their airways are larger and they have learned how to better manage the disease.

The largest demographic group suffering from asthma is women, who account for more than 55% of asthma cases in the United States. Two of the unique physiological factors at work in women might be obesity and hormone considerations. Research shows that the higher a woman's body mass index (BMI), the greater her chance of developing asthma.

Asthma rates in women increase around the time of puberty, suggesting that hormones may play a role. Many women with asthma notice perimenstrual asthma—an increase in symptoms immediately before and after their menstrual periods.

Asthma often goes undiagnosed and untreated in the elderly,

When to See the Doctor

An acute asthma attack can be life-threatening. Call your physician or proceed to the nearest emergency medical facility immediately. Symptoms of acute asthma attack include the following:

- Skin that has a bluish or gray tone
- Exhaustion
- Grunting during breathing
- Inability to speak
- Restlessness or confusion
- Oxygen-hunger—panting, unable to catch one's breath

because it is easily confused with other chronic conditions with similar symptoms such as congestive heart failure or chronic obstructive pulmonary disease.

Asthma can be controlled, but it cannot be cured. Susceptibility is believed to be inherited, but the tendency to actually get the disease depends on environment. Asthma attacks can be brought on by a number of chemical, microbiologic, physical, and immunological triggers, including exertion, upper respiratory infection, some medications, sulfites added to foods, pollution, cigarette smoke, cockroaches, dust mites, and pet dander.

In the United States, The Bronx in New York City is the epicenter of asthma. The rate of death from asthma is three times higher there than in the United States as a whole. Children with severe asthma have treatment regimens almost as complex as those of AIDS patients. Some researchers speculate that the high incidence of asthma in The Bronx may be related to the diesel fumes from the thousands of 18-wheelers that travel the Bronx Expressway. Even if this air pollution is not causing asthma, it is certainly provoking symptoms in people who have the disease.

Other asthma triggers—namely, cockroaches and dust mites—can be found in the inner city as well as the more pristine suburbs. The fecal material produced by dust mites is also highly allergenic. Dust mites need only heat, humidity, and dust (including shed human skin) to survive. It is estimated that 45% of the homes in the United States—44 million in all—have dust mites present in significant enough numbers to incite asthma in the homes' human residents.

In their search for the underlying cause of asthma, researchers are looking at the possibility that asthma has something to do with a slowly maturing immune system during the first few months of life. In people with this problem, the immune system learns to overreact to harmless allergens. People who develop asthma later in life may in fact have had a mild, undetected form of the disease all along.

A number of asthma specialists believe that the disease is a result of overcleanliness and overuse of antibiotics, which eliminate the need for a young immune system to practice fighting off microbial invaders. This theory could explain why children in the developing world—despite their exposure to various asthma triggers—tend not to develop the disease. Research also suggests that living close to the soil and to farm animals may be protective against asthma because such an environment helps program the young immune system not to overreact.

Diet and physical activity also may influence the incidence of asthma. Several studies have shown that the children of women who eat fish and leafy green vegetables have less asthma than do other children. And researchers speculate that children who are physically active outdoors take more deep breaths, and thus inoculate their lungs against microbes that could be asthma triggers for children who are less active or who primarily engage in indoor activities.

More than 250 substances in the workplace have been identified as asthma triggers. Work-related or work-aggravated asthma can be a manifestation of asthma that was undetected or in remission. New-onset asthma can be caused by ongoing exposure or even a single exposure to a respiratory irritant such as formaldehyde, latex, dusts from flour and grains, chlorine gas, or strong acids. Occupational exposure is the cause of 5 to 15% of new cases of asthma in working people.

A nondrug approach to control asthma relies on lowering the allergic provocations in the asthmatic's environment. Suggestions include the following:

- Remove pets from the home and thoroughly clean to eliminate their dander.
- Eliminate carpeting and drapes. Alternatively, vacuum often with a HEPA filter vacuum, which prevents dust particles from recirculating.
- Dust both vertical and horizontal surfaces weekly.
- Exterminate cockroaches. Avoid room foggers, which may worsen asthma.
- Keep indoor humidity below 50% year-round.
- Wash bedding weekly in hot water (130°F) and dry in a hot dryer.
- Replace bedding made of natural materials such as down and cotton with bedding made of synthetic fibers.

- Encase mattresses and pillows in mite-proof covers. Wash blankets and pillowcases once a week in hot water.
- Opt for leather furniture rather than upholstered pieces, since leather is an impervious material that is resistant to breeding dust mites.
- Open windows for an hour each day during dry seasons to improve ventilation.
- Clean mold off shower curtains, bathroom and basement walls, and other surfaces with a solution of bleach, detergent, and water.
- Use a dehumidifier if your basement is damp or musty.
- Never allow smoking in the house.

A nutritional supplement program to support asthma control may include the following:

- Vitamin B_6, 25 to 50 milligrams twice daily
- Vitamin B_{12} (sublingual), 1,000 micrograms per day
- Vitamin C, 1,000 to 3,000 milligrams per day, in divided doses
- Vitamin E, up to 400 IU per day
- Flavonoids, which are key antioxidants for asthmatics, such as quercetin, 400 milligrams before meals; grapeseed extract, 100 milligrams before meals; green tea extract (50% polyphenols), 200 milligrams three times a day
- DHEA (dehydroepiandrosterone; levels of which are decreased in asthmatics), up to 50 milligrams per day

Additionally, dietary changes that correlate to symptom improvement include the following:

- Reducing consumption of red meat, as beef contains arachidonic acid, a substance that promotes inflammation.
- Increasing the consumption of cold-water fish (salmon, mackerel, herring, halibut, and similar) that are high in anti-inflammatory omega-3 fatty acids. Omega-3 fatty acids contain eicosapentaenoic acid (EPA) and docosahexaenoic acid (DHA),

both of which are shown to improve airway responsiveness and respiratory function.

• Eliminating food allergens and all food additives. Coloring agents and preservatives (including sodium benzoate, sulfur dioxide, and sulfites) are major offenders.

There is some evidence that allergen immunotherapy can be useful for those whose asthma attacks are triggered by allergies. In some studies, immunotherapy has reduced or decreased the need for expensive medications and has improved control of asthma, especially when applied early in the course of the disease. New asthma medications in development include an antibody called anti-IgE that is administered via injection every two to four weeks, an inhaled drug that targets the start of the immune system reaction to allergens, and an asthma vaccine. Discovery of some of the genes that control asthma will lead to even more targeted treatments.

TUBERCULOSIS

Tuberculosis (TB), once known as "consumption," is highly contagious through coughing and sneezing. Infection is caused by the organism *Mycobacterium tuberculosis*. Inhaling just a single minute particle of TB bacteria can infect a susceptible person. Cattle are also susceptible and can transmit TB through nonpasteurized milk.

Tuberculosis is treatable if caught early, but nearly two-thirds of the people with active TB are not receiving treatment. Inappropriate or

TB Alert

For every case of TB that is not under medical control, that person infects an average of 10 to 15 people each year.

incomplete treatment is worse than no treatment at all, because this situation leads to the development of drug-resistant strains. According to the World Health Organization's Directly Observed Therapy Strategy (DOTS) program, treating a case of TB that is diagnosed early costs $20 to $40 per person, takes about six to eight months, and is without major side effects. Treatment for drug-resistant strains can cost $2,000 per person. The drugs are difficult to obtain, have serious side effects, and aren't as effective, and treatment can take up to two years.

There are approximately 20,000 cases of TB per year in the United States. The most unexpected place for overseas travelers to contract TB may not be a third-world country, but rather the plane that takes you there and back. With the incidence of tuberculosis on the increase worldwide, the World Health Organization has warned of the risk (albeit small) of contracting TB on a transatlantic flight. The CDC has identified cases of TB transmission on planes. These cases were not linked to cabin air quality or ventilation but rather to proximity to another passenger with TB and the duration of exposure to the TB pathogen. If you regularly travel internationally or live abroad for long periods of time, ask your doctor for a TB skin test every year.

In 1997, more than 1.9 billion people worldwide had active TB. The World Health Organization estimates that unless global control

High-Risk Groups for TB Exposure and Infection

- People who live or work in settings such as nursing homes, correctional facilities, homeless shelters, mental institutions, and drug treatment centers
- The elderly
- Individuals without access to health care
- People who abuse drugs and/or alcohol
- People who live with anyone experiencing the active stage of the disease
- Those who have emigrated from countries where TB is common
- People with weakened immune systems who are exposed to the disease

efforts are strengthened, by 2020 nearly a billion more people will be newly infected, 200 million will develop active disease, and 70 million will die. A major threat to TB control efforts in many countries is multidrug-resistant TB (MDR-TB), which is resistant to the two most important TB drugs, isoniazid and rifampin. MDR-TB has been identified in 104 countries. Few drugs are available to treat MDR-TB; in the past 25 years, only one new drug for this type of TB has been developed and none are currently in clinical trials.

During 1992–1993, the United States experienced a brief resurgence in the disease that reversed this country's downward trend. Since it coincided with an increase in HIV-positive individuals, experts thought that HIV and TB might be somehow linked. Now, however, it is believed that the primary correlation between HIV and TB is the fact that TB is a highly opportunistic disease easily contracted by people with weakened immune systems. Since 1993, TB rates have declined steadily. In 1998, thanks to substantial efforts among public health workers, only 18,361 cases of TB were reported, the lowest case rate in U.S. history and the sixth straight year of decline. Yet tuberculosis remains a persistent disease threat in the United States. Forty-three states and the District of Columbia have reported cases of drug-resistant TB, and the number of positive TB skin tests has risen in several of the states that have mandatory reporting laws (Missouri, South Dakota, and Indiana excluding Indianapolis). This could signal a growing population of still healthy people with latent TB who are at high risk of developing active disease—perhaps MDR-TB.

The Not-So-Friendly Skies

Airline travel is, from the standpoint of TB transmission, risky business. In recent news headlines, a Ukrainian airplane passenger infected 13 fellow passengers during a flight from Paris to New York, and a boy from the Marshall Islands who relocated to North Dakota infected 56 people at his home, school, and day care center.

The transmission of TB in office buildings increases in proportion to the amount of recycled (already breathed) air. Pilots, in cost-cutting tactics mandated by airline companies, restrict the fresh air intake

Beware the Air

- The chances of a passenger with TB being on a commercial airline flight is one in 9 million.
- The estimated risk of being exposed to TB on a commercial airline flight is one in 26,000.
- Aircraft HEPA systems allow for 50% air recirculation and permit air exchanges of between 6 and 20 times per hour.

Minimizing Your Chances of Contracting a Contagion While Aboard an Aircraft

- Always wash your hands with soap and hot water before touching your eyes, nose, and mouth, as well as before handling and consuming beverages or snacks.
- Coat the inside of your nostrils with an edible oil (almond, olive, or canola).
- Cover your nose and mouth with a water-soaked cotton handkerchief, which will help block the spread of germs

by turning off the plane's air packs (which cost just $80 per hour to operate) and mixing the precious fresh air with recycled cabin air. Clearly, it is entirely plausible that such a penny-pinching measure puts all air passengers at risk for contracting TB from a fellow traveler or cabin crew member. In 1995, the CDC reported that TB bacteria were transmitted from an infectious passenger with active TB to four other passengers during an 8½-hour domestic airline flight. Planes that recirculate air have HEPA filters that are supposed to filter out TB bacteria (HEPA systems are used in hospital settings for this reason). The CDC concluded that the 1995 incident resulted from being in close proximity to the passenger with active TB, causing the four people to inhale droplets produced when the infectious passenger coughed.

Signs and Symptoms of TB

◆ Early phase: no symptoms; if any symptoms, resembles flu.
◆ Second phase: low fever, weight loss, chronic fatigue, heavy sweating
  (especially at night).
◆ Later phase: cough with sputum that becomes progressively bloody,
  yellow, thick, or gray; chest pain; shortness of breath; sometimes,
  reddish/cloudy urine.
◆ Advanced phase: TB of the larynx occurs, making the patient unable to
  speak above a whisper.

Left untreated or improperly treated, TB may result in lung abscess; chronic obstructive pulmonary disease; spread of infection from the lungs to the bones, kidneys, intestines, spleen, and liver; respiratory failure.

The Tuberculin Skin Test

A positive tuberculin skin test means that you may have been exposed to TB and that your body has responded to the exposure. This does not mean that you have active TB. TB can remain latent for years: In the United States, only about 10% of people who test positive for exposure to the TB bacteria go on to develop active disease. Only a person in the active stage of disease can infect others. Anyone with active TB should postpone travel until his or her disease has become noninfectious.

If an airline becomes aware that someone with active infectious TB has flown on a flight longer than eight hours, the CDC suggests that the airline notify crew and passengers who may have worked near or been seated near the passenger with infectious TB. Note that the CDC's statements are recommendations, not mandates, and thus there are no measures for enforcement.

In the early stage, TB is not contagious. The CDC guidelines issued in 2000 for the treatment of latent TB in adults recommend 12 months of daily treatment with isoniazid. Once TB enters the second or later phases, where it is active, a combination of antitubercular drugs, administered for 9 to 12 months, can control the disease. It is imperative for patients under anti-TB therapy to follow their physicians' instructions on medication use precisely; otherwise, they risk relapse.

Promoting Immune Function and Lung Tissue Repair Naturally

While nondrug approaches are inadequate for treating TB, certain nutrients assist the body with tissue repair and enhance overall immunity.

MONONUCLEOSIS

Mononucleosis (also known as glandular fever), or "mono" for short, is an infectious, acute upper respiratory illness caused by the Epstein-Barr virus (EBV). This virus is a member of the same family of viruses that causes genital herpes, cold sores, chicken pox, and shingles (see Chapter 10). In mono, EBV infects the lymphocytes, or white blood cells, transforming the B cell into a reactive, malignant form. B cells circulate through the bloodstream, triggering responses from the immune system everywhere T cells find them. As T and B cells battle, we begin to feel worn down. Symptoms such as sore throat, fatigue, fever, swollen glands, and loss of appetite appear 30 to 45 days after exposure. The lymph nodes, responsible for producing T and B cells, may swell.

The most prevalent form of transmission of EBV is through the exchange of saliva; hence its moniker the "kissing disease." EBV incubates for 10 to 50 days before symptoms develop and is most contagious toward the end of that period. This is frequently before the infected person becomes aware he or she has contracted it. It is far too late to quarantine the person by the time mono can be confirmed.

Virtually everyone is exposed to the Epstein-Barr virus at some time during their lives. Studies show that up to 50% of college freshmen have mononucleosis antibodies circulating in their bloodstream, indicating previous infection during childhood. EBV tends to develop into mono in people who, for one reason or another, have a compromised immune system. EBV may be implicated in rheumatoid arthritis as well.

The mono infection can cause inflammation of the liver, leading to jaundice that may require hospitalization. It also can lead to a swollen spleen, which may rupture if subject to physical trauma. If there are no complications, the best treatment for mono is bed rest and plenty of liquids until the fever dissipates. Antibiotics are ineffective because mono is a virus; however, mono can lead to a strep infection in the throat, a condition that does require antibiotic treatment. Most people recover in six to eight weeks, but mono may return in a milder form in a few months. A person with mono may remain contagious for as long as a year. Eventually, the disease becomes dormant.

To avoid contracting mono, common-sense precautions include the following:

* Do not share eating utensils or cups.
* Do not kiss anyone who suspects they have mono, has been around someone else with mono, or is experiencing some of the symptoms of mono.

Some natural remedies shown to be helpful against mono include St. John's wort, echinacea, and astragalus. Milk thistle, garlic, lemon balm, ginger, elderberry, and turmeric, and the medicinal mushrooms reishi, shiitake, and maitake can help prevent the liver damage precipitated by mono. Vitamin C helps strengthen the immune system to fight the virus. During recovery and for two months thereafter, the infected person should avoid alcohol in order to allow the liver to recover and optimize its detoxification function.

MENINGITIS

Bacterial meningitis is caused by a meningococcus infection of the membranes around the brain and spinal cord. The infection is most often introduced through another body part, such as the lung, ear, nose, throat, or sinus. It is critical to identify meningitis in its early stages while it can still be treated with antibiotics. Unfortunately, its early symptoms—fever, neck stiffness, headache, sensitivity to light, and disorientation—are often mistaken for flu. A definitive diagnosis of bacterial meningitis is done with a spinal tap, which allows for microscopic analysis and culture of the cerebrospinal fluid.

Bacterial meningitis can be spread by kissing, sharing a drinking glass, or sneezing in close quarters. About 3,000 people contract meningitis each year in the United States, and as many as 13% of these victims die of the infection, often within 48 hours. Another 10% suffer devastating complications such as paralysis, hearing loss, speech impairment, and cognitive damage.

Each year, meningitis descends on college freshmen living in dorms across the United States. The CDC reports that the incidence of meningitis on campus doubled from 1991 to 1997, from 300 cases to 600. Students living in dormitories are almost three times more likely to contract bacterial meningitis than people in the general population, and freshmen in dorms have a sixfold greater risk than college students overall. Many campuses now warn students about bacterial meningitis on their preadmission health forms and recommend vacci-

Signs and Symptoms of Meningitis

- Fever, chills, sweating
- Headache
- Irritability
- Sensitivity to light
- Neck stiffness
- Vomiting
- Red-purple skin rash
- Confusion, lethargy, sleepiness, unconsciousness

Preventing Meningitis

Viral (aseptic) meningitis can be caused by polio virus, fungi (including yeasts), and autoimmune responses following viral illnesses. The best way to protect against viral meningitis is to keep current on immunizations for all viruses for which vaccines are available.

Meningitis Vaccine Under Fire

In late 1999, the British government instituted a mass national immunization effort to vaccinate all children under age 18 against meningitis, in a program that distributed more than 15 million doses. In October 2000, it was revealed that more than 16,000 adverse reactions, alleging the vaccines as the source, have been reported so far. Twelve people died after being vaccinated: Seven were a result of sudden infant death syndrome, and one of a convulsion experienced 10 days after vaccination.

nation. The vaccine is 70% effective in preventing the two strains of meningitis that cause most of the infections.

Bacterial meningitis is treated with intravenous antibiotics and corticosteroids. Absent of complications, recovery from meningitis takes about three weeks of close physician-supervised medical care. Nutritional supplementation is a way to support medical treatment, but is certainly not adequate as a replacement.

BUG-BUSTING BLOCKBUSTERS

An important theme in respiratory infection treatment is the enhancement of the immune system when infection strikes as follows:

- Vitamin C, 500 milligrams every two hours
- Bioflavonoids, 1,000 milligrams daily
- Vitamin A, up to 10,000 IU per day for five days (contraindicated in pregnant women and women of childbearing age not using birth control)
- Zinc, up to 30 milligrams per day
- Bed rest, to conserve your energy
- Increasing intake of hot caffeine-free fluids, such as hot broths and herbal teas, to help produce and expel secretions
- Limiting intake of simple sugars (including fruits and fruit juices) to less than 75 milligrams per day, to starve the bacteria that are infecting you

Chest percussion (see Chapter 17) is a technique that breaks up secretions and is particularly effective for loosening thick secretions in upper respiratory infection and asthma.

Postural drainage, which uses gravity to help drain secretions, may be helpful:

1. Apply a heating pad or hot water bottle to the chest area for 15 to 20 minutes.
2. Remove the pad or bottle. Place a few layers of disposable paper towels on an area of the floor near the side of the bed.
3. Lie on the bed, belly down, so that only your waist downward is firmly on the bed and your upper body half is over the paper towels.
4. Bend your forearms to the ground in a 90° angle to support your upper body.
5. Maintain this position for up to 15 minutes, and cough periodically to expectorate the secretions onto the paper towels.

For breathing exercises, see Chapter 17.

General Respiratory Therapies

- Products made from natural fruit enzymes such as papain and bromelain are used to break up thick mucus and reduce sinus inflammation.
- Consider taking 1,000 milligrams of N-acetyl cysteine (NAC)—an amino acid (protein building block) that breaks up thick mucus secretions.
- To soothe a sore throat, try gargling with 1 to 2 ounces of apple cider vinegar and a dash of salt mixed in 6 ounces of hot water.
- Oils of thyme, rosemary, peppermint, tea tree, eucalyptus, bergamot, black pepper, melissa, and hyssop inhibit most flu viruses. A 2% dilution makes an effective gargle or vapor steam. Steam treatment carries the oils directly to the sinuses and lungs and provides warm, moist air that helps to open nasal and bronchial passages. Essential oils can also be used in humidifiers or added to hot bath water.
- Natural inhalers made with essential oils can be found in health food stores. Commercial vapor balms also use essential oils. You can make the following vapor balm:
  - 2 teaspoons of peppermint oil
  - 3 teaspoons of eucalyptus oil
  - 1 teaspoon of thyme oil
  - 1 cup of olive oil
  - ¾ ounce of beeswax

Melt beeswax into olive oil over very low heat. Cool. Add oils and stir. Apply a few tablespoons to the chest, rubbing in a circular motion to promote the release of oil vapors. This mixture may be applied four to six times per day. Allow mixture to harden and store at room temperature.

7

More Than Skin Deep

Skin is the body's largest organ and normally it is alive with microorganisms. Bacteria, viruses, yeasts, fungi, mites, and insects find plenty of moisture and warmth, crevices to hide and breed in, and plentiful food in the form of dead skin and body excretions. The vast majority of these organisms are harmless, and some actually help control the numbers of bad bacteria. Given the chance, villainous microorganisms will invade the skin or enter the body through the skin. Your skin and mucous membranes are your primary barricade to invaders from the outside world.

There is a special interconnection between the skin and the immune system. After leaving the thymus, T cells (see Chapter 2) migrate to the skin's surface to receive special hormones produced only by skin cells. These hormones tell the T cells how to mature. Skin secretes an oil as well as a certain enzyme (also found in tears) that can kill microbes. So it's not a far reach to think that itching and scratching, the most common problems in all of dermatological care, may be symptoms of depressed immune function. Scratch an itch with a dirty fingernail and you've just compounded your immune problems severalfold.

HANDS

Your hand may contain as many as 200 million germs. Many of these organisms are resident flora—that is, they belong on the hand and usually crowd out other invaders. The more dangerous ones are the transient bacteria we pick up from our environment.

Antibiotics have made us complacent about one of the most effective anti-infection measures ever: handwashing. Research shows clearly that handwashing is essential for preventing the onset, or worsening, of several diseases:

- Skin conditions, including acne
- Allergies and asthma
- Athlete's foot
- Candida
- Colds and flu

Typical Germ Counts on the Hands of the General Population*

	MALE	FEMALE
Thumbnail	50–900 million	350,000–650,000
Index nail	800,000–1.1 million	850,000–17 million
Other fingernails	100–1.2 million	250,000–700,000
Palm	100–4,700	450–2.1 million
Back of hand	400–1,000	25–200

*Counts are per square centimeter (about the surface area of a shirt button).
Source: Adapted from K. Seaton, Life Health and Longevity, Scientific Hygiene Inc., 1994, p. 19.

- Pneumonia
- Worms

Under the fingernails, particularly the thumbnail, sufficient numbers of bacteria are present to overpower the strongest immune system. Of all the exposed parts of the body, the fingernail area is one of the places with the least efficient capacity to disinfect itself. Kenneth Seaton, who has conducted over a dozen years' worth of hygiene tests, reports in *Life Health and Longevity* that "we have convincing evidence that normal handwashing with bar or liquid soap . . . actually increases the number of germs under the fingernails in about 80% of cases." According to Seaton, few of us have adopted an effective system to clean under and around the fingernails. Additionally, he observes that while clipping nails close to the nail bed might improve the effectiveness of handwashing, doing so provides a passageway for germs to enter the body.

Handwashing by Health Care Professionals

A survey conducted by Medscape.com in February 2001 reports the following:

- 62% of health care professionals wash hands before seeing each patient.
- 20% wash hands just three to five times a day.
- Only 16% wash hands once an hour.
- 3% wash hands only at the start and end of the workday.

ABRASIONS

Cuts, rashes, and scratches compromise the skin's effectiveness as an infection blocker. Often, these can be treated with basic first aid. Do so promptly, following these general guidelines:

1. Allow the wound to bleed freely for several seconds to help clean it.

2. Gently cleanse the wound with mild soap and cool water to remove all dirt. For stubborn dirt and debris, use a 3% solution of hydrogen peroxide. Opt for an iodine-based product for stronger antiseptic action. (Before using any over-the-counter products such as hydrogen peroxide, cortisone creams, or antibacterial ointments, read the labels carefully.)
3. If the wound continues to ooze or bleed, apply pressure with a clean pad and the palm of your hand. Raise the injured area above the heart, over the head, to stop mild bleeding.
4. A light coating of triple antibiotic ointment can help speed healing and may prevent scarring.
5. Dress the wound and change the dressing daily for several days until a firm scab forms. Scabs act as protective barriers that prevent bacteria from entering the body.

Tetanus is an acute, often fatal disease caused by the toxin produced by the pathogen *Clostridium tetani*. Tetanus is characterized by general rigidity that starts as lockjaw and neck stiffness, and spreads through the entire body, accompanied by convulsive skeletal muscle spasms. To combat this disease, the tetanus shot (an antigen *C. tetani*) has been in use since 1924. Most often, by the time they are 7 years old, American children have been administered the combined antigen of diphtheria, pertussis, and tetanus (DTaP), in a series of spaced doses. The tetanus shot does wane, and most people fall below the optimal levels of tetanus antigen around 10 years after the last dose. As a result, booster doses of tetanus and diphtheria are required to maintain protection. The dose

Miscellaneous Mishaps

- Facial scrapes should be thoroughly washed to remove debris. Treat with antiseptic or antibiotic cream and do not bandage.
- Treat minor yet painful bruises by applying cold packs to reduce swelling.

When to See the Doctor

- If cuts, scrapes, or bruises are a result of a serious injury or accident
- If a wound was made by a sharp object you suspect was contaminated with rust or dirt
- If there is a foreign object embedded in your wound

The following are symptoms of infection and special situations requiring immediate medical attention:

- Heavy bleeding or bleeding that does not stop after applying pressure for 15 minutes
- Redness and tenderness at the wound site
- Oozing pus or red streaks radiating from the wound
- Fever
- Wounds with jagged edges that gape open
- Wounds more than 1 inch long with flesh protruding from them
- Wounds over a joint, on the face, or in the moist skin of the mouth, eyes, or genitals—places where healing is more difficult

Look to Your Kitchen and Medicine Cabinets for Quick Wound Remedies

Honey, toothpaste, and mud mask skin care products are all agents that, when spread on wounds, draw out water and body fluids to inhibit the growth of bacteria and fungi.

- Apply a thin layer of unprocessed honey (not pasteurized) to a cut or wound, two to three times a day until the wound has healed, and cover with a bandage.
- For superficial skin wounds, try dabbing on a small mound of toothpaste or mud mask product and leave uncovered. The paste or mud will dry, drawing out fluid or pus from the wound.

may be given sooner as part of wound management (in cases where the source of the wound creates an environment ripe for tetanus).

Myths and Truths About Wound Care

Throughout the centuries, everything from cobwebs to chloroform has been applied to cuts and sores. Scientific methodology now disagrees with the following:

- *Myth 1. Wounds should be left uncovered.* Although our medieval ancestors might have left wounds open to let bad humors escape, we now know that keeping a wound uncovered will make us susceptible to infection and will make the wound harder to heal by drying out the surface.
- *Myth 2. Heat helps wounds heal.* Wounds will dry out from heat from hair dryers or heat lamps, so don't use either if you want to promote the healing process. Wounds that dry out are susceptible to reopening and therefore are prone to exposure to bacteria and becoming (re-)infected.
- *Truth.* Moderate exposure (10–20 minutes daily) to sunlight can help speed wound healing. The light acts to stimulate metabolism and acts as a disinfectant.

BITES

Most bug bites are harmless, creating localized and minor swelling, redness, and itching. A small fraction of the population has allergies to the venom injected by the bug into the bite, characterized by difficulty swallowing, hoarseness, labored breathing, weakness, confusion, severe swelling, and a feeling of doom. Anaphylaxis (the most severe allergic reaction) can close the airway or trigger shock, resulting in unconsciousness.

To reduce your odds of being bitten by bugs, try these nontoxic approaches that produce scents that act as natural insect repellents:

- Calendula ointment.
- Brewer's yeast or garlic applied topically.
- Swimming in a chlorinated pool.
- Avoiding alcoholic beverages. These cause the skin to flush and blood vessels to dilate, making you a prime target for mosquitoes.
- Keeping ankles, feet, and toes covered. The same bacteria as found in Limburger cheese is the cause of foot odor, and this scent is a beacon that attracts dining mosquitoes.

After being bitten, wash the area thoroughly with soap and water. You can apply a topical anti-itch agent, such as the following:

- A paste made of 3 parts baking soda plus 1 part warm water, applied to the site of the sting for 20 minutes
- Meat tenderizer containing papain (a natural enzyme derived from papaya that can help break down the insect venom) mixed in warm water
- Calendula ointment, which also is an effective bug deterrent
- Calamine lotion
- Ice, if minor swelling occurs and is bothersome
- If outdoors, a dab of clay-containing soil packed on top of the sting, then covered with a bandage

For bites requiring special attention, do the following:

- Ant and mosquito bites: Wash thoroughly with soap and water, then apply a paste made of baking soda and water to suppress itching.
- Chigger bites: Brush and scrub the area well, then apply an ice pack to reduce swelling.
- Bee stings: Use tweezers to remove the stinger. To relieve the pain, apply a moistened gauze pad soaked in a tea of echinacea or yellow dock, or a poultice made with white oak bark, comfrey, slippery elm, or lobelia. Household ammonia applied immediately to a bite can help denature the poison and limit the pain.

Natural Ointments and Salves Soothe the Skin

- For dry itchy skin: black walnut, comfrey, echinacea, pokeweed, cloves
- For burns, blisters, insect bites, and bruises: echinacea, pokeweed, peppermint, lavender
- For inflammation: echinacea, red clover, burdock, milk thistle, hyssop, lobelia, pokeweed, black walnut, cloves, wormwood, lemon

Simply Irresistible

Researchers from the University of Durham in England and the Medical Research Council in Gambia report that mothers-to-be are bitten twice as often by mosquitoes as other women. The team speculates that metabolites exhaled by expectant moms serve as the dining call.

West Nile–Like Viral Encephalitis

Encephalitis is an inflammation of the brain caused by viruses and bacteria, including viruses transmitted by mosquitoes. West Nile encephalitis is an infection of the brain caused by West Nile virus, which is commonly found in Africa, West Asia, and the Middle East.

The U.S. version of West Nile virus is most closely related genetically to strains found in the Middle East. The CDC speculates that the virus has been in the eastern United States at least since the early summer of 1999. It was likely introduced to North America by international travel of infected persons to New York, importation (legal and otherwise) of infected birds, or migration of infected birds.

People contract West Nile encephalitis from the bite of a mosquito infected with West Nile virus. While infected ticks have been found in Asia and Africa, there is no proof that ticks play a role in U.S.

outbreaks. West Nile encephalitis is not transmitted from person to person, so kissing and touching an infected person, or contact with a health care worker who has treated someone with the virus, is safe. There is no current evidence that a pregnancy would be at risk due to infection with West Nile virus.

Symptoms of West Nile virus include headache, fever, rash, and swollen lymph glands. A severe infection can cause high fever, neck stiffness, disorientation, coma, tremors, and paralysis. In the elderly and people with compromised immune systems, the virus may cause life-threatening neurologic deterioration and muscle weakness. West Nile virus multiplies in the person's blood system, and, after reaching the brain, causes fatal disruptions of the central nervous system as well as brain tissue inflammation.

All residents of areas where virus activity has been identified are at risk of getting West Nile encephalitis. The virus has been most pronounced in the northeastern United States, particularly New York and Massachusetts. People age 50 and older are at the greatest risk for severe disease. The risk of infection only ends when mosquito activity ceases for the season during several days' worth of freezing temperatures. In locales where temperatures remain warm, West Nile virus can be transmitted year-round.

There is no effective treatment program for West Nile virus. In the 1999 New York outbreak, about 40% of the people experienced severe muscle weakness, and of that group 50% experienced flaccid paralysis. The CDC reports that up to 15% of people infected with West Nile virus will die.

There is no vaccine at the present time. In August 2000, a Massachusetts company was issued a federal grant of $3 million to develop one. Human testing could begin by spring 2002.

Experts at the CDC predicted that after the 1999 East Coast outbreak, West Nile virus would move south via the autumn migration of birds. To reduce the risk of contracting this virus, avoid contact with mosquitoes by doing the following:

* Staying inside at dawn, dusk, and early evening when mosquitoes are most active

- Wearing clothing that covers the skin—for example, a long-sleeved shirt and long pants
- Wearing light-colored clothing
- Applying insect repellent (sparingly) containing DEET (diethyltoluamide; follow product instructions for children)
- Spraying clothing with DEET-containing repellent

Killer Cousins

Two relatives of West Nile virus are St. Louis encephalitis and eastern equine encephalitis. Since 1964, there have been 4,437 reported cases of St. Louis encephalitis and 153 of eastern equine encephalitis.

Animal Bites

Animal bites and scratches, no matter how minor, can become infected and can spread bacteria to other parts of the body. Bites by animals, and humans for that matter, can transmit disease because the mouth is home to countless bacteria looking for new places to live.

All animal bites require some level of treatment, depending on the nature and severity of the wound:

1. If the bite is bleeding, apply pressure with a clean bandage or towel until bleeding stops. Use a clean latex glove to protect yourself from exposure to the blood, in the event that the animal carried a transmittable disease.
2. Clean the wound with soap and water, holding it under running water for five minutes.
3. Dry the wound and cover with sterile gauze.
4. Call your doctor. It may be necessary to administer antibiotics, a tetanus booster, or rabies vaccinations. Some wounds, particularly those on the face, may require special in-office care.

5. Involve your local animal-control authority to locate and confine the animal that caused the wound, particularly if the attacking animal was wild or behaving in a strange manner.

Reality Bites

Dogs attack more than one million Americans each year and are the most common type of animal bite. To protect you, your neighbors, and your pet, make sure you immunize and license Fido properly.

After an Animal Bite, See a Doctor If There Is . . .

◆ Swelling
◆ Pain
◆ Increased redness
◆ Drainage or discharge from the wound
◆ Fever
◆ Swollen glands
◆ Flulike symptoms

Human Bites

Human bites are more serious than animal bites. The sheer number and diversity of microbes in the human mouth outnumber that found in dogs and cats. *Eikenella corrodens,* which normally resides in the human mouth, frequently contributes to infections resulting from human bites. When *Eikenella* is present with other pathogens that are antibiotic resistant, it can spread aggressively. Another bacteria commonly found in the human mouth, *Veillonella parvula,* is a serious pathogenic agent when transferred.

Alert your doctor immediately if you receive a human bite. More importantly, a clenched-fist injury (resulting from punching someone in the mouth) carries a very high risk for deep-seated infection involving the tendon, bone, and joint. Antibiotics (the same ones used for treating infections in dog and cat bite wounds) may be necessary. Human bites, according to Boston Medical Center, should never be stitched up (sutured), as doing so may entrap infective microbes in the wound.

A First Aid Kit for Cuts, Scrapes, Bites, and Bruises

Assemble one kit for your home and one for each car, containing the following items:

- Sterile adhesive bandages in assorted sizes
- 2-inch sterile gauze pads (4–6 qty)
- 4-inch sterile gauze pads (4–6 qty)
- Hypoallergenic adhesive tape
- Triangular bandages (3 qty)
- 2-inch sterile roller bandages (3 rolls)
- 3-inch sterile roller bandages (3 rolls)
- Splints, ½ inch thick × 3 inches wide × 12–15 inches long
- Scissors, tweezers, needle
- Moistened towelettes
- Iodine-based antiseptic and hydrogen peroxide
- Sterile saline solution
- Thermometer
- Assorted sizes of safety pins
- Cleansing agent/soap
- Latex gloves (2 pair minimum)
- Eye goggles

STREPTOCOCCUS AND STAPHYLOCOCCUS

Boils

A boil is a localized, painful, burning infection on the skin surface. The medical term for a single boil is *furuncle,* and several furuncles connected with each other and hooked into the tissue just below the skin are called a *carbuncle.* Boils may appear anywhere on the body: A sty is a boil found on the eyelid.

A boil starts out as a red bump that slowly grows in size—some boils reach a half inch or more across. After several days, the boil becomes soft and pus-filled, with a yellow or white head in the middle of the surface. While sometimes difficult to resist, doctors recommend that boils be left alone: They will rupture on their own, drain themselves of the collected pus and blood, and begin to heal. Puncturing or squeezing a boil while it is still hard may make the infection worse. In some cases, your doctor may prescribe antibiotics. Nonprescription antibiotic creams or ointments are ineffective as topical treatments for boils.

Boils are caused by staphylococcus bacteria. Typically, the infection begins in a hair follicle and bores into the skin's deeper layers to produce the domed nodule. Staphylococcus bacteria are highly infectious. Once the boil is draining, keep it clean and covered with a dressing. Discard all dressings promptly and wash your hands thoroughly after touching the boil or the covering.

To relieve the pain associated with a boil, soak with warm water for 20 minutes three to four times daily. Make sure you wash your hands and wash towels promptly afterward.

To prevent boils, remember the following:

• Keep your skin clean and employ good washing hygiene (see this chapter's Bug-Busting Blockbusters).
• Don't share towels or clothing with anyone in your household who has a boil.

When to See the Doctor

- To drain a boil that measures more than a half inch across
- If you have a fever (over 100°F)
- If you get several boils at the same time
- If you get boils frequently

Cellulitis

Cellulitis is an insidious, noncontagious infection in which streptococcus and staphylococcus are most commonly implicated. Characterized by warmth, tenderness, and a localized redness that remains flat, cellulitis causes fevers, chills, tenderness, and general malaise. Cellulitis swelling grows rapidly within the first 24 hours of infection. An initial area is typically 1 to 3 inches in diameter. Frequently, a thin red line extends from the middle of the cellulitis area to the direction of the heart.

A 10-day course of oral antibiotics is the usual treatment mode for cellulitis. If the bacteria have entered the lymphatic system and bloodstream, hospitalization and intravenous (IV) antibiotics are necessary.

Get Treatment

Cellulitis on the face (erysipelas) may develop into brain infection or meningitis if prompt treatment is not obtained.

Important: Seek immediate medical attention for any infection that starts as a small localized incident but spreads quickly.

RINGWORM

Ringworm is not a worm but rather a fungal infection with ring-shaped lesions. The ringworm fungi feast on dead skin, hair, and nails. Poor hygiene and poor living conditions increase the chances of contracting ringworm. Ringworm is contagious via contact with infected surfaces such as towels, shoes, or shower stalls.

Signs of Ringworm

- Ringworm affecting the body: lesions that are flat, scaly, and red. The center of the ring clears as the scaly red edge advances.
- Ringworm affecting the scalp: round, sharply outlined areas where hairs are broken off just above the skin. Lesions can be both light and flaky, but moist and inflamed as well.
- Ringworm of the feet: more commonly known as athlete's foot. Causing minor scaling and cracking between the toes, athlete's foot can spread widely, become badly inflamed, or cause secondary infection if left untreated.
- Ringworm affecting the groin: more commonly known as jock itch. Occurring most commonly in men, it may be carried to the groin from the foot area.
- Ringworm affecting the nails: Known to doctors as paronychia, it is a commonly recurrent infection caused by a fungus or bacteria. In both cases, there is redness and swelling around the fingernail. Bacterial paronychia is curable with treatment in two weeks, whereas fungal paronychia is chronic and may require six months to heal.

When to See a Doctor

- You develop a fever.
- Lesions become redder, painful, and ooze pus.
- Pain or discomfort is not relieved by standard medical treatment.

Ringworm Prevention Tips

+ Maintain good personal hygiene.
+ Dry feet thoroughly after bathing or swimming.
+ Wear gloves when doing housework or gardening, and keep the insides
  of gloves dry.
+ Do not share hats, combs, or brushes.
+ Avoid tight shoes or underwear that may rub or chafe the skin.
+ Treat pets that have skin problems, since they may be ringworm
  transmitters.

Ringworm is treated with topical antifungal drugs. Treatment may continue after symptoms disappear in order to prevent recurrence. In widespread infections and nail infections, an oral antifungal may be prescribed. Be sure to launder promptly in hot water all clothing, towels, and linens that have touched those with ringworm lesions.

STUBBORN NAIL FUNGUS

Known by the medical diagnosis of onychomycosis, stubborn nail fungus affects 35 million people in the United States, and 90% of them have not yet sought medical attention. Caused by microorganisms called dermatophytes, nail fungus starts when these bugs find a way underneath the nail, where they begin to multiply. More often arising from trauma to the nail area (such as banging it, trimming too closely, or wearing shoes that cramp the toes) rather than from poor hygiene, nails weaken and become targets for infection.

Nail fungus rarely goes away with topical remedies and rarely resolves on its own. The most effective treatment is an oral antifungal prescription that may take up to three months to achieve its full effect in toenails, and up to two months for fingernails. Left untreated, nails

> ## Nail Fungus Prevention Tips
>
> ◆ Keep nails short and clean, and file them regularly to maintain a
>   manageable length.
> ◆ Clip toenails straight across to prevent them from becoming ingrown.
> ◆ Avoid trauma to and irritants (including polishes) on the nails.
> ◆ Wear cotton gloves for chores that do not involve water.
> ◆ Do not share nail grooming implements with others.
> ◆ Do not wear high heels or narrow-toed shoes.

may become painful and thick, requiring medical care for even the simple task of trimming.

LICE

Head lice infestation is second place to the common cold as the most communicable childhood disease. As many as 20 million people become infested by lice annually. Lice are wingless insects, about the size of a sesame seed. Lice survive by biting and sucking blood from the scalp, and the bites cause itching and red spots comparable to mosquito bites. Scratching lice bites can lead to secondary bacterial infections, with symptoms such as fever, achiness, and lethargy.

In 1997, the U.S. National Cancer Institute reported research that lindane, the active ingredient in lice poison shampoos at that time, was responsible for at least 70% of the reported serious health reactions to lice shampoos. Since then, lindane has been banned in 18 countries and severely restricted in 10 others. In the United States, the Food and Drug Administration (FDA) permits its pre-scribed use, but recommends it as a course of action when other treatments are ineffective. Today, lice shampoos contain pyrethrum- or permethrin-based pediculicides. There is a long list of cautionary statements associated with use of these products, so be sure to read package directions carefully and completely. One of the most important usage reminders is to wash objects treated with these pesticides well: A study by Rutgers University found residue in doses nearly 70 times in excess of Environmental Protection Agency (EPA) maximum exposure levels on toys and surfaces in a treated room. Just recently, the FDA approved a prescription-only malathion (0.5%) lotion.

The National Pediculosis Association averages 50 calls a day reporting failure of lice pesticide products. A study in Israel and one in the Czech Republic both demonstrate that increasing concentrations of permethrin are becoming routinely necessary to kill head lice, while a study by the Harvard School of Public Health reports that a sampling of lice could not be killed by any dose of permethrin exposure. A debate among pediatricians now rages concerning whether lice resistance exists, or if reinfestation as a result of incomplete or improper treatment of the initial outbreak is mistaken for resistance.

Lousy Statistics

- Lice can only survive 48 hours without a host.
- Lice do not like warm temperatures and will not harbor in body regions exceeding 75°F.

There is an effective natural treatment approach for lice. *Natural Health* magazine recommends this three-step program:

1. Mix together 2 tablespoons of olive oil, 10 drops of rosemary essential oil *(Rosmarinus officinalis),* and 10 drops of lavender essential oil *(Lavandula angustifolia).* Dampen the hair with warm water and massage the oil thoroughly into the hair and scalp. Cover with a shower cap and leave the mixture on the hair for one hour.

2. Add 3 drops of thyme essential oil *(Thymus vulgaris)* to 1 tablespoon of a shampoo that contains neem *(Azadirachta indica)*. Shampoo the hair, letting sit for five minutes before rinsing with warm water.

3. Rinse the hair and scalp with a mixture of 2 cups of warm water, 2 cups of vinegar, and 6 drops each of rosemary and lavender essential oils. Cover the hair with a shower cap for 15 minutes, then comb out with a lice comb. Rinse the hair and scalp again thoroughly with warm water.

This program can be repeated as necessary to kill any new lice that hatch.

Lice Aren't Nice

They wreak havoc on entire households, requiring us to do the following:

- Quarantine bedding, toys, and clothes of those infected. Deep clean with scalding water (140°F) and detergent. Discard any items for which you are unsure if cleaning was done adequately.
- Wash in scalding water all sports headgear, hats, combs, barrettes, scarves, and brushes in contact with the infected person.
- Vacuum carpets, upholstered furniture, car seats, and headrests in contact with the infected person. Discard the vacuum cleaner bag immediately.
- Shampoo the hair of infected family members with lice shampoo multiple times a day.

BUG-BUSTING BLOCKBUSTERS

Handwashing is one of the most important means of preventing
the spread of infection.

—Centers for Disease Control and Prevention

In the mid-1800s, the Hungarian physician Dr. Ignas Semmelweiss
noticed that fewer of his patients were dying once he instated a policy
of washing his hands and medical instruments between patient examinations. He proposed that his colleagues do the same, and was
viciously ridiculed for what was branded as an idiotic theory.

We now know that the simplest and cheapest way to prevent
infectious disease is through frequent and fastidious handwashing.
Otherwise, you risk infecting yourself from germs on objects touched
by others who might not be meticulous about their hygiene, and from
people you shake hands with or otherwise contact. When you subsequently touch your eyes, mouth, nasal passages, or open wounds, you
enable fast entry of microorganisms into your body—a process called
self-inoculation.

Penny Wise

Washing hands regularly costs less than a penny, which can prevent a $50 or
more office visit to the doctor to merely diagnose an infectious disease you
contract.

Wash your hands 10 times each day—double that if you're in an
environment where infectious germs abound (for example, proximity
to someone sick in the home or at the workplace, or physical contact

with objects touched by someone who is sick). It is especially important to wash hands in the following situations:

- Before, during, and after you prepare food (particularly raw meat, poultry, or fish)
- Before you eat
- Before inserting or removing contact lenses
- After you use the bathroom
- After you blow your nose, cough, or sneeze
- After treating a cut or wound of your own or someone else
- After handling animals or animal waste
- After changing a diaper
- After handling garbage
- When your hands are visibly dirty
- More frequently when you or someone in your home is sick

The CDC outlines the technique for proper handwashing as follows:

1. Wet your hands and apply liquid or clean bar soap. Place the bar soap on a rack that allows it to drain.
2. Scrub all surfaces, including wrists, palms, backs of hands, fingers, under the fingernails, and between fingers. Rub your hands vigorously together for 10 to 15 seconds.
3. Rinse well with warm water.

Spreading a Wealth of Germs

- A fresh paper towel is preferred to a cloth that is damp or has not been laundered recently.
- Wiping damp hands on clothes or hair can spread bacteria to other areas of the body.

4. Dry hands with a clean or disposable towel. Pat the skin rather than rubbing, to avoid chapping or cracking. Apply hand lotion if your skin is susceptible to drying out.

For improved efficacy of handwashing, use a product such as Natural Maxi-Cleanse Disinfectant Soap. Containing a blend of unique natural disinfectant agents in a fortified soap, this product is shown by laboratory testing to remove 99% of all germs from hands. The antibacterial agents in Natural Maxi-Cleanse Disinfectant Soap

A Graceful Exit

In a public setting, perhaps as important as proper handwashing is how you exit the rest room itself. To avoid recontamination by the same microorganisms you so diligently removed from your hands, remember the following:

- Use a clean, dry paper towel to grab doorknobs or to push doors open, and discard the towel promptly.
- Open doors with your elbows or feet—areas of the body less prone to spreading infectious disease.

Dirty Little Facts

An observational study of 7,836 U.S. adults conducted in August 2000 by the Handwashing Study prepared for the American Society for Microbiology reported the following:

- Only 58% of men washed their hands after going to the bathroom.
- 75% of women washed their hands after going to the bathroom.
- Fewer than 50% of food workers in inner-city restaurants wash their hands thoroughly or often enough to prevent contamination.

are natural: They will not harm the environment, nor will they contribute to the problem of antibiotic drug resistance. Natural Maxi-Cleanse Disinfectant Soap is available at the Anti-Aging Superstore at www.anti-agingsuperstore.com.

Perhaps just as important as washing your hands is properly drying them. Researchers at Auckland Hospital in New Zealand found that rinsed but undried hands can transfer tens of thousands of bacterial cells to food. Their follow-up studies found that drying hands for 10 seconds using a clean cloth towel followed by air drying for 20 seconds achieved a 99.8% reduction in the amount of bacteria moved from one place to another on the skin. The same technique also reduced the bacteria moved from human hands to food by 94%.

8

ABCs of Hepatitis

Hepatitis, a general term that refers to any inflammation of the liver, is a silent epidemic of enormous proportions. Nearly 47,000 cases of acute viral hepatitis were reported to the Centers for Disease Control and Prevention (CDC) in 1995 alone. Hepatitis is a real and present danger to anyone who does any of the following activities:

- Engages in casual sex
- Receives a blood transfusion
- Eats in restaurants
- Travels abroad

TYPES OF HEPATITIS

There are seven different strains of hepatitis, each identified by a letter, A through G (see the "Hepatitis by Type" table in this chapter). The most common forms are viral:

- Type A: spread through person-to-person contact and by ingesting food or water contaminated by sewage

- Type B: spread by sexual contact, blood transfusions, injections with nonsterile needles, bloodsucking insects, and from mother to newborn
- Type C: usually transmitted through intravenous drug use, blood transfusions, and other exposures from contaminated blood and blood products

Untreated or improperly treated hepatitis may become a chronic situation, persisting for more than six months and posing a notable public health threat due to the unwitting spread of the virus from people with untreated hepatitis via daily contact with others. Other complications include liver failure, cirrhosis (scarring) of the liver, liver cancer, and death.

BASICS ABOUT HEPATITIS A, B, AND C

Hepatitis A causes between 125,000 and 200,000 total infections annually in the United States, with a general upward progression in the number of cases during the past several years. Only two-thirds of those infected actually experience the classic symptoms of the disease, which means upwards of 40,000 active cases fail to be treated properly. There are large nationwide outbreaks every decade; the most recent occurred in 1989.

Hepatitis A, B, and C are NOT Spread By . . .

- Kissing and hugging (unless you are in contact with open sores on the infected person)
- Being coughed or sneezed on
- Sharing eating utensils or food

Blood, not saliva, is the body fluid involved in hepatitis transmission.

Hepatitis by Type

HEPATITIS	SYMPTOMS	INCUBATION	TRANSMISSION	TREATMENT	AT RISK
A	• None in children • In adults, flulike symptoms with nausea, fatigue, abdominal pain, appetite loss, diarrhea, jaundice, and fever over 6 to 12 months	Average 30 days	• Eating items contaminated with infected feces • Drinking water/ice contaminated with sewage; eating raw/ partially cooked shellfish from contaminated water • Eating fruits and vege- tables or uncooked food contaminated during handling • For men, having sex with other men	• Immuno- globulin 2 to 3 months before or 2 weeks after expo- sure offers temporary immunity. • Hepatitis A vaccine for long-term protection	Those who . . . • Are in contact with people from infected areas • Travel/work in infected countries • Engage in anal sex • Use intravenous drugs

(continued)

Hepatitis A virus is spread from person to person by putting something in the mouth that has been contaminated by the fecal matter of someone with hepatitis A. You can get hepatitis A from contact with a household member or sex partner with the disease. You cannot get hepatitis A from casual contact with an infected person. Hepatitis A kills 100 Americans annually.

(continued)

HEPATITIS	SYMPTOMS	INCUBATION	TRANSMISSION	TREATMENT	AT RISK
B	• Loss of appetite, nausea, vomiting, fever, fatigue, abdominal pain, dark urine or jaundice • No symptoms in some people	Can survive at least 7 days out of the body	• Exposure to infected blood, unpro- tected sex with an infected person, sharing contaminated needles, travel to countries with high rate of infection • Infected mothers may infect newborns.	• Interferon alpha-2b • For newborns, infants, and teenagers, the vaccine provides immunity for at least 5 years.	Those who . . . • Use intravenous drugs • Have multiple sex partners • Travel or work in developing countries • Received a transfusion before 1975

(continued)

Hepatitis A is preventable. Effective measures include the following:

• Hepatitis A vaccine: This vaccine does not contain live virus. The CDC believes that it protects those immunized for at least 20 years.
• Immunoglobulin, an antibody preparation, administered before and after known exposure (maximum protection provided if given within two weeks of exposure). Unfortunately, immuno- globulins are in short supply.
• Good hygiene and sanitation.

Hepatitis B is a serious disease that causes lifelong infection and cirrhosis (scarring) of the liver. It can become life-threatening. The disease strikes 140,000 to 320,000 people in the United States each

(continued)

HEPATITIS	SYMPTOMS	INCUBATION	TRANSMISSION	TREATMENT	AT RISK
C	• **More than half of those infected have no symptoms.** • Jaundice (yellowish eyes or skin), extreme fatigue, pain or tenderness in the right upper quadrant of the body (liver), persistent nausea or pain in the stomach, lingering fever, loss of appetite, diarrhea, dark-colored urine or light-colored stools • May also have hepatitis B	Can be as long as 28 weeks; averages 7 to 9 weeks	• Exposure to infected blood, sharing contaminated needles, sharing razors or toothbrushes with infected person	• Interferon alpha-2b, alpha-2a, or a combination of interferon and ribavirin • No vaccine	Those who . . . • Use intravenous drugs • Had a blood transfusion or organ transplant before July 1992 • Snort cocaine • Engage in unpro-tected sex with an infected partner

(continued)

(continued)

HEPATITIS	SYMPTOMS	INCUBATION	TRANSMISSION	TREATMENT	AT RISK
D	• Loss of appetite, nausea, vomiting, fever, fatigue, abdominal pain, dark urine or jaundice	Occurs only with hepatitis B virus	• Exposure to infected blood • Requires hepatitis B virus to replicate	• Interferon alpha for hepatitis B • No vaccine	Those who . . . • Use intravenous drugs
E	• Abdominal pain, dark urine, fever, jaundice, nausea and vomiting	2 to 9 weeks	• Water contaminated with fecal material (especially in developing countries), contaminated uncooked shellfish, fruits and vegetables	• Bed rest • No drug treatment or vaccine	Those who . . . • Are pregnant • Travel or work in developing countries
F	• Only a few cases have been described; may not be a distinct hepatitis virus				
G	• Similar to hepatitis C • Infection with hepatitis B, C, or both is common.		• Exposure to infected blood	• No proven treatment	

Who Should Receive Hepatitis A Vaccine?

- People traveling to, or working in, countries with high rates of the disease
- Children in communities with high rates of the disease and periodic outbreaks
- Men who have sex with men
- Illicit drug users
- People who may be exposed in the course of their work
- People with chronic liver disease
- People with clotting factor disorders (including hemophilia)

year, yet only 50% of those infected experience symptoms. Up to 10% of the total number of hepatitis B cases convert into chronic hepatitis annually, with the total number of chronic hepatitis B cases in the United States estimated at 1.25 million. Every year, hepatitis B infection kills 5,000 to 6,000 Americans as a result of its progression to chronic liver disease, including cirrhosis and primary liver cancer.

The incidence of hepatitis B increased through 1985 and then declined 55% through 1993 as a result of the wider use of the vaccine in adults, modification of high-risk behaviors, and possibly due to a decrease in the number of susceptible persons. Since 1993, however, the CDC has reported increases among sexually active heterosexuals, homosexual men, and intravenous drug users.

Hepatitis B is transmitted via contact with contaminated blood, sexual contact, and from infected mothers to infants. The disease is preventable by the following measures:

- Hepatitis B vaccine (available since 1982)
- Screening pregnant women so that infected newborns receive immediate treatment
- Routine vaccination of infants and 11- to 12-year-olds
- Vaccination of high-risk groups of all ages
- Screening of blood, organ, and tissue donors

Who Should Receive Hepatitis B Vaccine?

- Intravenous drug users
- Sexually active heterosexuals
- Men having sex with men
- Sexual and household members in contact with those infected
- Health care workers
- Infants and children of immigrants from countries with high hepatitis A rates
- Infants born to infected mothers
- Those living in poorer communities with inadequate sanitation
- Hemodialysis patients

Prior to the late 1980s, hepatitis C was so rare that it had no name and was not studied by medical researchers. Today, hepatitis C is the most common blood-borne illness in the United States. It is likely to increase, since most infected people have not been identified because they don't exhibit symptoms (see the "Hepatitis by Type" table in this chapter). You may be at risk for hepatitis C if any of the following items apply to you:

- You were notified that you received blood from a donor who later tested positive for hepatitis C.
- You injected illicit drugs, even if it was just once a long time ago.
- You received a blood transfusion or solid organ transplant before July 1992.
- You received a blood product for clotting problems, where the product was produced before 1987.
- You have been on long-term kidney dialysis.
- You have evidence of liver disease, such as persistently elevated ALT (alanine aminotransferase) levels.

Additionally, exposure may occur through the following:

* Occupational exposure (health care worker)
* Sharing a razor or toothbrush with an infected person
* Having tattooing or body piercing done with unsterile equipment
* History of cocaine or marijuana use (potential for exposure to open sores)
* Becoming sexually active at an early age
* Having had multiple sex partners
* History of sexually transmitted disease
* Serving time in prison

In 40% of cases, the specific mode of transmission of hepatitis C is unknown. Even more curious is that about 15% of those infected with hepatitis C are able to throw off the disease (scientists still don't know exactly how).

Hepatitis C infection is often discovered by chance, either during screening tests for blood donation or during a regular physical exam. Hepatitis C can infect the liver for as long as 20 to 40 years before being discovered. Currently, there is no vaccine to prevent hepatitis C. Researchers believe that the threat it poses to public health is as significant as the threat posed by HIV/AIDS. Although AIDS is more deadly than hepatitis C, hepatitis C affects four times as many Americans.

Treatment for hepatitis C by prescription drugs is debilitating,

Hefty Consequences of Hepatitis C

* Chronic infection results in more than 85% of cases.
* Chronic liver disease results in 70% of cases.
* Hepatitis C kills 8,000 to 10,000 Americans each year.
* One in five infected persons will wind up with cirrhosis (scarring of the liver) or liver cancer.
* Hepatitis C is the leading indicator for liver transplantation.

costly, and effective in less than 40% of cases. Recently, the National Institute of Diabetes and Digestive and Kidney Diseases launched an eight-year $28 million clinical trial to evaluate antiviral drug treatments for hepatitis C. Regular monitoring of blood levels of the liver enzyme ALT gauges progress of therapy. However, it is common for people with chronic hepatitis C to have ALT levels that periodically return to normal or near-normal. People with persistently normal ALT levels usually have a good prognosis. In a recent issue of *Health News*, Dr. John McHutchinson, medical director of liver transplantation at the Scripps Clinic and Research Foundation in La Jolla, California, recommends treating rather than waiting. "The analogy I think of is if a person tests positive for tuberculosis, you don't wait until there is a positive chest x-ray before you start treatment—you treat right away."

People suffering from any type of chronic hepatitis typically dete-

Be Good to Yourself and Others

If you have hepatitis C, you can avoid additional liver damage by following these guidelines:

• Avoiding alcohol
• Being vaccinated against hepatitis A and B
• Not starting any new medications
• Not using any over-the-counter herbal remedies or drugs without consulting your doctor

You can avoid transmitting the disease to others by doing the following:

• Not donating blood
• Not sharing toothbrushes, razors, or similar grooming items
• Covering cuts and sores
• If you are in a monogamous relationship, you and your partner don't have to make dramatic changes in your sexual practices. Your partner's risk of contracting the disease from you through sexual activity is low. If you are concerned, however, or if you have multiple sex partners, use a condom.

riorate to the point at which permanent and irreversible liver damage occurs. Of the 4 million Americans chronically infected with hepatitis C, 20% develop cirrhosis within 20 years. Fewer than half will live an additional five years after complications develop. Even after transplantation, only 6 in 10 will survive seven more years. The prognosis for hepatitis B patients who develop cirrhosis is more alarming: Only 50% will survive another five years, and so far, liver transplantation is very discouraging. In the 1980s, death occurred within 12 to 18 months of transplantation, and by the 1990s, many programs refused to offer transplants to patients with chronic hepatitis B.

THE NATION'S BLOOD SUPPLY

Every year, Americans donate approximately 12 million units of blood, which are processed into 20 million blood products. About 3.6 million Americans receive transfusions of these blood products annually. The FDA is responsible for regulating the blood industry, which includes the steps of collecting, processing, and distributing blood and blood products. Be mindful, however, that how a blood establishment is categorized decides how closely the facility is actively monitored. The nation's 1,000 licensed firms, engaged in interstate commerce, must report immediately to the FDA on breaches of safeguards and processing problems and accidents, and correct deficiencies. The several hundred blood establishments that are not engaged in interstate commerce and thus are not licensed—instead they are registered—are not required to immediately report problems, errors, or accidents to the FDA and simply do so annually as part of their FDA inspection.

The FDA believes that its "five layers of overlapping safeguards" are adequate protection of the nation's blood and blood products supply. They are as follows:

1. Donor screening: self-administered survey of health and risk factors, plus interview-administered questions regarding medical history.

2. Blood testing: Each unit of collected blood is tested for blood-borne infectious disease agents, including HIV, hepatitis, and syphilis.

3. Donor lists: Blood establishments are required to keep a current list of deferred donors—those temporarily excluded from giving blood for reasons such as having a temperature, cold, cough, sore throat, or taking certain medications on the day of donation.

4. Quarantine of untested blood: Blood products are not made available for general use until products are thoroughly tested.

5. Investigation of problems: including remediation of deficits found.

An independent panel of experts serving on the Blood Products Advisory Committee is responsible for continual review and update of requirements and standards for collecting and processing blood. Together with advances in technology and science, the FDA assures the American population that today's blood supply is as safe as today's regulations and processes can ensure. Yet, a clear but remote risk of transmission of serious blood-borne viruses such as hepatitis and HIV via blood and blood products exists. In the early 1970s, the risk of contracting some form of hepatitis from a unit of blood was as high as 6 to 8%. In 1995, the risk of contracting hepatitis B per unit of blood stood at 1 in 250,000, and the risk for hepatitis C was less than 1 in 3,300. The FDA anticipates that improvements in screening tests will continue to improve sensitivity of detection.

People Who May Not Donate Blood

People who have or had:

- Hepatitis after age 11
- Diabetes requiring insulin
- Used a needle to inject illegal drugs
- Done anything to put themselves at risk of catching or spreading AIDS:

    - Men who have sex with other men
    - Men who have sex with other men and with women
    - Men and women who perform sex in exchange for money or drugs
    - Men and women who receive paid sexual activities

- AIDS or positive HIV test
- Blood disease that keeps blood from clotting (hemophilia) and receive blood products as treatment
- History of cancer requiring surgery, X-ray treatment, or chemotherapy in past 10 years
- Malaria within last 3 years, or traveled to malaria risk area within past 12 months
- Taken oral antibiotics in last three days
- Close contact in past 12 months with someone who had hepatitis
- Had a tattoo,* ear or skin piercing,* acupuncture,* accidental needle stick, or come in contact with someone else's blood in past 12 months (*acceptable if performed using single-use, sterile, or properly sterilized equipment)
- Blood transfusion in past 12 months
- Been treated for syphilis or gonorrhea in past 12 months
- Sex in past 12 months with anyone who has AIDS or positive HIV test
- Are or have been pregnant in past six weeks
- Infection or disease for which they are taking prescribed medication at time of donation
- Recent flu, cold, sore throat, or fever

Heart, lung, kidney, or liver disease also may be exclusionary qualifications.

BUG-BUSTING BLOCKBUSTERS

The liver is one of the few body organs in which function can be restored if given an environment in which the body can stimulate tissue regeneration. Early detection, including regular screenings for at-risk populations for hepatitis, along with good personal hygiene and sanitation practices, can greatly reduce your chances for succumbing to the disease. Prompt and proper medical intervention can prevent you from converting an acute outbreak into chronic hepatitis.

Alternative approaches for hepatitis focus on either boosting liver and immune function or easing the symptoms of the disease or side effects of conventional treatment. When selecting an alternative treatment for hepatitis, be mindful of the following:

1. Liver disease impairs your body's ability to process certain dietary supplements, including vitamins and herbs. Without proper filtering of these substances by the liver, any dose may become toxic.
2. Beware of scams. There is no "cure" for hepatitis C, and many claims for the efficacy of alternative treatments for hepatitis A and B are unsubstantiated.
3. Check the credentials of the practitioner from whom you seek alternative treatment. Ask about education, licenses, and certificates.
4. Coordinate all alternative approaches through your primary care physician.

Nutrients with liver-protecting function include the following:

• Milk thistle (*Silybum marianum*) contains silymarin, a mixture of bioflavonoids that is the most potent liver-protecting substance discovered to date. On an intracellular level, silymarin inhibits liver damage in four key ways, and it stimulates the production of new liver cells. Studies demonstrate that administration of silymarin improved bilirubin levels (a by-product of the breakdown of red blood cells that, if not cleared, results in jaundice) of acute viral hepatitis patients in just five days. Dosing at 420 milligrams per day for 3 to 12 months in chronic viral hepatitis patients resulted in a reversal of liver cell damage, an increase in protein levels in the blood, and a lowering of liver enzymes, accompanied by an amelioration of discomfort and malaise associated with the condition. Select a standardized milk thistle extract (70% silymarin), or look for a new preparation, silymarin phytosome (silymarin bound to phosphatidylcholine), which has better absorption.

- Lipoic acid is effective in treating alcohol-induced liver disease, hepatic coma, and chemical poisoning of the liver. A daily dose for a year of 600 milligrams in a study conducted at New Mexico State University of three hepatitis C patients with advanced liver disease was able to promote regeneration of liver tissue.
- Selenium is a potent antioxidant that combats cell damage caused by free radicals associated with hepatitis C. The New Mexico State University study proved the effectiveness of a daily dose of 400 micrograms for a year.
- N-acetyl L-cysteine, an amino acid (protein building block), which successfully treats acetaminophen-induced liver toxicity, has important immune-enhancing and antioxidant properties.

[9]

Oral Infections

The mouth is often overlooked by medical practitioners as a source of infectious disease. An estimated 500 species of microorganisms live in the mouth, and each individual organism readily and rapidly reproduces in that warm, dark, moist environment and has direct access to your body through the mouth's highly absorbent tissues and the body's airways and digestive pathways. It is becoming very clear that the state of oral health may be a major single predictor of general health.

Kissing is a human expression of emotion enjoyed by people across the globe. Ranging from energetic to erotic, platonic to passionate, and speculated to be an ancestral evolution of a being's most primal need to contact something other than itself, kissing is thought to have evolved from the action of brushing face-to-face that is seen today among primitive cultures. As enjoyable as kissing might be, doing the salivary swap will exchange whatever is present, microbes and all, from kisser to kissee. The common cold and flu and mono—nicknamed the "kissing disease" (see Chapter 6), as well as the herpes virus and syphilis (see Chapter 10), can be readily transmitted through kissing. If kissing progresses to a more intimate encounter, there is a clear risk of transmitting hepatitis A, B, and C (see Chapter 8) as well as meningitis (see Chapter 6).

WATCH YOUR MOUTH

More than 80% of the adult population has some form of deterioration of the periodontium (the gum of the mouth), ranging from mild gum inflammation to full-blown periodontal disease that requires surgery.

The mouth is home to millions of microorganisms, most of which are harmless. Given certain conditions, some will cause infections such as tooth decay or gum disease, and through compromised gums, oral bacteria gain entry into the bloodstream to run amuck in the body. Comments Ira Shapira, D.D.S., assistant professor at Rush-Presbyterian–St. Luke's Medical Center Sleep Disorder Clinic (Chicago), "The area in the oral cavity affected by periodontal disease can measure as long as the distance from the ankle to the groin."

Because the gums and oral cavity are a major passageway through which bacteria can invade the body, dental infections have been identified as causes of the following:

- Heart disease: Bacteria hitch up with platelets to circulate through the body and may deposit into the vessels supplying the heart. In November 2000, researchers from the University of North Carolina at Chapel Hill reported finding severe gum disease in 85% of heart attack victims (as opposed to 29% in counterparts without cardiovascular incident).
- Stroke: The National Institute of Dental Research reports that 70% of the fatty deposits clogging the carotid arteries in stroke contain bacteria, with 40% of that bacteria originating from the mouth. Previous research shows that people with severe gum disease have twice the risk of stroke compared to people with good oral health.
- Lung diseases from pneumonia to chronic obstructive pulmonary disease: Extensive tartar buildup and plaque correlate to risk for chronic lung disease. Dr. Shapira explains, "Studies demonstrate an increased risk of lung infections,

abscesses, and upper respiratory infections in patients with gum disease."

- Diabetes: Diabetics with gum disease are three times more likely to have heart attacks than those without gum disease.
- Spontaneous preterm births: The National Institute of Dental Research reports that women with gum disease are seven to eight times more likely to give birth to premature low-weight infants.
- Tuberculosis: Primarily a phenomenon in developing countries, Dr. Shapira says that oral TB infects 2 billion people worldwide, accounting for 3 million deaths each year. Painful oral ulcerations are a hallmark symptom.

In August 2000, British researchers from the Centre for Applied Microbiology and Research at Porton Down announced that immuno-compromised dental patients may die if exposed to contaminated oral water sprays used in the course of routine dental treatment. Dr. James Walker and colleagues tested 52 of 55 water samples collected from 21 dental facilities across England and found that mycobacterium and legionella, both of which can cause life-threatening pneumonia, exceeded European drinking water safety limits. The findings were so clear that the British Dental Association alerted people with compro-mised immune systems, such as cancer patients and those with HIV infection.

Dr. Walker's study also identified oral streptococci in 10% of the 55 samples tested. The research indicates that the bacteria were sucked back into the tools and the dental unit water lines during vari-ous dental procedures. One physician reading the study results likened this to sharing spit with your fellow dentist visitors. Since bad news almost always comes in threes, we shouldn't be surprised to hear that Dr. Walker also observed total bacteria counts in dental unit water lines had exceeded acceptable levels in drinking water from 5 to 1,200 times. Dr. Walker and colleagues identified the source as bot-tled water utilized to supply the dental unit water lines.

As a result of this study, both the British Dental Association and the American Dental Association now advise dentists to use sterile water for immunocompromised patients and for those receiving surgery where the gum line is cut.

GUM DISEASE

Gingivitis is an inflammation of the gums and is considered to be an early stage of periodontal disease (a disorder affecting the infrastructure of the teeth, including the gums). Of adults age 65 to 74, 48% have gingivitis. Gingivitis is caused by plaque, deposits of bacteria, mucus, and food particles that accumulate on the gum area, causing swelling and bleeding. The gum erodes to form a pocket that entraps more plaque deposits. Gingivitis may also result from breathing through the mouth, fittings that fit poorly and irritate the gum area, or a diet consisting primarily of soft foods that do not work the teeth and gums.

When left untreated, gingivitis may progress to pyorrhea (periodontitis). Bacteria become trapped between the gum and teeth, causing infection. Pyorrhea may correlate to deficiencies of vitamin C, bioflavonoids, calcium, folic acid, or niacin. Bad breath (halitosis), as well as painful and bleeding gums, may follow. To avoid pyorrhea, be sure to do the following:

* Eat a properly balanced and nutritional diet.
* Limit intake of sugar.
* Practice good flossing and brushing techniques.
* Treat chronic illnesses, if any.
* Visit the dentist regularly for preventive checkups and cleanings.
* Do not smoke.
* Do not engage in illicit drug use.
* Do not drink alcohol excessively.

In extreme cases of pyorrhea, the bacteria invade the bony area that secures the teeth, causing abscesses that require surgery to remove infected tissue and reshape the bone.

Some medications prescribed for hypertension, antirejection (for recipients of organ transplants), and seizures can cause the gums to overgrow and become more vulnerable to infection. For women, estrogen loss is a strong predictor of gum disease. Research has shown that women who receive postmenopausal hormone replacement therapy (HRT) lose fewer teeth than women who do not.

Drugs prescribed for allergies, anxiety, depression, and hypertension can cause xerostomia (dry mouth—persistent lack of saliva), which can lead to mouth sores and difficulty chewing and swallowing. Saliva bathes the teeth to deliver calcium and other minerals, and keeps bacteria in check. If you are prescribed a medication that can cause dry mouth, tell your dentist. He or she may want you to use a high-fluoride toothpaste or mouthwash, a remineralizing solution to

Nutrients for Periodontal Disease

- Coenzyme Q-10, with numerous studies from Japan documenting its successful use in mouth and gum disease, 100 milligrams daily
- Vitamin C with bioflavonoids, to promote healing of bleeding gums, up to 6,000 milligrams daily for three weeks
  (*Important:* High-dose vitamin C should be administered only under a physician's supervision and should not be continued for more than two weeks.)
- Calcium, to prevent bone loss around gums, 1,500 milligrams daily
- Magnesium, a necessary mineral complement to calcium, 750 milligrams daily
- Vitamin A, to help heal gum tissue, up to 15,000 IU daily
  (*Important:* contraindicated in pregnant women or women of childbearing age not on birth control)
- Vitamin E, also helpful for healing gum tissue, 400 IU daily
- Folic acid, proven by numerous studies to reduce gingival inflammation: folic mouthwash (0.1% folic acid) far superior to supplementation at doses up to 5 milligrams per day
- Sanguinaria (bloodroot, *Sanguinaria canadensis*) mouthwash, possessing broad antimicrobial activity and anti-inflammatory properties
- Glutathione administered directly to the mouth, with antioxidant activity that neutralizes free radicals associated with periodontal disease

replace calcium and phosphate normally found in saliva, or a rinse to reduce levels of oral bacteria. Keep your teeth clean. To stimulate saliva flow, chew on sugarless gum or mints, ice chips, or one of the new gums specifically designed for dry mouth sufferers. Sour and bitter foods will also stimulate saliva flow. Avoid alcohol and select alcohol-free mouthwashes.

TOOTH DECAY

Tooth decay is one of the most costly infectious diseases in the United States: It is responsible for an estimated $50 billion in medical bills annually. *Streptococcus mutans,* the bacterium primarily responsible for tooth decay, enjoys sweet treats nearly as much as you do. The microbe, which most of us have in our mouths beginning by age 3, uses sugar to produce lactic acid, which erodes the dental enamel, thus causing cavities (dental caries). In March 2000, scientists at the University of Florida College of Dentistry developed a technique that swaps the pathogenic strain of *S. mutans* with a version that has its lactic acid–producing mechanism crippled. This technique may lead to methods in which scientists will be able to swap bacteria that cause infections with nonpathogenic counterparts.

In July 2000, researchers at the University of Minnesota found that chewing gum containing xylitol, a substance that comes from the bark of birch trees, may reduce the risk of tooth decay by suppressing levels of *S. mutans* bacteria in the mouth.

Infection Danger

University of Rochester scientists have confirmed that *S. mutans* can travel from the mouth via the bloodstream to lodge in the heart, creating a danger of life-threatening infection.

Natural Dental Care Products

* Toothpaste: Baking soda–based toothpastes may contain herbal extracts such as green tea, tea tree oil, or neem to kill bacteria and inhibit plaque from sticking to teeth; calcium carbonate to gently whiten teeth; and natural mint oil flavorings. Natural toothpastes contain no added colorings or artificial sweeteners.
* Mouthwash: Hydrogen peroxide–based mouthwash, some with added zinc, helps control bacterial growth in the mouth.
* Anticavity gel: A fluoride gel applied to the teeth enhances remineralization and helps prevent cavities.

Nutrients to Protect Your Teeth

* CoQ10: may decrease the depth of the periodontal pocket (the pocket of gum where bacteria create infection)
* Grapefruit seed extract: acts as an antimicrobial against as many as 800 different bacteria
* Apple: contains cysteine proteinase inhibitor, which inhibits a potent gum-damaging enzyme excreted by oral bacteria

BAD BREATH

An estimated 60 million Americans suffer from chronic oral malodor, called halitosis. According to an article in a 1996 edition of the *Journal of the American Dental Association,* the source for bad breath in 85% of people is inadequate oral hygiene, in which the tongue serves as a breeding ground for bacteria. The germs generate foulsmelling sulfides and fill the mouth with noxious gases such as hydrogen sulfide (rotten eggs smell) and methyl mercaptan (barn animal odor).

While brushing teeth reduces mouth odors by 25%, cleansing the tongue by scraping reduces them by 75%, removing the germs as well as food debris on which the bugs feed. Studies show that tongue scraping is 700% more effective at removing odor-causing bacteria than simply brushing the tongue with a toothbrush or using a mouthwash. Together, brushing and tongue scraping will reduce mouth odor by 85%.

Dentists and oral hygienists recommend that we clean our tongues twice a day in conjunction with brushing. The process takes less than 30 seconds and is invaluable for general oral health.

Scrape Away the Smells

Tongue scraping will do the following:

• Inhibit formation of dental plaque by as much as one-third
• Remove the white coating often found on the tongue (see Chapter 16) by 40%
• Improve taste sensation

CANKER SORES

Canker sores, known to physicians as aphthous ulcers, are small and painful ulcers that occur in the lining of the mouth. Forming suddenly as a red, ulcerated spot with a yellowish border, canker sores can be as tiny as a pencil point dot or as large as a quarter, persisting from a few days to several weeks. Canker sores that occur in conjunction with lesions on the genitalia, conjunctivitis (eye inflammation), arthritis, or diarrhea may indicate autoimmune disease. Canker sores may be contagious if caused by a virus.

Canker sores are opportunistic. Prevention is very important as follows:

Is It a Canker Sore or a Cold Sore?

Canker sores are found on the tongue, the soft part of the gums, and the inner cheeks and lips. Cold sores (fever blisters) appear on the hard part of the gums and outer part of the lips, and are caused by herpes simplex virus (see Chapter 10).

Natural Treatment of Canker Sores

- Deglycyrrhizinated licorice (DGL), a special extract of licorice found to promote healing: Chew one or two 380-milligram tablets 20 minutes before meals.
- Zinc lozenge, to promote local relief and speed healing time: Take one every three to four hours.
- Vitamin C, taken at first sign of lesion to quicken healing: 500 milligrams daily.
- Vitamin B complex, taken at first sign of lesion to quicken healing: once daily.
- L-lysine (proven effective in treating herpes cold sores), taken at first sign of lesion to quicken healing: 500 milligrams daily.
- Powdered probiotics, which begin to rebalance the bacteria growth in the mouth immediately. Before each meal (three times a day), take ½ teaspoon each of Lactobacillus acidophilus, Bifido bifidum, and Lactobacillus bulgaricus, mixed in an 8-ounce glass of distilled water. Swish the mixture in your mouth for a few seconds before swallowing.
- Mouth rinse made of equal parts of sage and chamomile, boiled in water and allowed to cool, rinsing four to six times a day; or rinse mouth with solution of ½ teaspoon of salt in 8 ounces of water, three times a day.

- Maintain the normally alkaline environment within the mouth, where friendly bacteria prevail.
- Limit your sugar intake to minimize the overgrowth of both good and bad bacteria.

* Avoid factors that increase vulnerability to developing canker sores:

  * Hot, spicy, acidic, or salty foods
  * Food allergies and/or leaky gut (see Chapter 4)
  * Yeast (see Chapter 5)
  * Nutritional deficiency
  * Poor oral hygiene
  * Stress
  * Fatigue
  * Viral infection

The reason why we get canker sores is not well understood. They can be managed by antibiotics, anti-inflammatory agents, immune modulators, or anesthetics. You can clean sores with a cotton swab dabbed in 2% hydrogen peroxide. Stubborn canker sores often respond to prescription-strength tetracycline paste applied directly to the sore.

BUG-BUSTING BLOCKBUSTERS

Try the following helpful hints for a smile with style:

* Use a soft toothbrush. A hard toothbrush abrades dental enamel and gum tissue.
* Select a fluoride toothpaste that bears the American Dental Association seal of approval. The mechanical action of brushing is more important than the type of toothpaste you select. The American Dental Association instructs us to do the following:

  * Place your toothbrush at a 45° angle against the gums.
  * Move the brush back and forth gently in short (tooth-wide) strokes.
  * Brush the outer tooth surfaces, the inner tooth surfaces, and the chewing surfaces of the teeth.

- Use the "toe" of the brush to clean the inside surfaces of the front teeth, using a gentle up-and-down stroke.

- Brush twice a day for two minutes each session. Brush or scrape your tongue to remove bacteria and freshen your breath.
- If using an abrasive toothpaste—such as one designed to lighten smoking stains or a whitening product—alternate use with a standard tartar-control toothpaste every few days.
- Floss daily, especially between meals, to stimulate gums.
- Use the right mouth rinse: While studies show that most over-the-counter antiplaque rinses and antiseptics are only about 20% effective in reducing plaque that causes gingivitis, anticavity rinses that contain fluoride are clinically proven to fight up to 50% more of the bacteria that cause cavities.

Think of your toothbrush as a biohazard, carrying diseases that can't wait to leap into your mouth. The toothbrush offers plenty of food and water and an effective delivery system for influenza virus, herpes simplex 1, streptococcus, staphylococcus, candida, gingivitis, and bacteroids. Pets as well as pests (bugs and rats) have an affinity for trying human toothbrushes on for size. Consider these tips to keep your toothbrush a friend:

- As recommended by the American Dental Association, change your toothbrush every three to four months. From the standpoint of an infectious disease potential, we suggest shopping for a nifty new toothbrush every month (even this isn't foolproof, as one in five brand-new brushes straight out of the package have been found to be contaminated with *Staphylococcus epidermidis*).
- Be mindful that the microorganisms in toothbrushes are not effectively killed by most means that we'd otherwise think would destroy them. A reasonable regimen for brush bug-busting includes a 30-second flush in running tap water before

and after brushing, flicking the bristles dry after the second rinse. You might also try a 30-second dunk in hydrogen peroxide or an antiseptic mouthwash before use. Boiling and microwaving will kill the minimum number of bugs to claim your brush is "safe," but doing so often mangles the toothbrush so that it can't be used anymore. People suffering from chronic diseases should not use electric-powered brushes, particularly with old bristles. Doing so presents an increased chance for reinfection, as well as for infecting others, by leaving germs on the unit.

• Don't store your toothbrush anywhere near the toilet. Keep the toilet seat down, especially when flushing. Every time you flush, bugs can be propelled from the toilet into the air, and a soft toothbrush could break their fall.

• Don't store your toothbrush in the medicine cabinet, as it is a dark, wet, warm environment in which germs will breed even quicker.

Fluoride Toxicity

• Take care not to swallow anticavity rinses, as they contain sodium fluoride, which can build up and lead to fluoride toxicity.
• Per U.S. Federal Drug Administration rules, new labels on toothpaste warn that too much toothpaste can poison small children. In reality, a child would have to eat more than a whole tube to experience the most mild of symptoms, including nausea. Nevertheless, low-grade buildup of fluoride may lead to toxicity.

To soothe a sore mouth, do the following:

• Open a capsule of vitamin E oil and rub the oil on inflamed gums to promote healing.
• Clove oil rubbed on a tooth can ease toothache.

When to See the Doctor

- If you have fever above 101°F
- If sores do not improve within 10 days of treatment
- If pain becomes excruciating or is not relieved by analgesics
- If you experience significant weight loss (5 pounds or more) since first onset of canker sore

Be on the lookout for these early warning signs of gum disease:

- Gums that bleed when you brush
- Red, swollen, and tender gums
- Persistent bad breath
- Loose or separating teeth
- Receding gums
- Changes in the way your teeth fit together when you bite

[10]

STD Fundamentals

You're not just sleeping with one person, you're sleeping with
everyone they ever slept with.

—*Dr. Theresa Crenshaw, American Association of Sex Educators, Counselors, and
Therapists, interviewed in January 1987 by NBC-TV*

A TRIAD OF DISEASES WITH A COMMON
VIRAL BASIS

There is mounting evidence to support the theory that sexually transmitted diseases (STDs), autoimmune deficiency syndrome (AIDS), and
chronic fatigue syndrome (CFS) are all caused by the same combination of two particular viruses. The new model of STD/AIDS/CFS pro-
poses that the human herpesvirus 6, variant A (HHV-6A), is the primary
virus that causes cell destruction in AIDS. This theory advances the
notion that human immunodeficiency virus (HIV) is not an independent
cause of AIDS. According to Mark Konlee, editor at the nonprofit organization Keep Hope Alive Limited (www.keephope.net), long-term HIV
nonprogressors are absent of the HHV-6A infection, while active
HHV-6A, along with HIV, is present in nearly 100% of the lymph nodes
of those who have progressed to AIDS. Additionally, HHV-6A is rarely
found in the general population not affected by either AIDS or CFS.

From Pigs to People

In the 1970s, when the United States was at the height of its strategic conflict with the communist-controlled nation of Cuba just 90 miles south of Florida, the Nixon administration ordered the release of African swine fever virus in Cuba in hopes of crippling the country's second largest industry (pork production). Fidel Castro proceeded to slaughter over 500,000 infected pigs. What if the germs unleashed by the United States against Cuba had come from an African boar that was infected not only with African swine fever virus but with HIV and HHV-6A as well? With the flood of Haitian migrant workers who handled pig processing in Cuba landing in boatloads on U.S. shores, Americans would become unwitting recipients of, quite literally, a dose of our own medicine. If Mark Konlee's proposition is correct, then the international AIDS epidemic was instigated by the United States in a covert episode of biowarfare.

Konlee challenges HIV experts, who hold steadfastly that HIV evolved from simian immunodeficiency virus (SIV) in chimpanzees. He questions how SIV could have evolved in African chimps into HIV and directly caused a worldwide AIDS epidemic, which, these same experts agree, initially began in Haiti.

It is established that flu viruses can be transmitted between humans and pigs, and that the virus evolves in one species to infect the other, mutating and infecting over an extended period of time. Since the medical community agrees on that relationship, the second question posed by Konlee for HIV experts is how did HHV-6A that came from swine get together with HIV to cause AIDS in the first place. The prevailing explanation that can be supported from scientific data is that HIV is a virus that promotes HHV-6A to become activated and cause either AIDS or CFS.

RISKY BUSINESS

Sexual promiscuity does indeed correlate to the incidence of STDs. The Safer Sex Institute categorizes sexual activities on a continuum from high risk to risk-free. Activities at the top carry a high risk of STD transmission, especially for the receiving partner. Upper-middle-range activities carry a minimal or indeterminate risk, and lower-middle-range activities carry a theoretical risk. Activities at the bottom are completely safe.

HIGH RISK ↑ Unprotected anal intercourse

Unprotected vaginal intercourse

Sharing needles (for drug use, body piercing)

Sharing implements that draw blood (whips, knives)

Unprotected oral sex on a menstruating woman

Unprotected oral sex on a man with ejaculation

Unprotected oral-anal contact

Getting urine or feces in mouth, vagina

Unprotected stimulation with fist or fingers

Unprotected oral sex on a man without ejaculation

Unprotected oral sex on a nonmenstruating woman

Sharing uncovered sex toys

Anal intercourse with a condom

Vaginal intercourse with a condom

Oral sex on a man using a condom

Oral sex on a woman using a latex barrier

Oral-anal contact using a latex barrier

Stimulation with fist or fingers using a glove

Petting, hand-genital contact

Deep (French) kissing

Spanking, whipping that does not break the skin

Bondage and discipline play

Masturbation (alone or with partner)

Hugging, touching

Massage

Talking dirty, phone sex, fantasy

LOW RISK ↓

ALL ABOUT STDS

Sexually transmitted diseases (STDs), formerly known as venereal diseases, are named as such because they are spread through sexual contact in which the recipient is exposed to semen, blood, or vaginal fluid. The latest estimates indicate that there are 5 million new cases of STDs each year across the nation. There are more than 20 diseases that are sexually transmitted. Recent studies show that both ulcerative (causing sores) and nonulcerative STDs seem to enhance susceptibility to HIV infection as well as the ability to transmit the virus. A person with genital lesions from herpes, for example, is 100 times more likely to contract HIV during a single sex act than someone who has never had an STD. With new cases of HIV occurring at a rate of about 40,000 per year, proper detection and prevention are critical to prevent an STD from placing you at an increased risk for HIV.

STDs are a significant public health problem because they are difficult to track, typically lacking a well-defined and obvious set of symptoms. The United States lacks a widespread screening program, and state laws on reporting to health departments vary greatly: Chlamydia, gonorrhea, syphilis, hepatitis B, and chancroid are reportable STDs in most, but not all, states. Although some STDs, such as gonorrhea, are at all-time lows, others, such as chlamydia, continue to spread.

While the vast majority of Americans consider HIV/AIDS to be the most notorious of all STDs, the average adult is far more likely to contract one of the lesser-known STDs for which there are no coordinated prevention efforts. In a survey conducted by the Kaiser Family Foundation, women were asked to name the two most common STDs: Only 13% named human papilloma virus (HPV) and only 3% named trichomoniasis (see Chapter 5). Yet these two diseases are typically responsible for about two-thirds of all new cases of STDs that occur in the United States. HPV is more common among women entering college than are all other STDs combined. STDs are most effectively

Losing Odds in Getting Lucky

A study of 665 southern California college students published by the *New England Journal of Medicine* (March 15, 1990) found the following:

- 34% of men and 10% of women have told lies in order to have sex.
- 68% of men and 59% of women have been involved with more than one person whom their current partner doesn't know about.
- 47% of men and 42% of women would understate the number of previous partners in order to convince someone to have sex.

treated with antibiotics and other drugs, while natural remedies boost overall immune function or modulate the severity of symptoms.

If you suspect you have an STD, take care of yourself and your partner by doing these things:

- Seeing your doctor as soon as possible to begin treatment. The sooner you receive treatment, the better your chances for recovery (if the STD is curable), and you can minimize long-term complications, as well as reduce the chance of infecting others.
- Avoiding sexual contact with anyone until your doctor confirms that you do not have a contagious disease.
- If you do have an STD, urging your sex partner(s) to be tested as soon as possible—for their own sake and to ensure that you are not reinfected.

The Most Common STDs (other than HIV)

STD	INCIDENCE (ESTIMATED NUMBER OF NEW CASES A YEAR)	PREVALENCE (ESTIMATED NUMBER OF PEOPLE CURRENTLY INFECTED)
Chlamydia	3 million	2 million
Gonorrhea	650,000	Not available
Syphilis	70,000	Not available
Genital herpes (HSV-2)	1 million	45 million
Human papilloma virus (HPV) infection	5.5 million	20 million
Hepatitis B	120,000	417,000
Trichomoniasis	65 milion	Not available

Source: American Social Health Association.

Teenagers and young adults are at high risk for contracting STDs because they are more likely than other age groups to have multiple sex partners and to engage in unprotected sex. Chlamydia and gonorrhea are the most common curable STDs among teens, but if these diseases are left untreated, they can result in severe health consequences later in life.

Most STDs can be transmitted from a mother to her fetus and can result in fetal death, premature birth, or serious long-term problems for the child. Untreated syphilis and herpes can cause mental disorders and death, while gonorrhea and chlamydia can cause premature birth, eye disease, and pneumonia in infants.

Top Five STDs

DISEASE	CAUSE	CONSEQUENCES	TREATMENT
Human papilloma virus (HPV)	Viral infection	Increased risk of cervical cancer	No cure; warts removed by surgery or medication
Trichomoniasis	Parasitic infection	Complications during pregnancy	Antibiotics
Chlamydia	Bacterial infection	Pelvic inflammatory disease; infertility	Antibiotics
Genital herpes (HSV-2)	Viral infection	Recurrent sores; complications during pregnancy	No cure; antiviral drugs can reduce lesions
Gonorrhea	Bacterial infection	Pelvic inflammatory disease; tubal pregnancy; infertility	Antibiotics

Chlamydia

The fastest-growing and most commonly reported infectious disease in the United States, chlamydia may be one of the most dangerous of all STDs because it often strikes without symptoms. While more than 660,000 cases of chlamydia were reported in the United States in 2000, its asymptomatic nature has public health officials estimating the actual number as 3 million new cases.

Chlamydia is a bacterial infection caused by *Chlamydia trachomatis*. It can be transmitted during vaginal, oral, or anal sexual contact with an infected partner. It is readily cured with antibiotics (azithromycin, doxycycline, and erythromycin).

- Up to 40% of women with untreated chlamydia will develop pelvic inflammatory disease (PID), from which 20% will become infertile.
- Women infected with chlamydia have a three- to fivefold increased risk of acquiring HIV, if exposed to it.
- Chlamydia has been linked to squamous cell cervical cancer.

Symptoms of Chlamydia

WOMEN	MEN	COMMON
• Burning/itching in vaginal area • Unusual vaginal discharge • Redness/swelling/ soreness around vagina • Bleeding between periods	• Discharge from penis • Burning/itching around opening of penis • Pain/swelling in testicles	• Painful/frequent urination • If eye infected, can become swollen and red

* A pregnant woman may pass the infection to her newborn during a vaginal delivery.
* Among young men—a population that is seldom screened for chlamydia—the disease may cause urethral infection or epididymitis (an inflammation of a part of the male reproductive system located near the testicle, characterized by pain and swelling of the scrotal area). Left untreated, epididymitis can cause male infertility.

Screening for chlamydia in women has become easier with the introduction of a urine-based test. The CDC recommends that all sexually active teenage girls be tested for chlamydia twice a year.

Natural Remedies

* Follow a light diet of fresh fruits and vegetables plus lots of fluids for several days during treatment.
* Herbal remedies containing echinacea, saw palmetto (berberine), goldenseal, and cranberry extract may be helpful.
* Bromelain, a compound of enzymes derived from pineapple, exerts an anti-inflammatory effect and increases the absorption of the prescription antibiotics amoxicillin and tetracycline.

Human Papilloma Virus

HPV is probably the most common STD among the young and sexually active. The CDC estimates that approximately 20 million Americans are infected with HPV, with 5.5 million new infections each year.

Unfortunately, most people have never even heard of HPV, and many do not understand the health risks associated with it. There are more than 100 different types of HPV. Of these, about 25 cause genital warts, while 20 types cause infection without symptoms (subclinical infection), which can lead to cancer. HPV subclinical infection is more common than genital warts and currently there is no treatment. The persistent cervical infection that accompanies HPV-16 is the single most important risk factor for cervical cancer. Recent research suggests that HPV-16 also may cause malignant tumors on the tonsils.

Condoms can reduce, but not prevent, the spread of HPV. There is a 60 to 90% chance that the partner of someone with genital warts is also infected with HPV. Anal mucosa is very receptive to the HPV virus; thus, anal intercourse is especially dangerous without a condom. But because the virus lives over the entire genital region, HPV also can be spread during nonintercourse sexual activity, or between parts of the body not protected by a condom during intercourse—for example, from the base of the penis and the scrotum to the vulva. In addition, tampons can transport the virus from the labia to the vagina.

To confirm a diagnosis of HPV in women, your physician will conduct a colposcopy, where a magnifying-like instrument is used to view the vagina and uterine cervix. The doctor will identify invisible lesions by applying vinegar (acetic acid) to areas of suspected infection. If you are scheduled for a colposcopy, verify that the vinegar test will be utilized—otherwise, find a new doctor.

Symptoms of HPV

- Warts start as small, painless, hard spots that often originate at the bottom of the vaginal opening. Typically, they are thin, flexible, solid elevations of skin, taller than they are wide, and resembling flesh-colored cauliflower. Growing on stalks or in clusters, genital warts may also be flat and white, pink, or brown.
- Most of the time, those infected with genital warts do not report pain, but sometimes the warts are associated with itching and irritation, and pain or burning with intercourse.
- Warts most commonly appear on the vulva, cervix, penis, scrotum, groin, thigh, vagina, and anus. They may sometimes be confused with hemorrhoids.
- Growths can cause itching/pain/bleeding (rare).
- Infrequently, genital warts can grow in the throat.

External genital warts may be eradicated with topical solutions, and small warts may be removed by cryosurgery (freezing) or electro-cautery (burning), both in-office procedures. However, standard medical approaches often do not eradicate the virus. A study from San Francisco physicians confirms that genital wart infections may persist for as long as 10 years. While direct injections of interferon may be used to treat recurrent warts, it is not a curative method.

The following natural approaches can be helpful in raising the efficacy of conventional medical genital wart treatment:

- Vitamin A, which helps normal cell reproduction, prevents invasion of the area by bad microbes.
- The herb lomatium is an antimicrobial that slows the progression of warts, and the herb thuja relieves burning pain from the warts themselves and as a side effect of standard treatment.
- Tea tree oil, containing 48 compounds, enables a broad-spectrum bacteriocidal effect: Apply full-strength directly to genital warts two to three times a day.

Genital Herpes (HSV-2)

The word *herpes,* derived from the Greek word meaning "to creep," was coined during the height of the Roman Empire when it spread rapidly and rampantly. Herpes simplex virus (HSV) exists as HSV-1 and HSV-2. Ninety percent of infections caused by HSV-1 are oral; 90% of infections caused by HSV-2 are genital. Genital herpes affects an estimated one in four Americans, or 45 million people each year.

The herpes virus likes to take residence in the mucous membranes of the mouth, nose, ears, throat, genitals, and anus. The cervix and urethra are also favorite places, along with any region where sweating is common, such as the upper thighs, underarms, hairline, lower back, scrotum, and buttocks.

The first indicator of herpes is tenderness and redness of a watery bump or blister. The blister phase may be so mild and quick that it goes unnoticed. Afterward, sores or lesions develop at the site of the blister.

Rub on the Red

Resveratrol, a compound found in red wine and mostly known for its protective effect against heart disease, has been modified by Northeastern Ohio University researchers to advance the development of a topical gel that can be used to inhibit herpes virus replication. As with the naturally occurring compound, the synthesized one inhibits DNA (deoxyribonucleic acid) synthesis of the herpes virus—even drug-resistant strains. The researchers are also working on a version that can be added to birth-control foams or condoms to prevent the transmission of HSV-2.

Forever Yours

Once infected, the herpes virus remains in the body for the rest of one's lifetime. After the outbreak, the virus takes up residence in a state of suspended animation deep in the spinal nerves. Through a process of viral shedding, meaning that the virus is alive and risk of transmission is high, the herpes carrier remains capable of transmitting the disease even if he or she shows no symptoms.

Herpes lesions are painful, sore, and tender to the touch, and may cause difficulty in urination if affecting the genitourinary (GU) tract.

The herpes virus is readily transmittable from active lesions and body fluids, including saliva and sex fluid. Touching a sore and then touching another part of the body, or someone else, transmits it. For this reason, infected persons should wash hands with disinfectant soap frequently.

Herpes symptoms can be treated; the disease cannot be cured. After an initial episode, herpes can recur—on average about four times per year—sometimes triggered by surgery, illness, stress, fatigue, skin irritation such as sunburn, diet, or menstruation. Episodes may

Cold Sores

Caused by herpes simplex virus 1 (HSV-1), cold sores (also called fever blisters and known to doctors as herpes simplex labialis) affect an estimated 50 million Americans. Cold sores appear on or in the mouth as painful red blisters and can last for a week to 10 days. They are contagious. They can also appear in the genital area. Outbreaks can be triggered by stress, menstrual cycle, cold or fever, or exposure to the sun. There may be an itch or a heightened sensitivity in the affected area just before an outbreak.

Ice can ease the pain and reduce swelling. University of Texas researchers discovered that aspirin (125 milligrams daily) helped herpes cold sore sufferers recover in just five days (compared to nine days in their nonaspirin counterparts). Prescription medications can speed healing, and, if used soon enough, prevent development of sores. In summer 2000, an over-the-counter topical cream containing 10% docosanol was approved for treatment of cold sores. The docosanol inhibits viral entry into cells, but does not act directly on the virus.

Vitamin C, 600 milligrams orally each day, may reduce the healing time of herpes sores by half. Topical application of vitamin C, zinc, or lysine also may reduce healing time. A cream containing a 1% lemon balm extract may speed healing. Laboratory studies have shown that lemon balm, licorice, and garlic inhibit HSV-1 and may be used internally as well as in creams, oils, and compresses.

To help prevent recurrence of cold sores, take a daily lysine supplement (500 milligrams to 1,000 milligrams). Eat foods high in lysine such as kidney beans, split peas, and corn. Avoid foods rich in arginine (seeds, nuts, peas, and chocolate), as it interferes with the absorption of lysine.

Replace your toothbrush after having a cold sore.

decrease over time, but the virus is transmissible between episodes when no symptoms are present.

Antiviral therapy is recommended for an initial genital herpes outbreak. Daily suppressive therapy of HSV-2 with acyclovir, famcyclovir, or valacyclovir can significantly reduce the frequency of recurrence. Currently, researchers are working on human application of transfer factor (a substance extracted from leukocytes that confers immune sensitivity) taken from calves immunized with HSV-1 and HSV-2.

The Herpes Cycle

In a primary herpes episode, lesions can persist for 7 to 12 days, followed by a crusting or scabbing period. Pain and tenderness may be experienced until the infection clears within 10 to 21 days. At that time, crusts or scabs will be completely formed. Secondary symptoms—fever, headache, muscle aches, pain or difficulty with urination, vaginal discharge, and swollen glands in the groin—may accompany the primary herpes outbreak.

Frequently, a new series of lesions may begin within the first or second week of a primary outbreak. Recurrent episodes are less severe, less extensive, less painful, and of shorter duration.

Methods of Transmission of Herpes 1 and 2

- Skin-to-skin contact from an active lesion
- Kissing, via saliva
- Sexual intercourse
- Oral sex
- Occasional cases traced to close nonsexual contact, such as sporting events in which skin may become scraped and come into contact with the competitor's exposed herpes lesions
- Rarely transmitted by contact with toilet seats or in hot tubs frequented by an infected person

A team of researchers from Washington University School of Medicine and St. Louis Children's Hospital cultured samples of HSV-1 and HSV-2 with zinc. They found that zinc gluconate and zinc lactate inactivated all of the HSV-1 isolates by more than 97.5%. Zinc was less effective on the HSV-2 samples. Zinc is suspected to work by blocking a glycoprotein that the herpes virus uses to penetrate and enter cells. High-dose zinc, applied topically, may become a new and effective treatment.

The amino acid lysine—found in fish, poultry, eggs, dairy products, potatoes, and brewer's yeast, and available as a dietary supplement—can help to control stress-related herpes recurrences. Contrarily, the amino acid arginine may aggravate herpes, so it may be prudent to minimize consumption of chocolate, peanuts, almonds, cashews, walnuts, sunflower and sesame seeds, and coconut. Herbs that strengthen the immune system—goldenseal, echinacea, and ginseng—are helpful. Licorice and tea tree oil have been used with varying results, but melissa (lemon balm) is demonstrated by clinical studies as useful in speeding healing and shortening outbreaks. When lesions appear, aloe, goldenseal, or lavender salves can be applied directly.

Gonorrhea

After being on the decline since the late 1980s, gonorrhea infection rates rose nationwide in 1998. Officials cite an increase in risky sexual behavior as the cause. Infection rates are highest among females between the ages of 15 and 19 and males between 20 and 24.

Gonorrhea, caused by the *Neisseria gonorrhoeae* bacterium, is highly contagious. It is spread by contact with secretions of an infected person: Unprotected sexual intercourse is the primary mode of transmission. It can affect the penis, anus, vagina, throat, and eye. Gonorrhea is a major cause of pelvic inflammatory disease, infertility, and tubal pregnancy among women. In men, gonorrhea can cause sterility. Any damage gonorrhea causes before treatment is permanent.

When gonorrhea bacteria enter the bloodstream, it leads to systemic infection. Patients may experience fever, rash, and joint inflammation. Doctors can confirm the systemic presence by testing fluid removed from affected joints.

If detected early, gonorrhea can be easily cured by a course of antibiotics. But over the past decade, it has become resistant to penicillin and tetracycline. Herbal remedies containing echinacea, saw palmetto (berberine), goldenseal, and cranberry extract may provide relief from symptoms but are not a treatment. Those with gonorrhea

Symptoms of Gonorrhea

WOMEN	MEN	BOTH SEXES
• Yellowish vaginal discharge	• Yellowish discharge from urethra	• Discharge/itching with rectal infection; pain during bowel movements
• Burning/pain when urinating	• Painful/frequent urination	• Sore throat
• Need to urinate frequently	• Blood in urine	
• Burning/itching in vaginal area	• Swollen glands in groin	
• Redness/swelling/ soreness of vulva	• Redness on tip of penis	
• Pain in pelvis/ abdomen during sex		
• Abnormal vaginal bleeding		

should follow a light diet of fresh fruits and vegetables plus lots of fluids for several days during treatment.

Syphilis

Once a major cause of cardiovascular and neurological disease, the introduction of penicillin has nearly eliminated syphilis. Every 7 to 10 years, however, it reappears. An estimated 70,000 cases are diagnosed annually. The disease causes genital ulcers that dramatically increase the likelihood of sexual HIV transmission. It can also cause severe neurological problems in people whose immune systems are depressed. An infected woman can pass syphilis to her fetus during pregnancy.

Syphilis is usually treated with penicillin, administered by injection. Other antibiotics can be used for patients allergic to penicillin. Some

Symptoms of Syphilis

PRIMARY STAGE	SECONDARY STAGE	LATENCY	TERTIARY STAGE
• Open red sore (chancre) that forms at point of contact with syphilis bacteria (lips, tongue, eyelids, face, chest, fingers, breasts, anus, mouth) —Men: on penis, inside urethra, on scrotum —Women: inside/outside vagina, on cervix, inside urethra • Chancre disappears on its own after a couple of weeks.	• Within six months, measles-like rash all over body • Fever/fatigue/ flulike symptoms • Swollen glands	No symptoms	• Blindness • Mental illness • Tumors • Stroke

people, however, do not respond to the usual doses of penicillin, so it is important that people being treated for syphilis have periodic blood tests to check that the infectious agent has been completely destroyed. In all stages of syphilis, proper treatment will cure the disease, but in late syphilis, damage already done to body organs cannot be reversed. Everyone diagnosed with syphilis should be tested for HIV. If the initial test is negative, they should be retested in three months.

Chanchroid

Although chancroid is not widespread in the United States, it has the potential to cause large outbreaks. It causes disfiguring genital ulcers and may contribute to increased HIV transmission. According to the most recent data available, four states account for 85% of all reported chancroid cases: California, New York, South Carolina, and Texas.

Chancroid can be treated with antibiotics. People diagnosed with chancroid should be tested for both syphilis and HIV. If these tests are negative, they should be repeated in three months.

For STDs, nondrug therapies should be undertaken only in consultation with a qualified health care professional who coordinates these approaches with drug treatment. Discuss supplementation with the following:

- Butylated hydroxytoluene (BHT): An over-the-counter antioxidant, BHT has been widely used to prevent outbreaks of herpes and may be an effective alternative for treatment of HIV as well as CFS by tackling the levels of human herpesvirus 6A (HHV-6A).
- DHEA, the master hormone involved in dozens of life-giving body functions, modulates the metabolic processes that become overexcited when blood levels of DHEA are low. Administering DHEA (injections under the skin) enhances immune resistance to viral and bacterial infection by counteracting the inflammatory, immunosuppressing reaction caused by glucocorticoids.

Human Immunodeficiency Virus/Acquired Immunodeficiency Syndrome

HIV/AIDS was first identified in 1981 and since then has become a worldwide pandemic. In 1983, researchers established that the HIV-1 virus, and its less common counterpart, HIV-2, are the cause of AIDS.

In the United States, as of 1998, an estimated 800,000 to 900,000 people were infected with HIV, of which 200,000 didn't yet know it. Worldwide, the United Nations AIDS program (UNAIDS) estimates that approximately 47 million people have been infected with HIV since the start of the global epidemic. Through December 2000, an estimated 21.8 million children and adults had died, and an estimated 36.1 million people were living with HIV infection or AIDS. UNAIDS estimates 5.3 million new HIV infections occurred in 2000. This represents almost 16,000 new cases per day. An estimated 3 million adults and children died of HIV/AIDS in 2000.

While the death rates from AIDS are declining (dropping to 21% in 1998), the demographics of the epidemic are shifting. The majority of new cases arise from two sources: injection drug use and heterosexual spread. With regard to the latter, risky behavior by men and women under age 25 is responsible for half of new HIV infections.

A positive HIV test (HIV+) does not necessarily mean that a person has AIDS. In fact, an HIV-positive person may never progress to full-blown AIDS, which is a diagnosis given when an HIV-infected person develops one or more of the 29 AIDS indicator conditions (viral, bacterial, fungal, parasitical, mycoplasmic, and neoplastic) identified by the CDC. An HIV-positive person who does not have a serious illness can be diagnosed with AIDS based on the results of a blood test that measures the immune system's T cells.

Recommendations on HIV Testing

HIV infection usually is diagnosed by using HIV-1 antibody tests. HIV is detectable in at least 95% of people within six months after infection. The CDC recommends testing for HIV-2 at blood banks or when special circumstances mandate the test—for example, when the potentially infected person is from a country where HIV-2 is endemic or is the sex partner of someone from such a country. It is also a good idea to test for HIV-2 when tests for HIV-1 are negative, but HIV infection is strongly suspected nonetheless.

HIV infection can weaken the immune system so much that it has difficulty fighting off certain opportunistic infections. Infections that a normal immune system easily controls may become life-threatening to someone with HIV/AIDS.

Among people who are HIV positive, about half develop AIDS within 10 years of becoming infected. This prognosis, however, can vary greatly from person to person depending on many factors such as overall health and lifestyle.

There are medical treatments that can slow the rate at which HIV weakens the immune system, and other treatments can prevent or even cure some of the illnesses associated with AIDS, though they do not cure AIDS itself. The earlier HIV infection is detected, the more options there are for treatment, and thus the greater the likelihood for control.

HIV Transmission: Facts and Fallacy

HIV is spread by the following:

* Sexual contact with an infected person
* Sharing needles and/or syringes with someone who is infected
* Transfusions of infected blood or blood-clotting factors

Babies born to HIV-infected women may become infected before or during birth or through breast-feeding. Health care workers have been infected with HIV after being stuck with needles contaminated with HIV-infected blood. A study by a group of CDC authors who looked at data on percutaneous injuries from 1995 through 1999 found that 60% of the injuries were preventable, in 33% of the cases the use of needles was unnecessary, and 39% could have been prevented by using a safe-needle alternative. The odds of HIV-infection after a needle stick are significantly less if the patient is in the early stages of infection. Prospective studies conducted by the CDC put the risk after a percutaneous exposure to HIV-infected blood at 3 in 100. Risk of transmission from exposure to fluids or tissues other than HIV-infected blood is negligible, and the transmission when HIV-tainted blood gets into an open cut or a mucous membrane of a health care worker stands at about 9 in 1,000.

HIV has been transmitted between family members living in the same household, but these transmissions likely resulted from contact between infected blood and a family member's skin or a mucous membrane—in much the same way a health care worker might contract the infection from exposure to infected blood. There is no known risk of HIV transmission to co-workers or consumers in businesses such as food service or personal care.

Instruments that penetrate the skin, such as those used in tattooing, body piercing, and acupuncture, should be used once and disposed of, or thoroughly cleaned and disinfected with bleach after each use. There have been no reported incidences of HIV infection related to body piercing or tattooing. The hepatitis B virus, however, is much more readily transmitted via these activities.

Food workers with the HIV virus need not be restricted from work as long as they don't have other infections (for example, diarrhea or hepatitis) that are known to spread via unsafe food handling. Personal care workers—barbers, hairdressers, manicurists, cosmetologists, massage therapists, and so forth—should follow precautions

HIV and the Nation's Blood Supply

Nearly all people infected with HIV as a result of blood transfusions received those transfusions before 1985, the year in which HIV testing began for all donated blood. The U.S. blood supply has been screened for antibodies to HIV-1 since March 1985 and HIV-2 since June 1992. By government mandate, blood and blood products that test positive for HIV are removed from the supply stream and safely discarded.

The CDC estimates that 1 in 450,000 to 1 in 660,000 donations per year are infectious for HIV but are not detected by current antibody screening tests. In August 1995, the FDA recommended that all donated blood and plasma also be screened for HIV-1 p24 antigen. The CDC cites improvements in processing methods of all blood products for reducing the number of infections.

issued by the CDC regarding cleaning, disinfecting, and disposing of instruments, although there has been no evidence of transmission from a personal services worker to a client or vice versa.

Concern has been expressed that HIV may be transmitted via air, water, or insects (for example, mosquitoes). Research has shown that HIV does not survive well in the environment and it is unable to reproduce outside its living host except under laboratory conditions. HIV does not survive or reproduce in insects, nor do insects inject their own or a previously bitten person's or animal's blood when they bite their next victim. To date, no new modes of transmission have been confirmed.

There have been reports of blood-to-blood HIV transmission by human bite. Biting, however, is not a common means of transmission. HIV has been found in small amounts in the saliva, tears, and sweat of some AIDS patients, but there has been no reported transmission via these means. It is important to remember that just because HIV is found in small amounts in a body fluid does not mean it can be transmitted via that fluid.

Treatment Options

As of fall 1999, 16 HIV drugs were licensed by the Food and Drug Administration. Unfortunately, some people do not respond to these drugs, cannot tolerate their toxic effects, or are not compliant with complicated dosing schedules. Moreover, the virus can hide in reservoirs (probably nonactive T cells resting in the brain, intestines, bone marrow, and genital tract) below the immune system's radar screen where the drugs cannot reach it.

Resistant strains of HIV are emerging in 1 to 5% of newly infected people. Drugs currently in use attack HIV after it has entered a blood cell. The next wave of drugs, called fusion or entry inhibitors, will prevent HIV from entering cells, thus interfering with its ability to multiply. Researchers are also seeking ways to boost the activity of the thymus gland, which produces the immune system's T cells and which slows down with age.

Nutritional Supplementation for HIV/AIDS

NUTRIENTS AND OTHER FACTORS	POTENTIAL BENEFITS AND MECHANISMS OF ACTION
B vitamins (folic acid, B_6, and B_{12})	◆ Deficiency common in HIV-positive people. ◆ Can cause increased homocysteine level, leading to accelerated deterioration of immune system and increased replication of HIV. ◆ May slow progression to AIDS; may help reduce psychological stress.
Vitamin A	◆ Important for function of T cells and B cells. ◆ May be depleted in HIV infection due to chronic infections and impaired food intake and absorption. ◆ Deficiency may be a marker for risk of mortality in people with AIDS.
Carotenoids	◆ The greater the immune impairment, the greater the beta-carotene deficiency. ◆ May increase glutathione concentration.
Vitamin C	◆ Deficiency common in HIV-positive people due to greater free radical load. ◆ May slow decline or even improve T-cell count (lab tests). ◆ May be used to treat early lesions of Kaposi's sarcoma.
Vitamin D	◆ Serum levels important marker for immunodeficiency.
Vitamin E	◆ Deficiency common in HIV-positive people due to greater free radical load.
Selenium	◆ Deficiency common in HIV-positive people. ◆ May increase glutathione concentration, boost efficacy of AIDS vaccines and other treatments, and reduce toxicity of drug treatments. ◆ May increase energy, reduce gastrointestinal problems and skin infections, prevent weight loss, and improve mood.
Zinc	◆ Deficiency common in HIV-positive people. ◆ Important for maintaining immune function. ◆ May boost efficacy of zidovudine (AZT). ◆ May reduce development of Kaposi's sarcoma and other infections.
CoQ10	◆ Deficiency common in HIV-positive people. ◆ May increase T cells.

(continued)

(continued)

NUTRIENTS AND OTHER FACTORS	POTENTIAL BENEFITS AND MECHANISMS OF ACTION
Glutathione	• Deficiency common in HIV-positive people. • Supplementation may prolong survival.
N-acetylcysteine	• Helps body synthesize glutathione.
L-glutamine	• Increases immunoglobulin A (IgA) levels.
Pycnogenol (pine bark extract of flavonoids)	• Boosts activity of natural killer cells that slow progression from HIV to full-blown AIDS (in animal models).
Carnitine	• Deficiency common in HIV-positive people. • May inhibit destruction of white blood cells. • May improve lipid metabolism.
Maitake	• May boost activity of T-helper cells that slow progression from HIV to full-blown AIDS.
Licorice	• Shown to limit replication of HIV in the lab setting.
Garlic	• Anti-HIV properties are found in raw garlic, due to its content of a compound called ajoene, a fusion inhibitor. Three cloves of raw garlic daily, blended with cold-pressed olive oil (and fresh parsley to deodorize the garlic), may begin to restore natural killer cell function (see Chapter 2).
Cayenne	• Consumption of cayenne and other hot peppers correlate to a lower death rate from AIDS in the United States. May function by modifying immune response to HIV.
Vinegar	• A study from Glasgow, Scotland, found that both white and brown (malt) vinegars were able to inactivate HIV in heroin users. The vinegar was administered with heroin in a ratio of 1:3 in water.

Nutritional Support for HIV

No nutrient can kill HIV, but a number of nutrients can help HIV-positive people feel better and stay healthier. Because wasting syndrome (excessive weight loss and recurrent diarrhea) is common in people with AIDS, it is important to consume enough protein and calories.

Because HIV/AIDS is a very complex disease, nutritional supplementation should be supervised by a physician.

Natural immunity to HIV/AIDS may be conferred as a result of high levels of immune-boosting cells, specifically the immunoglobulin A (IgA) and killer T cell CD8. Increased levels of IgA and CD8 can be promoted by increasing cytokines, which are chemical messengers that control immune response. Consider the following to increase levels of cytokines:

- Minimize consumption of white and simple sugars: Sweets and processed foods containing empty carbohydrates weaken the function of macrophages and NK cells, and weaken the body's resistance to infections.
- Minimize consumption of trans-fatty acids. Found in most heated and processed vegetable oils and margarines and in foods cooked or prepared with them, trans-fatty acids weaken immune function by distorting the shape of the membranes of CD8 cells.
- Correct intestinal permeability and leaky gut (see Chapter 4).
- Consume cold-water fish (salmon, sardines, mackerel, halibut, and trout). The omega-3 fatty acids reduce levels of tumor necrosis factor (which throws off normal cellular health) and

Bites That Fight

The bite of a tiny Southeast Asian insect larva known as a chigger could hold the key to developing a low-cost treatment for AIDS. In the August 2000 issue of *The Lancet,* a U.S. Army doctor working in Thailand reported finding consistently lower levels of HIV in blood of AIDS patients who caught scrub typhus, a fever caused by a parasite transmitted in chigger bites. This phenomenon was observed within two weeks of contracting scrub typhus, and while viral load tended to increase after two more weeks, the HIV load was still lower than when the patients originally were admitted for treatment of the typhus.

support T-helper (Th1) cytokine production (which promotes cell-based mediated immunity).

* Consume oleic acid, found in cold-processed olive oil, green and ripe olives, filberts, hazelnuts, almonds, and almond oil. Do not consume products that are heat-treated or roasted, as these processes reduce the omega-3 content.

The search for an AIDS vaccine continues amidst a growing complacency about the threat of HIV/AIDS. Public health officials

STD Awareness Quiz

1. True or False: If you have one STD, you are more than likely to catch another.
   True. Because bacteria and viruses weaken the skin in the genital area, it's easier for subsequent bugs to gain entry.

2. True or False: Having a lesion or sore is the clearest indication that you have an STD.
   False. The most common STDs, especially HPV, chlamydia, and herpes, produce no obvious symptoms in up to three-quarters of those infected. Painful urination in gonorrhea or a chancre in syphilis, not a sore, are telltale signs.

3. True or False: At-home testing is available for HIV, chlamydia, and HPV.
   False. The only approved home testing kit is for HIV.

4. True or False: There is a vaccine available for herpes but not for chlamydia.
   False. No vaccines are available for chlamydia or herpes.

5. True or False: Women, as a group, are experiencing the fastest growing rate of HIV infection.
   True. Women now account for 22% of the total AIDS cases reported to the CDC. AIDS-related infections rank fourth among the leading causes of death in women aged 25 to 44.

If you answered fewer than all five correctly, we strongly recommend that you reread this chapter and carefully study the information available from the organizations listed in the Resources section for this chapter in Appendix B.

Immune System Restoration as Innovative HIV/AIDS Treatment: A Call for Research Support

The authors have had personal experience with a scientific/research medical establishment that values profit over patients' lives.

In HIV/AIDS, it is important to develop a treatment alternative that is less toxic than AZT, provide a treatment that is efficacious despite the onset of new drug-resistant viral strains, and offer a method for long-term control of the virus. The authors of *Infection Protection* are inventors of a new medical technology known as Hyper-Augmentative Immune Therapy (HAIT), a technique that achieves all of these goals.

HAIT is a multistep treatment protocol that stimulates the immune system and then collects, optionally concentrates, and stores components of the stimulated immune system for later infusion into the patient:

- Phase I involves raising the patient's immune system to a highly stimulated level and harvesting and storing immune components of the stimulated immune system. The raised immune system not only has enhanced abilities to fight disease, but also provides the immune components for later use. Immune system stimulants utilized may include organ extracts and immune-boosting herbs and nutrients ranging from astralagus to medicinal mushrooms.
- Phase II involves treatment (drugs, surgery, chemical, or other method) for antiviral replication inhibition, thereby depleting the burden of the virus within the body.
- Because a common side effect of these treatments is a weakened immune system, stored immune components obtained through Phase I are reinfused into the patient as Phase III.

In HIV/AIDS, the combination of these complementary treatments will destroy enough of the viruses to significantly delay the debilitating effects of the viral infection. HAIT returns the individual to the typically early-disease stage of low virus concentration and few, if any, symptoms. It is possible that the combination of the augmented immune system, along with antiviral drug-induced depletion of the viral load, may eradicate the virus altogether or alternatively place it into remission. Phases I and III may also be effective against secondary diseases plaguing immunocompromised patients.

HAIT-type devices have been utilized with success in cancer treatment at Kyoto Prefectural University of Medicine in Japan, but no one has yet attempted it for HIV or other infectious diseases. This nontoxic treatment could have lifesaving value to millions of HIV-infected individuals as well as many others with life-threatening infectious diseases. If you know a philanthropist who would care to conduct this important research, please contact Dr. Klatz at drklatz@worldhealth.net.

are directing efforts toward disease prevention. The *proper* and *consistent* use of condoms for vaginal, anal, or oral intercourse greatly reduces the chance of acquiring or transmitting all STDs, including HIV. Although there are many types of condoms on the market, only latex and polyurethane condoms provide a highly effective barrier to HIV.

CHRONIC FATIGUE SYNDROME

It may be the most common health complaint of the late twentieth and early twenty-first centuries: fatigue. Everybody is exhausted.

Continuous, incapacitating, inexplicable fatigue is your body's way of saying something is seriously wrong. Most people with CFS

Just How Tired Are You?

To establish a diagnosis of CFS, most physicians refer to the following working case definition issued by the U.S. Centers for Disease Control and Prevention:

1. A patient must have debilitating fatigue that reduces activity to less than 50% of the patient's previous activity levels for six months' or longer duration; and

2. Concurrently experience four or more of the following persistent symptoms:

   - Sore throat
   - Forgetfulness
   - Impaired memory or concentration
   - Tender lymph nodes
   - Muscle discomfort or pain
   - Multijoint pain (without swelling or redness)
   - Headaches of a new type, pattern, or severity
   - Unrefreshing sleep
   - Postexertion malaise lasting more than 24 hours

experience an acute onset of severe fatigue after a viral or flulike ill-ness or a physical trauma. After several months, they may feel better and then plateau at a level where they can function but do not feel well. In about a third of cases, the onset of CFS is gradual rather than sudden. Cognitive problems such as forgetfulness and an inability to concentrate are common complaints whether onset of the condition is fast or slow. In addition, existing allergies may become worse. Most people with CFS improve in 5 to 10 years, but even so-called recov-ered patients can relapse.

Although it has no distinctive diagnostic markers and manifests no unique abnormalities in a physical exam or in blood tests, CFS was recognized as an illness by the CDC in 1988. More than 500,000 Americans have been diagnosed with CFS. Two million more may have the condition and not know it. CFS can strike any-one of any age. For unknown reasons, it is more common in women (55 to 60% of people with CFS are women). Unfortunately, although CFS is officially recognized as a medical condition, many people still believe it is nothing more than depression or a psycho-somatic phenomenon.

Before diagnosing CFS, your doctor must disqualify all other potential causes for CFS-like symptoms. Fatigue-producing diseases include cancer and anemia, as well as thyroid dysfunction, hepatitis, tuberculosis, Lyme disease, substance abuse, sleep apnea, autoim-mune disease, and HIV/AIDS. CFS is diagnosed only after ruling out these conditions, and if supported by a complete physical exam and medical history, as well as a thorough battery of blood tests, including microorganism assessment.

Although the cause of CFS is still unknown, researchers speculate that it is a multifactorial immune system disorder triggered by an infection such as Epstein-Barr virus, herpes simplex, or human her-pesvirus. On the other hand, although viruses are common in people with CFS, they may be markers for the illness rather than triggers. There is no evidence to support the view that CFS is a contagious dis-ease.

Nonviral CFS triggers may be food allergies, nutritional deficien-cies, overgrowth of intestinal pathogens (candidiasis), stress, and exposure to toxic environmental chemicals. Some researchers believe that chronic fatigue syndrome, chronic Lyme disease, fibromyalgia, and Gulf War syndrome may be caused by persistent bacterial infections. All of these conditions share the same hallmark symptoms: fatigue, muscle pain, and cognitive dysfunction.

There are no proven treatments for CFS, but there are some measures you can take to help relieve your symptoms:

- Eat a balanced diet with plenty of fruits, vegetables, and grains.
- Boost protein intake: Try kefir, tofu, plain yogurt, canned sardines or canned salmon, almonds, and walnuts.
- Avoid salt: It reduces energy production by causing cells to direct their resources to process sodium.
- Eliminate all potential allergens—food, medicine, and environmental.
- Generally, avoid activities that tire you. However, aerobic exercise, as long as overexertion is avoided, may be helpful.
- Aspirin or ibuprofen may help relieve flulike symptoms.
- Antidepressants may help you sleep and relieve muscle pain.
- Injections of gamma globulin may help boost your immune system.
- The following dietary supplements may counter fatigue by helping cell mitochondria produce more ATP (adenosine triphosphate, also known as cellular energy):
  - Nicotinamide adenine dinucleotide (NADH), up to 10 to 20 milligrams daily
  - Alpha lipoic acid, up to 300 milligrams daily
  - Carnitine, up to 3 grams daily
  - CoQ10, up to 100 milligrams daily
  - Cold-processed whey proteins
- Cayenne as a dietary supplement can increase body temperature, promote appetite, and improve general immune function.
- Although there are no clinical studies proving their effectiveness, acupuncture and acupressure may be helpful in relieving symptoms.

• Mind-body therapies, including tai chi, meditation, relaxation, guided imagery, and yoga, promote restfulness.

CFS by Any Other Name

Chronic fatigue syndrome may be called the following names:

- Chronic fatigue immune dysfunction syndrome
- Chronic EBV (Epstein-Barr virus; see Chapter 6)
- Yuppie flu
- Chronic viral syndrome
- Postviral fatigue syndrome

BUG-BUSTING BLOCKBUSTERS

Be Sexually Savvy

Twenty years ago, practicing safe sex meant taking precautions against becoming pregnant. Today it means minimizing contact with fluids involved in sex (saliva, blood, vaginal secretions, semen, and sometimes urine and feces) to limit the odds of contracting a variety of debilitating and life-threatening diseases. With respect to infectious disease, there is no such thing as safe sex—the best we can all expect of ourselves and our partners is *safer* sex.

Basic Reminders
• The safest sex is with a disease-free partner in a mutually monogamous relationship.
• Choose your partner carefully. Avoid high-risk groups such as intravenous drug users, men who have sex with other men, and people of either gender with a history of incarceration or who are sex partners to inmates. Anal intercourse is the riskiest activity for sexual transmission of HIV infection.

- When you and your partner are at the point in your relationship when you think having sex is imminent, use your brain, not your sex organs, to make an informed decision. Have an open discussion about sex before you engage in intercourse.
- Know your partner's sexual history. You are at risk if your partner has had sex with anyone else in the past three to five years.
- Conduct a cursory check of your sex partner for warning signs of STDs. Look for open sores and vaginal warts in women, genital warts in men, and anal warts in both sexes. Feel whether lymph nodes (neck and armpit nodes are easiest to find) seem swollen. The lower right side of the abdominal area, where the bulk of the liver is located, as well as the area just below the bottom of the rib cage where the spleen is found, should not be tender to the touch.
- Have regular medical checkups. Seek medical attention immediately if you suspect you have been exposed to an STD.

Being Condom-Compliant

- Say no to casual sex or to a male partner who refuses to wear a condom.
- Latex condoms, when used properly and carefully for every sexual activity, can reduce (not eliminate) the risk of contracting and transmitting an STD.
- Spermicidal foams, jellies, and creams (especially those containing nonoxynol-9) and a diaphragm may offer added protection when used with a condom. Don't assume that a spermicide will protect you from disease.
- If using a lubricant with condoms, choose a water-based product (such as K-Y Jelly), since petroleum-based ones may dissolve the latex in the condom and weaken it.

Being Sex Savvy Doesn't Stop with Condoms

- Immediately before and after sexual activity, urinate and wash the genital area with plain unscented soap and water to help remove bacteria from the urinary tract.

Humdrums on Condoms?

If you or your partner resists using condoms consistently and properly because of the commonly heard complaint that condoms make sex less pleasurable by reducing sensation, there are ways to put some zest back:

- Foreplay fun: Tease and tantalize until both you and your partner approach climax, and neither of you will notice the condom.
- Experiment with a variety of condoms (keeping in mind that latex is shown to be the most effective barrier for STDs): Ribbing or ridges will increase stimulation for your partner, and flavored or colored condoms can make oral sex a refreshing experience.
- Lube job: Spread some water-based lubricant on the head of the penis before slipping on the condom to enhance the sensation for the condom wearer.

- Do not have vaginal sex after anal sex unless you wash the area thoroughly and repeatedly first. Feces harbor many organisms that can infect the vagina, and even microscopic amounts can lead to serious infections, including pelvic inflammatory disease and sterility.
- Never share condoms. Make sure sex toys are washed well with soap and water and then with 3% hydrogen peroxide solution, or disinfected with bleach, and dried thoroughly between uses.
- Use a lubricant product such as Saf-T-Sex-Lube, a long-lasting sexual-aid lubricant that may help protect against STDs by preventing skin irritation, bruising, cuts, abrasions, and scrapes that would allow bacteria to have access to capillary blood vessels. Most STDs will not penetrate intact skin. Saf-T-Sex-Lube protects skin with skin-healing agents and a long-lasting, highly efficient skin lubricant that actually forms a protective coating atop the skin. This product contains a number of natural antibiotic and antiseptic ingredients as well [not evaluated by FDA and no claims of efficacy are made].

> ### The National Organization for Women
> ### reports the following relating to birth-control methods:
>
> • The condom fails 14.2% of the time.
> • The diaphragm fails 15.6% of the time.
> • Spermicide fails 26.3% of the time.

Saf-T-Sex-Lube is available at the Anti-Aging Superstore at www.anti-agingsuperstore.com.

• Always wash towels and bedsheets promptly. Never reuse towels on your face or hands that were used to wash up after sex.

• Women should follow the tips on avoiding a vaginal infection discussed in Chapter 5.

• If you and your partner are involved in a monogamous relationship, continue precautions until both of you have had a thorough checkup and have been given a clean bill of health.

Reminders for Safe Sex with an HIV-Positive or AIDS Partner

• So long as the uninfected partner does not get body fluids from the infected partner on broken skin, touching and kissing are safe activities.

• No cases of AIDS have been attributed to kissing, including deep (French) kissing—unless one partner has open sores or bleeding gums.

• Use the same precautions against AIDS that are recommended for STD prevention.

Note: At the Thirteenth International AIDS Conference held in July 2000, a team of researchers from Howard Brown Clinic in Chicago reported that the contraceptive gel nonoxynol-9 may actually increase transmission of HIV. Use of topical gel microbicides may increase the chances of genital ulcers in women. In the absence of the physical protection against contact with semen that is provided by a condom, the genital ulcers may serve as the transmission route for the HIV virus.

Important: A lubricant may be a good idea because irritation and abrasions allow microscopic cuts and rents in the skin, thereby allowing HIV-infected fluids to penetrate. Lubricants can protect against cuts and scrapes and also provide an added barrier against STD penetration. Always wash thoroughly with soap and water immediately following sex.

[11]

Pets Our Pets Don't Need:
Zoonotic Diseases

*During the course of our efforts on behalf of the American Academy
of Anti-Aging Medicine (A4M, www.worldhealth.net) to advocate the
research and application of methods that extend human longevity, it
is one of our greatest privileges to meet the best and brightest for-
ward-looking minds in the medical profession. As a natural extension
of the field of life-extending, life-enhancing health care for humans,
antiaging medicine is now a high-growth niche of veterinary medicine. A leader in this newly emerging veterinary specialty is Carol
Osborne, D. V.M., founder and director of the American Pet Institute
and PAAWS and the first veterinarian to be board certified by the
American Board of Anti-Aging Medicine. In this chapter, she writes
about zoonosis—the dangers of the transmission of animal diseases
to people. Dr. Osborne practices in Chagrin Falls, Ohio.*

OVERVIEW

Currently, there are over 200 kinds of zoonoses, or animal diseases
that are transmissible to people and thereby pose a significant infectious risk to human health. Domestic animals, including dogs, cats,
cattle, horses, poultry, sheep, and swine, can transmit a variety of diseases to humans. People interacting with wildlife such as bats, birds,

Diseases That Can Be Transmitted from Pets to People

DISEASE	WHICH PETS CAN GET THIS DISEASE?	HOW DOES IT GET FROM PETS TO PEOPLE?	WHAT HAPPENS IF I GET IT?	TIPS FOR PREVENTION
Toxoplasmosis: an infection caused by a single-celled parasite called *Toxoplasma gondii*	Most pets can carry this disease, but only cats shed the infection. Cats get it by eating rodents, raw meat, cockroaches, or flies, or by contacting infected cats, infected cat feces, or contaminated soil.	It is rare for people to get this disease from cats. However, pregnant women and anyone with reduced immunity should take precautions. Toxoplasmosis can be transmitted to humans by (1) eating undercooked meats or unwashed fruits and vegetables, or (2) not washing your hands after gardening, playing in the sandbox, or cleaning out the cat's litter box.	If you are healthy, the symptoms may be fever, malaise, or lymph node enlargement. If you are pregnant and it is your first exposure, the consequences range from birth defects to possible fetal abortion/ death. If you have a compromised immune system, toxoplasmosis can lead to potentially life-threatening central nervous system disorders.	(1) Practice careful hygiene around litter boxes. (2) Keep children's sandboxes covered. (3) Keep your cat from hunting. (4) If you are pregnant, don't handle cat litter; let someone else clean the litter box. (5) Cook meats well; wash your hands after handling raw meats; wash fruits and vegetables. (6) Wear gloves while gardening.
Roundworms (*Toxocaral larva migrans*): Many species of worms, often in the intestines	Dogs are the most likely to become infected.	People can get roundworms from the fecal matter of dogs. Most often, these are young children who eat dirt or sand in which round-worm eggs are found because of dog stool left on the soil.	Larvae of roundworms can hatch in the gut. Although they don't complete their life cycle in humans, roundworms can migrate in the body and cause damage to the retina of the eye.	(1) Make sure puppies are dewormed. (2) Always clean up your dog's stool. (3) Make sure young children don't eat dirt.

(continued)

(continued)

DISEASE	WHICH PETS CAN GET THIS DISEASE?	HOW DOES IT GET FROM PETS TO PEOPLE?	WHAT HAPPENS IF I GET IT?	TIPS FOR PREVENTION
Parrot fever (psittacosis): a bacteria-like organism that causes pneumonia called *Chlamydia psittaci*	Pet birds and wild birds can carry and spread psittacosis.	People catch psittacosis from contact with infected bird droppings.	Although usually mild or moderate in character, human disease can be severe, especially if untreated in elderly persons.	(1) Don't expose your pet bird to other birds. (2) Keep the cage clean and wash your hands thoroughly with soap and water after handling the bird and the cage.
Hantavirus: a common virus in deer mice that attacks the lungs	Hantavirus is an airborne virus. It can be spread to humans who sweep up deer mouse droppings. A dog or cat cannot spread the hantavirus from a rodent to a person.	Hantavirus is carried by deer mice but not by field mice. Deer mice are most common in rural areas; most city mice are field mice.	This virus usually starts with flulike symptoms such as headache, muscle pain, and fever. It may progress to something more serious, including death.	Take precautions when cleaning up mouse droppings. (1) Soak mouse droppings with disinfectant. (2) Wear gloves and a protective face mask if you are likely to be exposed to high levels of contamination or in spaces with little ventilation. (3) Pick up the mouse droppings without sweeping or vacuuming. (4) Hantavirus requires immediate and aggressive treatment.

(continued)

(continued)

DISEASE	WHICH PETS CAN GET THIS DISEASE?	HOW DOES IT GET FROM PETS TO PEOPLE?	WHAT HAPPENS IF I GET IT?	TIPS FOR PREVENTION
Rabies: a virus that attacks the brain	Carriers of significance include raccoons, bats, and skunks. Pets can become infected with rabies when bitten by these animals.	Rabies is transmitted to humans through the bite of an infected animal whether wild or a pet.	Immunization can be given after a bite has occurred, and a physician should decide when this is appropriate. Once symptoms have developed, death is imminent.	The best protection for pets and people is to immunize all pets and avoid handling wild animals.
Cat scratch disease (bartonellosis): a bacterial infection that causes skin infections	Cats pick up the bacteria under their claws.	Because their claws are thin and sharp, cat scratches inject bacteria under the skin. If an infected cat licks an open cut, sore, or lesion, transmission can also occur.	If scratch wounds are not cleaned properly, the skin can become infected. In rare cases, more serious complications can arise.	(1) Teach your cat not to scratch you. (2) Clean lesions thoroughly with soap and water. (3) Consult your physician to prevent infection.
Salmonella: bacteria that cause severe diarrhea; a common cause of food poisoning	Chicken eggs can carry salmonella. Pets, birds, and reptiles can also be carriers.	Pets that carry salmonella don't get sick from it, but people do. People get it from direct contact with their pets or from cages, living areas, or bird feeders contaminated by salmonella.	Salmonella can cause severe vomiting and diarrhea.	(1) Clean your pet's cage and living area thoroughly. (2) Wash your hands well with soap and water after handling pets. (3) Keep reptiles away from young children and infants.

(continued)

(continued)

DISEASE	WHICH PETS CAN GET THIS DISEASE?	HOW DOES IT GET FROM PETS TO PEOPLE?	WHAT HAPPENS IF I GET IT?	TIPS FOR PREVENTION
Kennel cough (*Bordetella bronchiseptica*): an infectious disease of the airways	Dogs are most susceptible. Cats are also susceptible. The disease is transmitted by direct contact with other infected dogs.	Kennel cough rarely spreads to people. Whooping cough is caused by related bacteria but does not spread from pets to people.	The symptoms are similar to those of a cold or bronchitis.	The best prevention is through immunization and by keeping your dog away from areas of concentrated canine population. Kennel cough is treatable with antibiotics.

insects, opossums, and rodents are at risk of catching one of 42 diseases. Effective control of these diseases in animals is paramount to their control and prevention in people.

Medical doctors and veterinarians are required to report certain diseases to local health authorities. Infectious diseases that threaten our economic welfare, such as mad cow disease, tuberculosis, and brucellosis, must be reported within 24 hours.

Report Animal Bites

- Bites that break the skin should be reported to local health authorities, especially if they were caused by an animal that is not your own, if they are serious, if they involve the head or neck, if the bite was unprovoked, or if the animal's behavior was abnormal.
- Rabies is potentially fatal, and specific protocols available from your local health department will be effective if implemented quickly.

Zoonotic Diseases in the Immunocompromised

Individuals with reduced immunity, including cancer therapy patients and HIV-positive people, are more susceptible to zoonoses and should take extra precautions around pets.

According to a recent survey, the two disease agents of greatest concern for immune-compromised individuals are salmonella species and *Toxoplasma gondii*. Veterinarians consider salmonella to be the leading zoonotic problem of the two. Because of the high incidence of salmonella in reptiles, most vets recommend that immune-compromised people should not own reptiles. Physicians listed *Toxoplasma gondii* as their greatest concern, and many medical doctors advise against pet cat ownership in immunocompromised patients.

In both situations, however, contact with pets is not the only or even the most important source of infection for people. Contaminated foods are the most common source of transmission of salmonella. Ingestion of undercooked meat and the handling of raw meat are much more important in the transmission of *Toxoplasma gondii* than contact with infected pet cat feces. In addition, up to a quarter of the lamb and pork we eat already contains infective *Toxoplasma* tissue cysts. Cat ownership has not been associated with an increase in *Toxoplasma*-positive blood tests (seroconversion) among HIV-infected people.

ZOONOSIS FOCUS

Toxoplasmosis

Toxoplasmosis is the most common parasitic infection in the world, affecting an estimated 2 billion people, or about one-third of the world's human population. This parasite is responsible for over 3,000 human infant infections, transmitted from mother to unborn baby during pregnancy. Signs can occur at birth, during the first few weeks or months of life, or several years later. The majority of cases appear at puberty. The most common signs involve the eyes and/or the nervous system, and result in mental retardation. Deafness, fevers, liver dysfunction, skin rashes, and respiratory disease in a variety of combinations can also occur. In people with compromised defense systems, the disease is much more severe and often fatal.

Toxoplasmosis is an infection caused by a single-celled parasite named *Toxoplasma gondii*. It is found throughout the world. More than 60 million people in the United States probably are infected with the *Toxoplasma* parasite, but very few have symptoms because the immune system usually keeps the parasite from causing illness. Cats are the primary reservoir of infection and frequently spread the disease to other animals and people.

Humans risk transmission by petting cats' fur contaminated with feces or handling the litter of infected cats. People can also become infected by eating raw or undercooked meat. The initial infection in humans is mild and resembles a cold, so most people don't even know they've become infected.

To minimize exposure risk, women considering having children should discuss toxoplasmosis with their obstetricians and should be aware of the following:

• A blood test can determine whether you have already been exposed.

Just Dropping By

In February 2000, researchers from Albert Einstein College of Medicine in New York reported that an elderly woman taking immunosuppressant drugs following a kidney transplantation became infected by *Cryptococcus neoformans* that was very likely transmitted from her pet cockatoo. The type of *C. neoformans* found in the woman was identical to that found in the bird's droppings. The team believed that the woman's infection was caused by inhaling *C. neoformans* spores from the droppings.

* If pregnant and testing positive, your doctor may prescribe a combination of antibiotics, which has a success rate of reducing fetal infection by 50%.
* A negative blood test means you are at greater risk of transmitting toxoplasmosis to your baby if you become infected during your pregnancy.

To minimize human exposure risk (especially for pregnant women), be mindful of the following:

* Don't let pet cats hunt. Keep them indoors or put a bell around their neck to decrease successful predator skills.
* Wear rubber gloves when handling potentially contaminated soil—in the garden, flower beds, children's sandbox, and litter box.
* Test household cats for the disease prior to your becoming pregnant.
* Avoid handling the litter box and have someone else change the litter box daily or every other day.

And the Cat Came Back . . . It Just Wouldn't Go Away!

* Cats infected with toxoplasmosis may first experience lethargy, depression, appetite loss, and fever. Pneumonia with severe respiratory distress is the classic sign in most cats. Vomiting, diarrhea, blindness, seizures, and loss of coordination occur when the infection spreads to other organs (the liver, pancreas, eyes, and brain).
* Cats already infected with feline leukemia virus or feline immune deficiency virus can be predisposed to develop toxoplasmosis.
* An exact diagnosis requires microscopic examination of infected tissues.
* Treatment with antibiotics is generally effective in cats. No vaccine is available to prevent the infection or disease.

- Wash all uncooked fruits and vegetables well before eating them (in case of cat fecal contamination).
- Wash your hands well after contacting soil, cats, uncooked meat, fruits and vegetables, and unpasteurized dairy products.
- Don't eat raw or undercooked meat, and don't consume unpasteurized dairy products.
- Cook all meat to 158°F (70°C) for 15 to 30 minutes before eating.

Ticks and Lyme Disease

Ticks are external parasites that suck blood from other animals to survive. They are most prevalent in wooded rural areas but can be found anywhere animals live. Ticks bite dogs, cats, livestock, snakes, squirrels, turtles, ducks, robins, and people. Most ticks are just a nuisance, but some transmit disease.

When you're in an area that may have ticks, such as when hiking or camping in the woods, check yourself, your children, and your pets carefully within 12 hours. Most ticks don't carry disease, and if those that do are removed in less than 12 hours, it is unlikely that you and/or your family or pets will get a disease.

Tick-ing Time Bomb

The number of annually reported cases of Lyme disease in the United States has increased about 25-fold since national surveillance began in 1982.

Proper Tick Removal Nothing can prevent ticks from attaching to pets or people. The key is to remove the tick promptly. If you are bitten by a tick, do the following:

- Remove it immediately by grasping it with tweezers and pulling it straight out. Wear rubber gloves to remove it.

  • If part of the tick's head remains, use a sterilized needle to
    remove it, just as you would a splinter.
  • Don't squeeze the tick. Doing so can cause the contents of
    the tick's body to be injected into the person or pet, and if
    the tick is carrying a disease, the individual can become
    infected this way.

 • Disinfect the bite area with hydrogen peroxide or rubbing
   alcohol.
 • Seal the tick in a container with a little rubbing alcohol and
   take the tick to a physician for identification.

Lyme Disease Lyme disease is the most commonly reported tick-
borne disease in the United States. The multisystem illness is caused
by a microscopic organism (a spirochete) called *Borrelia burgdorferi* and
is transmitted by Ixodes ticks.

Lyme disease is a complex illness that affects dogs, cats, other animals, and people. It was first recognized in the United States in 1975
when a cluster of rheumatoid arthritis cases appeared in the town of
Lyme, Connecticut. The outbreak occurred mostly in children, and

Tick Tock

The following life cycle of the tick plays an important role in determining when
disease can be transmitted:

  • Ticks lay eggs in the spring; one month later, larvae emerge. The larvae
    feed once in the summer on small mammals (such as rodents), especially
    the white-footed mouse, then survive the winter.
  • The next spring, the larvae molt into nymphs. Nymphs feed on dogs, cats,
    deer, and people in the late spring and early summer. Nymphs are tiny
    and are therefore difficult to detect in your pet's fur.
  • In the fall, nymphs molt into adult ticks and feed on larger mammals, such
    as white-tailed deer. They mate, lay their eggs, and die.

the first signs were rashes, headaches, and joint pains during the summer months. By 1994, 48 states and the District of Columbia had reported Lyme disease in resident populations. According to the Centers for Disease Control and Prevention (CDC), there were more incidents of Lyme disease reported in 1997 than measles, mumps, rubella, whooping cough, cholera, tetanus, diphtheria, and meningitis combined.

Deer ticks, black-legged ticks, and western black-legged ticks become infected with the Lyme disease bacteria when they feed on the blood of an infected animal, most notably the white-tailed deer, the white-footed mouse, other mammals, and birds. The ticks must be attached to the host for at least 24 hours to become infected with Lyme disease.

About 85% of people infected with Lyme disease get a characteristic rash. However, many people do not recall being bitten because the tick is so tiny and the bite is relatively painless. Diagnosis is not only based on the history of the tick bite but also on symptoms and ruling out other diseases that may have similar symptoms. In February 1999, the U.S. Food and Drug Administration (FDA) approved a new blood test that can be performed at the doctor's office and provides results within an hour. The test searches for antigens produced by the *B. burgdorferi* bacterium and is recommended for use as a supporting mechanism for clinical diagnosis.

Early Lyme disease readily responds to antibiotic therapy. If untreated or inadequately treated, the condition can progress weeks,

Theoretically Possible

In theory, Lyme disease could spread through blood transfusions or other contact with infected blood or urine. Theoretically, people could get Lyme disease from the air, food, water, sexual contact, or direct contact with wild or domestic animals, too. To date, the CDC has not documented any cases of Lyme disease contracted by these methods.

months, or years after the tick bite occurs, transforming into late-stage Lyme disease, which includes arthritic, neurologic, and cardiac complications.

In December 1998, the U.S. FDA licensed the first vaccine to help prevent Lyme disease. It stimulates the human immune system to produce antibodies against *B. burgdorferi*. The vaccine induces antibodies to enter the tick and kill the bacteria. Two injections are administered in the winter months, and a final third injection is given a year later. Studies find the vaccine only 50% effective after the first two injections, while the third injection generates 80% effectiveness for the entire series.

The Lyme vaccine is approved for people aged 15 to 70 who live in grassy or wooded areas. The FDA is quick to warn that the vaccine will not prevent all cases of Lyme disease, and that it is not known how long protection against Lyme disease will last.

Ticks in Pets

If Lyme infection does occur, the disease affects the skin, joints, and nervous system. In cats, signs are generally more vague than in dogs, but arthritis with fever, lethargy, and appetite loss may occur two to five months after initial exposure. Treatment is with antibiotics given for two to four weeks, and your pet may suffer relapses.

Since nothing can stop ticks from attaching, prompt removal and prevention of exposure to ticks in the first place are the solutions. In the past, insecticides applied to the coat as a spray, powder, or dip killed the ticks, but their protection was short-lived, and repeated treatments were necessary in high-risk areas. New monthly medication prescribed by your vet can be given to cats and dogs as a pill or drops. These new products are easier to administer and far more effective than those previously available. Be mindful that cats are very sensitive to insecticides, and only products specifically labeled for cats should be used. Your vet will be able to recommend the best product for your pet.

Experts recommend that protection should be the first and primary line of defense against Lyme disease. Follow these tips:

- During the height of Lyme season (May through August), avoid wooded and grassy places (including lawns and gardens) where deer ticks roam.
- Wear long pants and long-sleeved shirts when frequenting wooded and grassy areas.
- Tuck pant legs into socks or boots, and tape the area closed.
- Wear light-colored clothing to help you identify ticks trying to attach.
- Spray insect repellent containing diethyltoluamide (DEET) on exposed skin (other than the face). Treat clothing with permethrin, which kills ticks on contact. (Use these products sparingly around children.)
- Walk in the center of trails to avoid overhanging grass and brush.
- Shower after all outdoor activities.
- Check for what appears to be a speck of dirt anytime you've been outside.
- After your pet comes in from outside, check from head to paw for all types of ticks; if found, remove promptly and correctly.
- If your dog goes roaming in the wilderness frequently, consider getting it vaccinated. There is no vaccine currently available for cats.

Bull's-Eye

In people, early-stage Lyme disease is usually marked by a telltale skin rash (erythema migrans), appearing between three days and one month after the tick has bitten. It starts as a small red spot at the site of the bite. As it enlarges, the center of the rash may clear, resulting in a bull's-eye appearance. Common sites are the thigh, groin, trunk, and armpits. The rash is often accompanied by flulike symptoms such as fever, fatigue, and muscle pain. Other early signs are secondary skin lesions and facial paralysis.

Timing Is Everything

Administration of the Lyme vaccine should occur such that the second and third doses are given before the beginning of the *B. burgdorferi* transmission season. In the northeastern United States, where Lyme disease is rampant, this equates to the month of April.

Rabies

Rabies, found in the saliva of an infected animal, can cause brain and central nervous system dysfunction, and, if left untreated, can lead to death. It can be spread to humans through a bite by an infected animal, or by coming into contact with their saliva. Contact with a dead animal infected with rabies can also result in human transmission.

The most common carriers of rabies with which humans may come into contact are bats, cats, cattle, coyotes, dogs, foxes, skunks, and raccoons. It is sometimes found in rabbits, mice, squirrels, rats, and possums.

Rabies is on the increase in the United States, reaching epidemic levels across the Southeast, Middle Atlantic, and Northeast. A new process involving a single dose of rabies immune globulin and five injections of human diploid cell rabies vaccine simplifies the previously cumbersome antirabies procedure.

To protect against rabies, do the following:

• Vaccinate all pets yearly.
• Never approach a stray cat or dog.
• Stay away from wild animals.
• Report wild animals that allow a human to approach to a close distance to your local animal-control office.

Fleas

Fleas are the most common cause of itching and skin irritation in cats and dogs. While there are more than 200 species of fleas in the United States, the main troublemaker for pets is the cat flea *(Ctencephalides felis)*. Feeding on cats, dogs, and humans, these wingless insects will most likely choose pets because they provide a warm and fur-protected breeding ground. Fleas suck blood, and may cause anemia and transmit tapeworms. Fleas live primarily in the environment, not on your pet. They only stay on your pet long enough to get a blood meal. Then they jump back to the ground and lay more eggs. The presence of just one flea on your dog means a thousand more are around the corner; that's why prevention is so important.

Over half of all skin allergies in dogs are due to fleas. The allergy is actually a reaction to a protein component of the fleas' saliva, and constant itching may be the first sign of infestation. These allergic dogs scratch themselves until their skin is raw. Most will end up with areas of hair loss and secondary bacterial skin infections. In humans who are allergic to fleas, a single bite can cause itching for up to 14 days.

Signs of fleas in pets include itching, especially at the base of the tail, and tiny black specks in the fur that look like dirt. To confirm that this "dirt" is flea dirt, place it on a moist cotton ball. Flea dirt will turn red because of the blood it contains. Once your pet has been diagnosed with a flea problem, you need to treat all of the pets in the home and the home itself by doing the following:

- Vacuum carpets and throw away used vacuum bags so that flea eggs do not hatch in the bag.
- Use insect-growth regulators such as fenoxycarb or methoprene to treat carpets for up to 18 months. As an alternative, you can sprinkle borax onto the carpet, then vacuum (borax will protect against fleas for up to one year).
- Wash your pet's bedding with hot soapy water.

• Bathe all the animals living in your home. Use a flea shampoo with pyrethrins or d-limolene as the active ingredient.
• Apply a treatment containing nematodes—live microscopic worms—to your yard. Nematodes will eat the larval and pupal forms of fleas as well as those of 250 other pests. Be sure to treat the dark, damp areas of your yard, which provide a haven for breeding fleas.

Prevention is the key to flea control. Your vet can prescribe the most appropriate product for your pet. Many new over-the-counter monthly products are available. Regardless of the product used, prevention should start in the spring, when the outdoor temperature reaches 65° to 70°F on a regular basis.

Preferred Seating

• In dogs, fleas prefer the area from the base of the tail up the back (the "flea triangle").
• In cats, fleas prefer the head and neck.
• In people, fleas bite the ankles and lower legs.

Ringworm (Dermatophytosis)

Ringworm, or dermatophytosis, is the most common fungal infection of dogs and cats. The incidence is three times higher in cats than in dogs and prevails in warm, humid climates. Ringworm is an infection of the hair and hair follicles caused by certain types of fungi called dermatophytes. In cats, over 90% of cases are caused by the *Microsporum canis* fungus. These fungi live on keratin, found in the superficial layers of the skin, hair, and nails. Pets with ringworm usually have lesions on their heads and/or faces, although lesions on other body parts may occur.

Ringworm is easily spread to other animals and people (see Chapter 7). Children and young animals are most susceptible. The classic ringworm lesion looks like a circular patch of skin with no hair or broken hairs. The edges are generally red, scaly, and crusty. Long-haired cats, less than a year old in multicat environments, are at highest risk. Ringworm is spread by contact with an infected cat, infected hairs, or skin scales shed into the environment.

Cleaning up the contaminated environment, while extensive and costly, is the most effective postinfection approach to reduce the chances of reinfection. Be sure to wear rubber gloves and wash your hands well to avoid spreading ringworm to yourself and/or other family members, and proceed as follows:

- Dispose of all pets' bedding, brushes, blankets, scratching posts, and similar items.
- Contaminated items you can't dispose of must be disinfected. Wash in a solution of hot water and iodine soap, then soak them in the same solution for one hour. Rinse them with a solution of 1 part chlorine bleach to 10 parts water, and air-dry them in sunlight.
- Dry-clean drapes.
- Steam-clean carpets.
- Clean floors and walls with chlorine bleach.
- Vacuum and disinfect all heating and cooling vents.
- Change air filters weekly.
- Disinfect your pet's carrier and your car or van and cat flaps.

Healthy Carriers

Some cats with ringworm are "healthy carriers." They carry and spread the infection but show no signs themselves.

To help prevent ringworm outbreaks, vacuum your home daily and clean your pet's cage daily.

Anthrax

Anthrax is caused by an organism that lives in the soil and has been recognized for centuries. Sudden death in domestic livestock is the rule. Today, livestock in high-risk areas are vaccinated to prevent anthrax.

In humans, the death rate in untreated cases exceeds 90%. Aerosolization of these bacteria poses a terrorist threat (see Chapter 1).

Parrot Fever

Parrot fever (psittacosis) is caused by bacteria called *Chlamydia psittaci.* It is an occupational hazard to workers in the pet bird industry as well as to owners of pet birds. Preventive measures require imported birds to be routinely quarantined, placed on the antibiotic chlortetracycline for 30 days, and leg-banded. The leg band allows the bird to be traced to its site of origin should a problem occur. These bacteria cause death, without signs, in psittacine birds, pigeons, and poultry. Treatable with antibiotics, the disease can range from a flulike illness (with fever and coughing) to acute pneumonia in people.

Salmonellosis

Salmonellosis is a bacterial infection causing severe diarrhea and occasionally death in pets. In 1975, pet turtles were the number one source of human infection. The sale of turtles with shells less than 4 inches in diameter has since been banned in the United States. Pet iguanas have recently become an important source of salmonella in people. Salmonella is also found on freshly laid eggs. This problem has been effectively controlled by pasteurizing egg products. Humans are treated with antibiotics, and infants and small children are frequently hospitalized to receive antibiotics intravenously.

Cat Scratch Disease

Cat scratch disease is caused by an organism called *Rochalimaea hense-lae*. Each year, approximately 22,000 people in the United States are diagnosed with cat scratch disease. It causes a severe necrotizing inflammation of the lymph nodes and can be fatal.

Studies have determined that the cat flea *Ctenocephalides felis* carries the bacterium *Rochalimaea henselae*. (*Note:* The cat flea also infects dogs and may be referred to as the dog flea.)

Antibiotic therapy (doxycycline or erythromycin) for up to three months usually clears the infection in people who are not immunocompromised. Individuals with compromised immune systems may or may not respond to therapy.

With 57 million cats living in over one-third of U.S. households, the potential for infection is vast. Proper flea control in cats, and particularly in kittens, will reduce the number of fleas as well as the potential risk of transmitting this disease (see discussion on fleas). Tips for prevention include the following:

* Teach your cat not to scratch or bite you.
* Provide a scratching post.

Leptospirosis

Two types of leptospirosis can affect people:

1. Weil's disease, caused by the bacterium *Leptospira icterohaemorrhaguae*. This serious and sometimes fatal infection is transmitted to humans by contact with urine from infected rats.
2. *Leptospira hardjo* is transmitted from cattle to humans.

Both diseases start as a flulike illness with a persistent and severe headache. Weil's disease may progress to jaundice. Anyone who is exposed to rats, rat or cattle urine, or fetal fluids from cattle is at risk. Farmers are now the main group at risk for both Weil's disease and cattle leptospirosis. Others at risk include vets, meat inspectors, butchers, slaughterhouse and sewer workers, and workers in contact with canal and river water.

The bacteria can enter your body through cuts and scratches and through the lining of the mouth, throat, and eyes, and after contact with infected urine or contaminated water, such as in sewers, ditches, ponds, and slow-flowing rivers. Rat urine may also contaminate animal feed on farms. Follow these tips for prevention:

• Get rid of rats. Don't touch them with unprotected hands.
• Consult your vet about the cattle infection.
• Cover all cuts and broken skin with impervious protection (first aid plaster, gloves, etc.) before and during work where you may be exposed to these bacteria.
• Wear protective clothing.
• Wash your hands after handling any animal, or any contaminated clothing or other materials, and always before eating, drinking, or smoking.
• Report any illness to your doctor. Leptospirosis is much less severe if it is treated promptly.
• Vaccinate pet dogs for leptospirosis annually.

In humans, leptospirosis may occur in two phases: After the first phase, with fever, chills, headache, muscle aches, vomiting, or diarrhea, the patient may recover for a time but become ill again. If a second phase occurs, it is more severe; the person may have kidney or liver failure or meningitis. This phase is also called Weil's disease, and may last from a few days to three weeks or longer. Without treatment, recovery may take several months. Leptospirosis is treated with antibiotics, such as doxycycline or penicillin, which should be given early in the course of the disease. Intravenous antibiotics may be required for those with more severe symptoms. The illness caused by *Leptospira hardjo* may also be greatly shortened by appropriate antibiotic treatment.

Feline Pneumonitis

Chlamydia psittaci is a microscopic bacteria-like organism that lives in the tissues of the cat's eye called the conjunctiva. Chlamydial infection causes a syndrome called pneumonitis and usually affects the respiratory system and/or the eyes. The most common sign is runny eyes due to conjunctivitis, an eye infection, beginning most often in one eye and spreading to involve both eyes. Chlamydia can also cause mild to severe respiratory disease, with signs ranging from sneezing and a runny nose to fever, pneumonia, and diarrhea. Antibiotic eye ointments are effective treatments. A vaccine for chlamydia is available. It does not provide complete protection but will decrease the severity of infection.

Safe TLC for Kitty and Owner

Chlamydial infections can be spread to people, so be sure to wash your hands well after administering treatment, especially eyedrops, to your cat. Humans can develop a mild form of the disease called chlamydiosis, which is treatable with a course of tetracycline.

Tularemia

Rabbit droppings may contain the bacteria that cause tularemia, a disease that is fatal in about 5% of untreated animals. People can be infected without having direct contact with the rabbit or droppings. Much like Lyme disease, it may be contracted via a bite from a flea or tick that has bitten an infected rabbit. In summer 2000, a death on Cape Cod in Massachusetts was attributed to complications resulting from tularemia.

Tularemia causes enlarged red spots on the skin, swollen lymph nodes in the groin or armpits, headache, muscle pains, conjunctivitis, shortness of breath, fever, chills, sweating, weight loss, and joint stiffness. Some people may develop walking pneumonia. Antibiotics are used to eliminate the infection.

Hantavirus

Hantavirus is contracted by direct contact with the fresh or dried droppings, urine, or saliva of rodents infected with the virus—for example, by touching a surface such as a tool or furniture where the virus has been deposited and then touching your nose, eyes, or mouth. Hantavirus also may be transmitted via inhaling tiny droplets from rodent droppings, urine, or saliva or via rodent bites. Researchers believe that 10 to 15% of the mouse population carries hantavirus. The western deer mouse, white-footed mouse (common in the eastern United States), and Texas cotton rat and rice rat are the most common carriers of hantavirus.

Most cases in humans have been acquired in rural settings, but everyone is at risk, since many homes, garages, sheds, and abandoned dwellings house rodents. People are typically exposed when they do the following:

- Disturb rodent-infested areas while hiking and camping
- Work in spaces that are or have been rodent infested
- Clean out areas in the spring where rodents may have lived in the colder months
- Come in contact with more rodents in the fall as mice seek shelter indoors

Infection with the hantavirus leads to an often fatal infection of the lungs called hantavirus pulmonary syndrome. Its initial symptoms, which last from several hours to several days, include fever, headache, shortness of breath, severe muscle aches, coughing, vomiting, and abdominal pain. Victims rapidly develop respiratory failure and in more than 40% of cases they die within several days.

Hantavirus cannot be prevented any other way than by avoiding contact with rodents. Ways to keep your home free of rodents include the following:

- Keep all food and garbage in metal or thick plastic containers with tight-fitting lids.
- Never leave pet food and water out overnight.
- Wash dishes and cooking utensils after use and clean spilled food from counters and floor immediately.
- Dispose of trash and clutter.
- Stuff steel wool or concrete in cracks, chinks, and holes larger than a quarter inch in diameter. Mice can squeeze through a hole the size of a dime.
- Place 3 inches of gravel under mobile homes.
- Place metal roof flashing around the base of wooden, earthen, or adobe structures.
- Use spring-loaded traps with covers or set traps in bags to minimize contact with dead rodents. Keep traps out of the reach of children and pets. (Experts advise against using humane traps; release the mouse and it will come right back.)
- Spray rodents found in traps with household disinfectant or a 10% bleach solution. Wear gloves when emptying traps. Disinfect or dispose of the gloves.
- Use EPA-approved rodent killers in dark corners such as behind the stove, refrigerator, washer, and dryer. Keep rodenticides out of the reach of children and pets.
- Use rodent traps inside barns and sheds.
- Don't touch mice that the cat kills—inside or outside the house.
- Move wood piles, vegetable gardens, trash cans, and animal feed at least 100 feet from the house. Hay bales, wood piles, and trash cans should be at least 1 foot off the ground.
- Encourage natural predators such as owls.
- Cover backyard sandboxes with plywood when not in use.
- Don't allow children to play in basements or attics, under porches, in crawl spaces, or around wood piles.

- Forbid children to play with cute (and potentially deadly) baby mice they may discover.
- Air out cabins and seasonal retreats before anyone enters. Douse any areas of mouse infestation with a 10% solution of chlorine bleach. Wear boots, gloves, mask, and protective clothing while cleaning up rodent waste. Use wet paper towels; bag and discard them.

BUG-BUSTING BLOCKBUSTERS

It is important to do all you can to prevent disease problems that threaten both human and animal health. Some helpful approaches include the following:

- Adopt your pet from an animal shelter, or purchase it from a reputable pet store or breeder.
- Do not take in a wild animal.
- Do not approach an unfamiliar animal.
- Teach your children to tell you if they are bitten or scratched by an animal, familiar or otherwise.
- Arrange for new pets to be examined immediately by a veterinarian.
- Abide by the routine preventive care program set by your vet.
- Get your pet dewormed.
- Immunize your pet against rabies. Doing so not only protects your pet from rabies but reduces the odds that you'll contract it if your pet is bitten by a rabid animal.
- Feed your pet a balanced diet.
- Do not allow your pet to eat raw food or to drink from the toilet.
- Clean the pet's living area at least once a week. Bury the feces, or place it in a plastic bag and dispose of it.
- Clean kitty litter boxes daily. Place dirty litter in a plastic bag. *Note:* Pregnant women should never change the cat litter box,

as bacteria in the waste may lead to complications with pregnancy or birth defects.

• Cover children's sandboxes when not in use, to prevent them from being used by pets or other animals as a waste area.

• Teach children not to consume dirt.

• Wash hands with soap and water immediately after handling or cleaning up after animals.

[12]

Immunization

The most common immunizations are called vaccinations. The painful prick of a syringe delivering vaccinations to infants through elementary schoolers has been a perennial right of the youth of this nation. The U.S. vaccination policy is a control measure that prevents the rampant outbreak of many infectious diseases. In certain areas of the world where visitors may be at high risk of acquiring specific pathogens, travelers may receive vaccines to protect themselves, as well as others who would unwittingly be exposed to the pathogens by the traveler. The word *vaccination* actually means inoculation with vaccinia, which is the virus that causes cowpox. That vaccine, now more than 200 years old, was a medical miracle at the time and was so successful that no American today even needs the smallpox vaccine.

Vaccines are not without risk. The Vaccine Adverse Event Reporting System received 11,000 complaints last year, about 15% of which were of serious magnitude. Consider the following:

- There is a negligible possibility for vaccines containing live but weakened viruses (oral polio, measles, and mumps) to trigger the disease rather than prevent it.
- It was discovered recently that the rotavirus vaccine causes bowel prolapse, prompting the temporary withdrawal of the vaccine.
- DTP, an old vaccine for diphtheria, tetanus, and pertussis, is

associated with convulsions. DTP was replaced by DtaP in the early 1990s.

- In July 1999, the American Academy of Pediatrics and the U.S. Public Health Service urged discontinuation of mercury as a preservative in vaccines, after it was proven that accumulated mercury could cause neurological damage.

When Vaccines Go Awry

In 1960, government researchers discovered that when hamsters were injected with a polio vaccine that had been cultured in green-monkey kidneys, the hamsters developed tumors. Further investigation led to the discovery of SV40, a cancer-causing monkey virus. In 1961, the federal government ordered all vaccine manufacturers to screen for SV40, but never recalled existing stocks of vaccine. As a result, between 1955 and 1963, 98 million Americans were inoculated with the potentially virus-laden vaccine.

Subsequent research showed that SV40 did not cause cancer in human beings. This research, however, turned out to be less rigorous and lengthy than some scientists believed necessary to rule out a link between SV40 and human cancer. Additional research revealed a connection between the monkey virus and the slow-growing (10 to 20 years) cancer mesothelioma in humans. SV40 is also associated with bone, brain, pituitary, and thyroid tumors.

Today's *injected* polio vaccine is produced using monkey cells in a different way and is said to be free of viral contaminants. The *oral* vaccine is still produced using monkey kidneys. Regulations issued by the CDC state that American children should receive only injected vaccine. Scientists have recommended that older polio vaccine stocks—from the 1960s, 1970s, and 1980s—be screened for slow-growing strains of SV40.

RECOMMENDED IMMUNIZATIONS

Most vaccines are delivered via injection, with several shots needed for full protection. For some diseases, booster shots in childhood and preteen years are warranted. Over the last decade, the number of immunizations received by children in the United States has more than doubled. Children now receive 18 shots before they start first grade. (That number used to be 21 before the controversial rotavirus vaccine was implicated in a bowel obstruction known as intussusception, or bowel prolapse.)

Supporters of vaccines maintain that benefits far outweigh the risk of getting the natural disease. For example, varicella (chickenpox) is now the number one cause of vaccine-preventable death in children in the Western world.

Recently, the CDC recommended that all children living in states with high rates of hepatitis A be vaccinated against the disease. These states include Arizona, California, Washington, Oregon, New Mexico, Utah, Colorado, Idaho, Nevada, Texas, and Oklahoma.

With so many children vaccinated, adults are becoming more vulnerable to vaccine-preventable diseases. Between 50,000 and 70,000 Americans die every year from flu, hepatitis B, pneumococcal pneumonia, and meningitis—more than the number of people killed in auto accidents each year or the number who die from AIDS. Adults are also vulnerable because, a growing body of evidence indicates, the immune-enhancing effects of immunization may eventually wear off.

Vaccine-Preventable Diseases

- Hepatitis A
- Hepatitis B
- Diphtheria
- Tetanus
- Pertussis
- *Haemophilus influenzae,* type B (meningitis)
- Polio
- Measles
- Mumps
- Rubella (German measles)
- Chickenpox
- Rotavirus (temporarily suspended)

DISEASE UPDATE

The CDC tracks the incidence of once common diseases preventable by vaccine. Its 1999 report concluded the following:

- The transmission of indigenous measles—that is, measles that originates in the United States—is no longer occurring.
- The transmission of indigenous rubella is down dramatically in the United States. Since a second dose of the vaccine was recommended, the number of cases reported in 1998 was at an all-time low of 606 versus 5,000 in 1990.
- Pertussis is running slightly higher than it has in the recent past. Cases are stable or down among children under age 5 (the target vaccination population), but up among children 10 to 14 and among adults. Many parents, fearful of adverse events associated with vaccinations, are refusing to immunize their children, so we are now seeing a growing pool of "susceptibles" within the general population.
- Cases of varicella (chickenpox) were down considerably where the CDC monitors incidence closely. There is still concern that a large number of unvaccinated children may reach adulthood without developing chickenpox and could be vulnerable to a serious epidemic of the illness.
- The end of paralytic polio is within reach. All cases since 1979 have been vaccine related. Oral polio vaccine, which contains live virus, was phased out in 2000—but not in developing-world nations where eradication is still under way.
- In 1998, 150 cases of the meningitis causing Hib (*Haemophilus influenzae* type b) infection were reported to the CDC and only a third were confirmed. Before the 1990s, Hib was the leading cause of bacterial meningitis. Since then, new vaccines being given to all children as part of their routine immunizations have reduced the occurrence of meningitis due to *H. influenzae*.

In light of this success, the CDC warns against parents presuming "herd immunity"—that is, expecting that your child's playmates are vaccinated and therefore believing that this will keep your child from acquiring an immunizable disease. The greater the number of "exemptors" (children who for medical, religious, or philosophical reasons are not vaccinated), the greater the risk to the nonexempt population.

ANTHRAX

At a lengthy and emotional congressional hearing in October 2000, a series of men and women serving in active military service testified to suffering adverse reactions following administration of the anthrax vaccine. The troops suffered from a variety of ailments from severe weight loss to loss of consciousness, and some families charge that the deaths of their loved ones were a consequence of the vaccine.

The bacterium *Bacillus anthracis* (anthrax) has a highly variant incubation period before the virus becomes active. Exposure to aerosol anthrax spores could cause symptoms as soon as two days after exposure, but illness could develop as late as eight weeks afterward. Left untreated, 90% of people exposed to anthrax will die, most within one to three days. Antibiotics can significantly reduce the risk of death, but only if given within the first few days of symptoms.

The FDA acknowledges that the squalene molecule linked in a recent Tulane University report to Gulf War illness has been found in the anthrax vaccine, but the FDA claims it is present in quantities no greater than occurs naturally in the human body. The FDA states that anthrax vaccine manufacturers do not add the toxic compound to the vaccine, and that it is present naturally in the vaccine. Although as of fall 2000 there were more than 1,500 reports of adverse reactions filed, the FDA contends that reports received since the government began immunizing active-duty troops are insufficient evidence of significant safety concerns with the vaccine.

BUG-BUSTING BLOCKBUSTERS

When compared to the potential for widespread outbreaks and when assessed in a cost-benefit analysis on quality-of-life issues (rather than solely on an economic basis), the approved childhood vaccines are instrumental for promoting both public and personal health. Follow national guidelines for both childhood and adult immunizations for everyone in your family, and ask about receiving vaccines that help to protect you and others from pathogens you may incur while traveling abroad.

Even though risks associated with immunizations may be small, risks do exist, and it takes years for adverse effects to be discovered and properly addressed. Polio, the most studied and safest of all vaccines, caused paralysis in 49 people who were healthy when immunized and another 40 who came into contact with someone recently immunized. Researchers are continually exploring changes in the composition and administration of vaccines to lower the rate of unintended adverse effects. Be an informed consumer of health care, and make it a point to know the benefits and consequences of vaccination.

The Elixir of Life: Water

Humans can go days, even weeks, without food. Deprived of water, life can end within three days. Water composes more than half our bodies, one-quarter of our bones, and one-third of our brains. Water is present in every cell and tissue of the body and facilitates every bodily function, including respiration, digestion, cognition, and immunity. Taking steps to make certain the quality of the water you consume is "grade A" is one of the most inexpensive yet most critical ways you can boost your resistance to infectious disease.

WATER CONTAMINANTS

We hear it every day, from our doctors and at our fitness clubs: Drink at least eight 8-ounce glasses of water daily. But, do you know for certain that what you're drinking isn't causing more harm than good? The tap water you drink may have passed through as many as five human bodies before you drink it! Today, virtually everyone in the United States has one or more toxic chemicals lodged in fatty tissue as a result of the everyday consumption of water.

In fact, for many Americans, tap water exceeds the legal limits for dangerous contaminants such as parasites, bacteria, and chemicals. New agricultural and industrial toxins are being introduced to the water sup-

Don't Tap the Tap

In the United States, 53 million Americans drink water from municipal water supplies containing potentially dangerous levels of chloro- and fluorochemicals, lead, fecal bacteria, as well as pesticides and other impurities associated with cancer and metabolic dysfunction.

Bottled and filtered water are better than tap water. Consider installing a water filtration system in your home, particularly for drinking and cooking needs. To make the most appropriate selection (based on contaminants present, daily use volume, and convenience), ask for recommendations from your plumber or local water department.

In 1990, about 210 million Americans had their water delivered from a public-supply system. The remaining 43 million people in America drank from privately supplied water sources; 97% of these sources were private wells. Private well water poses the risk of containing elevated levels of pesticides, which are utilized to control the insect population, and hazardous chemicals that are improperly stored or disposed of. Over time, both of these contaminants can leach into water sources by migrating from the soil surface. In the absence of the government patrolling the public water-supply system, well users must be particularly vigilant about their water source. Well owners must regularly monitor for excesses of the Environmental Protection Agency's (EPA) Lifetime Health Advisory for water contaminants regulated by the Clean Water Act. Exposure to several hazardous chemicals together may multiply the effects of any single chemical. If elevated contaminant levels are found, it is the well owner's responsibility to contact the state or county health officials to correct the problem.

Inhaling steam vapors containing toxic metals is just as detrimental as consuming them. Consider installing a whole-house filtration system that purifies water in your bathrooms.

Distilled, sterile water is best, as it has the maximum ability to eliminate toxins from your body and is devoid of other substances and minerals. If you drink only sterile distilled water, however, you lose both the beneficial minerals and toxic (heavy) metals by excretion through urine. If your diet is not balanced with five or more servings of fruits and vegetables a day, add a quality daily multimineral dietary supplement.

ply at an alarming rate. In addition, scientists have identified bacteria usually found only in human feces in deep ocean waters, the result of human sewage disposal. That some of these bacteria are resistant to antibiotics is a clear sign that they originated in humans who were taking the drugs. In an ocean upwelling, these dormant pathogens can be brought to the surface—sometimes miles from their original dumping site.

Each year, as many as 7 million people suffer gastrointestinal effects from drinking water (an especially dangerous threat for the very young and very old and for people with compromised immune systems). And, in some places, experts speculate that contaminated water may cause birth defects, miscarriages, and cancer.

The three most common water contaminants are cryptosporidium, lead, and chlorine. Cryptosporidium is a parasite from animal fecal matter that can cause even people with strong immune systems to suffer severe diarrhea and vomiting. In 1993, cryptosporidium contaminated the Milwaukee city water supply, sickening more than 400,000 people and killing 70. In 1998, children playing in a public fountain at a Minnesota zoo were infected. The source of the contamination may have been a child in diapers who played in the fountain. Even though the fountain water was recirculated through a sand filter and then chlorinated, the pathogen survived.

Millions of Americans are exposed to water that violates the EPA's 15 parts per billion limit for lead. Excessive exposure to lead can cause high blood pressure, anemia, kidney damage, and mental retardation. The most common sources of lead in drinking water are the lead pipes and solders commonly used before 1982.

Since the early 1900s, chlorine has been used by water-treatment plants to kill disease-causing bacteria. Chlorine itself poses few direct health risks, but chlorine reacts with organic material in water to produce cancer-causing by-products. It can also react with acids in water to form trihalomethanes (THMs), which have been linked to miscarriage and various cancers.

BUG-BUSTING BLOCKBUSTERS

Stay alert to the quality of your water supply. The CDC reports that 900 deaths and one million cases of intestinal malaise each year are attributable to water-borne organisms.

The Environmental Working Group reports that 14 million people drink water contaminated with five of the most toxic herbicides. By doing so, 3.5 million people in our largest cities are at a cancer risk 10 times greater than the general population.

Most municipalities chlorinate water to kill dangerous microbes. Chlorine by-products thus wind up in the water supply of 100 million people, causing about 10,000 incidences of bladder cancer each year.

First thing in the morning, run the cold water for at least 30 seconds before ingesting, cooking, or offering a bowl to your pet. Many home plumbing systems are copper-based, and the minerals normally present in water may cause copper to leach from pipes as it sits overnight.

Ask your local water department to provide you with a copy of the most recent analysis of your water supply. Discuss your concerns relating to pesticides, radioactivity, and industrial wastes with the water department management or your town officials.

Contact the bottler of your bottled water product to ask for a copy of a complete independent analysis. There are over 450 bottling facilities in the United States producing more than 700 different brand labels of bottled water, creating a $2.2 billion industry (1990 estimates). Unsubstantiated health claims about bottled water are unlawful. All bottled water must come from a government-approved source, which must be inspected and the water sampled, analyzed, and found safe and sanitary with or without treatment. For additional bottled water information, contact the International Bottled Water Association in Alexandria, Virginia.

In the event of a natural disaster, which may compromise your access to water from your tap or bottle source, follow these techniques to purify water for drinking:

- Boiling: vigorously, for 10 minutes.
- Bleaching: Add 10 to 20 drops of household bleach per gallon of water, mix well, and let stand for 30 minutes. A slight smell or taste of chlorine indicates water is good to drink. (*Note:* Do not use scented bleaches, color-safe bleaches, or bleaches with added cleaners.)
- Tablets: commercially available purification tablets.
- Solar disinfection, known as SODIS: a new technique developed by researchers at the Swiss Federal Institute for Environmental Science and Technology in Duebendorf in which clear plastic bottles are filled with water and left in the sun. The heat warms the water, and the combination of warm water and ultraviolet radiation kills most microorganisms. The institute's tests showed that 99.9% of the *Escherichia coli* in a sample of contaminated water were killed when the sun heated the water beyond 122°F (50°C). At that temperature, disinfection takes about an hour, but placing a corrugated metal sheet under the bottle can shorten the time. Additional tests demonstrate SODIS as an effective approach for killing the cholera bacterium, *Vibrio cholerae,* and that it could inactivate parasites, including the diarrhea-causing cryptosporidium. The institute is widely promoting SODIS in Asia and South America.

[14]

Who Says Cleanliness Is
Next to Godliness?

If, as the saying goes, cleanliness is next to godliness, then why aren't more soap company executives being sainted? America's bug-busting frenzy has resulted in the lucrative and enormous markets of antibacterial cleaners as well as antibiotics. But it's now becoming less clear whether they have helped humankind or helped the germs.

ANTIBIOTICS

Under normal circumstances, the immune system should be able to destroy whatever pathogens cross its path. When you become ill with an infection, it is not because of the pathogen per se but rather because your immune system didn't work the way it should have.

In 1900, there was no such thing as an antibiotic. One hundred short years later, we are inundated with them—and the bacteria they were designed to fight are still smarter. Humans lived for millions of years without antibiotic drugs, which were not introduced until the 1930s and 1940s. Prior to that time, people relied on antimicrobials such as colloidal silver, antiseptics such as alcohol, and various plant extracts that boosted the body's own defenses (see Chapter 17).

Beginning with the introduction of the germ theory of medicine at the French Academy of Sciences in 1878 and accelerated by the use of antibiotics, many people began to believe that their health was beyond personal control. The quest to cure disease with drugs and technology has spawned a multibillion-dollar pharmaceutical industry. Yet, the drug pharmacopeia is not brimming with immune-stimulating drugs. There are quite a few nutrients and herbs that can bolster a faltering immune system. Be mindful that antibiotic supplements can be potentially toxic at pharmacological doses (a large dose that acts like a drug), so consult your physician before self-prescribing.

We have imbued antibiotics with an almost magical power, but as medical historians note, many infectious disease rates were on their way down prior to the introduction of antibiotics—thanks in large part to improved nutrition, sanitation, and personal hygiene. When penicillin was introduced during Word War II, it was heralded as nothing short of a medical miracle. Thousands of soldiers who would have died from their infected wounds were saved; thousands more who contracted venereal disease could be sent back to the front much faster. Soon pharmaceutical companies began mass producing the drug, and it wasn't long (1943) before the first penicillin-resistant microbe emerged, *Staphylococcus aureus*, which can cause pneumonia, meningitis, toxic shock syndrome, and other infections when it grows out of control.

Almost 25 years later, another penicillin-resistant bug emerged—pneumococcus. The pace has quickened since then. Less than 10 years later, during the Vietnam War, penicillin-resistant gonorrhea was iden-

Antibiotics Garnish Food

The antibiotics that enter your body aren't always from the drugstore. Some are from the grocery store. Of the 50+ million pounds of antibiotics produced in the United States each year, 40% are administered to livestock animals to keep them healthy and promote weight gain. The quinolone group of antibiotics is responsible for a drug-resistant microbe that is passed directly to consumers who eat undercooked meat.

tified among American military personnel serving in Southeast Asia. Only 7 years later, *Enterococcus faecalis,* which causes an intestinal infection in hospitalized patients, joined the ranks of microbes that could beat penicillin.

By 1998, a few strains of enterococcus had become resistant to the drug of last resort, vancomycin. Over the next few years, the frequency with which vancomycin-resistant enterococcus was found in hospitals increased more than 2,000%. *Streptococcus pneumoniae* has developed several antibiotic-tolerant strains: Unable to grow in the presence of antibiotics, they wait until treatment is ended to repopulate.

Antibiotic resistance is a result of human complacency. By the

How Smart Are You About Antibiotics?

Questions for You to Answer

True or False: Antibiotics kill viruses.

False. Viral infections are not helped by antibiotics.

True or False: Antibiotics kill bacteria.

True. Killing bacteria is what antibiotics are designed to do.

True or False: Antibiotics are a strong form of aspirin.

False. Aspirin relieves fever and inflammation.

True or False: Antibiotics should be given for colds and flu.

False. Both colds and flu are typically caused by viruses (see Chapter 6).

Questions About Your Doctor

Yes or No:

Does your doctor prescribe antibiotics over the phone? _____

Does your doctor authorize an antibiotic refill without seeing you? _____

Has your doctor told you that antibiotics are harmless and have no side effects? _____

Does your doctor dismiss your concerns about antibiotics? _____

Does your doctor prescribe one type of antibiotic after another in an attempt to find one that works? _____

If your answer is yes to even one of these questions, you have reason to be concerned about your doctor's liberal use of antibiotics.

early 1980s, infectious disease appeared to be under control, thanks to the more than 150 antibiotic drugs available (based on just a few basic chemicals). Drug companies halted their research programs on infectious disease and focused on viral disease. Bacteria, however, continued to proliferate into strains that now defy drug treatment. Most of the microbes that cause serious infections are resistant to at least one, if not several, of the antibiotics once used to treat them.

We urge you to refrain from running to the doctor's office in quest of antibiotics for every ailment large and small. These drugs set the process of natural selection in motion that creates resistant strains in the population of bacteria that normally inhabit the body. Antibiotics also upset the natural balance of bacteria in the gut (see Chapter 4). They kill beneficial bacteria that help keep "bad" bacteria and opportunistic infections at bay. Moreover, harmless bacteria that become drug resistant can also pass that resistance along to infection-causing microbes.

In 1998, the Institute of Medicine announced that the percentage of antibiotics prescribed inappropriately ranges from 20 to 50%. The Centers for Disease Control and Prevention (CDC) estimates that a third of all antibiotic prescriptions are unnecessary. Doctors commonly prescribe antibiotics for colds and acute bronchitis (see Chapter 6), largely to appease complaining patients. It is rare for drugs to be of help, as colds and bronchitis are viruses, not bacteria. Ear infections (otitis media) among children are the leading cause for the

Antibiotics and Contraceptive Failure

A review by the AMA's Council on Scientific Affairs published in July 2000 identifies the very popular antibiotics amoxicillin, ampicillin, metronidazole, and tetracycline as drugs that may potentially decrease the effectiveness of oral contraceptives. Surveys in some doctors' offices indicate that about 1.6% of women experienced failure of oral contraception while on antibiotics. Physicians are urged to counsel women taking both at the same time to use nonhormonal contraceptive methods (such as condoms).

office-based prescription of antibiotics. Antibiotics are prescribed to prevent mastoiditis, an infection of the mastoid bone, which may be unnecessary. More than three-quarters of these children with ear infections have food allergies—in many of whom controlling the latter cures the former.

Experts agree that antibiotics should be restricted to patients who have bacterial infections and should not be given to patients to prevent infection, such as surgical patients or children who are prone to recurrent ear infections. Responsible prescribing also means giving narrow-spectrum, or targeted, antibiotics—that is, those that attack a few known types of bacteria—as appropriate.

For years, the physician's drug of last resort for treating infection has been vancomycin. Proven to wipe out nearly every pathogen, we are now witnessing one of the greatest public health nightmares. Enterococcus, for years a feeble bacterium always eradicated by vancomycin, has emerged in a new lethal strain. Vancomycin-resistant enterococcus (VRE) is untreatable given the medical knowledge of today. If it progresses to circulate in the infected person's bloodstream, it is deadly. Nearly all cases of VRE are caught by people being treated for other diseases in hospital intensive care units.

Medical professionals and public health officials are frightened

Survival of the Fittest

Drug resistance is a textbook lesson in evolution. Technically, antibiotics don't cause drug resistance, but they create an environment in which resistance can happen. When you take an antibiotic, some of the bacteria may be able to survive the attack because they are just that much stronger and able to alter themselves in some way. Surviving bacteria are left to multiply. Hence, when you are taking antibiotics, it is critical to take the complete course of the drug (7 to 10 days or even longer), thus giving it time to act on the stronger microbes and prevent them from flourishing. As many as 50% of all people using prescription antibiotics do not complete a full course of treatment.

about VRE because bacteria are known to pass along their drug-resistant genes to other kinds of bacteria. VRE is on the rampage in U.S. hospitals. It is absolutely essential that you take measures to stay as healthy as possible and out of the hospital. Not only do an inordinate number of people die in hospitals, but you can pick up a load of incurable microorganisms set on eating you (see Chapter 15).

If VRE were to pass its resistance gene to a more widely circulating pathogen, such as staphylococcus or streptococcus, be prepared to walk around in full-body contamination suits, lest you risk succumbing to the impending widespread death curse.

Frankenstein Proportions

♦ At least 30 seconds of vigorous handwashing is required to remove VRE.
♦ A small sample of VRE can survive on an object (such as a doorknob, tray table, or cup) longer than 24 hours without degradation.

PHAGES

Phages are viruses that thrive by consuming bacterial cells. Likely the most simple and most common organism on Earth, phages grow wherever bacteria grow. Like any virus, when not in contact with a cell, phages lie dormant. But they can launch a successful multiwave attack against bacteria, and they are harmless to human cells.

Discovered at the Pasteur Institute in 1917, and first administered given the medical knowledge of the early twentieth century, the effectiveness of phages was sporadic, so once penicillin and other antibiotics were released in the 1930s onward, phage use dropped to nearly nil. However, with the recent and mounting concerns over antibiotic resistance, scientists are revisiting the use of phages. Indeed, some American scientists predict that within three to five years, phages will be used routinely in American hospitals when all else fails.

Phage Facts

- Phages are about one-fortieth the size of most bacteria.
- Phages have one of the most basic constructs of all organisms on Earth.
- When the Western world abandoned phage therapy in the 1930s, work continued in the former Soviet Union. The Eliava Institute of Bacteriophage, Microbiology, and Virology reported in 1985 that the phages produced there were 80% more effective against enterococcus than antibiotic treatment.
- The tailed phage is the most studied bacteriophage. These phages are so common that if all of them were gathered up and put on a scale, they would outweigh the world population of elephants by 1,000-fold.

ANTIMICROBIALS

While hospitals have been using antibacterial soaps for more than 30 years, only in the past decade have antibacterial products hit the consumer market. Stroll down the household and personal care products aisles at the supermarket these days, and you'll see that virtually every

Tips on the Wise Use of Antibacterial Agents

- Wash your hands often, using regular soap.
- Use bleach and chlorine cleaners to disinfect surfaces.
- Use products containing the antibacterial agent triclosan judiciously.
- Wash fruits and vegetables thoroughly.
- Rinse animal foods in running water.
- Don't be lured by household items advertised as containing antibacterial agents (for example, toys, cutlery, cutting boards, fabric, countertops, toilets). Cleaning items in hot water and using bleach, then letting them air-dry, is effective.
- Wash clothes in hot water and use bleach whenever possible.

Pick Soap That Won't Make People Sick

Generic liquid dishwashing soap is up to 100 times more effective than antibacterial soaps in killing respiratory synctial virus, which can cause life-threatening respiratory diseases. The virus is problematic in settings that provide care to large groups of people or groups that are sick or have compromised immunity, including hospitals, nurseries, day care centers, and nursing homes.

---

cleaning agent has an antimicrobial or antibacterial version. Antimicrobials are broad-spectrum germ-fighting chemicals that target bacteria and other microorganisms. Antibacterials are more specific antimicrobials that target only bacteria.

But using these agents instead of regular soap offers no guarantees. In one study, generic dishwashing soap was up to 100 times more effective than antibacterial soap in killing a virus that causes infant pneumonia and bronchiolitis. Prolonged use of antimicrobial products may lead to the evolution of organisms that can withstand antimicrobials when they are really needed.

Scientists at the University of London maintain that without the exposure to the bacteria that were once a part of everyday life, the body's defense mechanism loses some of its ability to fight illness and may become more prone to attacking itself. An increasingly hygienic environment may be the underlying cause of recent skyrocketing rates

---

Soap Shopping

+ More than 75% of all liquid hand soaps and nearly 30% of bar soaps contain antibacterial agents.
+ In 1998 alone, manufacturers sold $400 million worth of antibacterial hand cleanser.

of asthma, allergies, and immune system disorders. According to the hygiene hypothesis, encounters with infection or with harmless microbes called mycobacteria early in life appear to train the immune system not to attack the body's own tissues and not to react to harmless environmental triggers such as pollen. In an overly antiseptic environment in which all microbes—good and bad—are killed, the immature immune system doesn't have the opportunity to practice fighting bacteria.

An antibacterial kills bacteria on your hands and on surfaces the way an antibiotic kills disease-causing bacteria in your body. And like an antibiotic, when an antibacterial is overused, the target bacteria undergo genetic changes that make them resistant to the antibacterial. As a result, bacteria become even harder to kill than their original counterparts. To make matters worse, Tufts University researchers believe that once bacteria—for example, food-borne *Escherichia coli*—mutate, they can share their DNA with other bacteria—for example, those that cause a disease such as tuberculosis—thus making the latter bacteria resistant to treatment as well.

Volleying the Blame

The Alliance for the Prudent Use of Antibiotics believes that antibacterial soaps are dangerous. In 1998, the group's president, and Tufts University professor, Dr. Stuart Levy, issued a warning that triclosan, a potent antibacterial agent found in many consumer cleaning products, creates an environment where resistant, mutated bacteria are more likely to survive. His statement is supported by research published in August 2000 by St. Jude Children's Research Hospital in Memphis, Tennessee, which warned that triclosan as an ingredient in household cleaning products will lead to resistant strains of everyday germs, and that such formulations are not supported by scientific research.

The advocates for the soap products industry, the Soap and Detergent Association and the Cosmetic, Toiletry, and Fragrance Association, responded that the entire problem of resistance was created by physicians' overprescribing of antibiotics.

BUG-BUSTING BLOCKBUSTERS

Prudent Patients

The 10 rules of antibiotic use are as follows:

1. Do not demand antibiotics from your physician.
2. Do not take an antibiotic for a viral infection such as a cold or the flu.
3. Do not save some of your antibiotic for the next time you get sick.
4. Do not take an antibiotic that was prescribed for someone else.
5. Take antibiotics exactly as the doctor instructs.
6. Tell your doctor if you might be pregnant before you are prescribed antibiotics.
7. Tell your doctor if you are following a special diet.
8. Tell your doctor if you have experienced a previous adverse reaction to the antibiotic prescribed.
9. Ask the doctor if the drug will interfere with the effectiveness of another medication (especially if you're taking birth-control pills).
10. Wash your hands properly and frequently to reduce the chance of spreading your infection to others.

Prudent Physicians

In 1997, North Carolina instituted new statewide guidelines to reduce vancomycin-resistant enterococci (VRE). Other hospitals, as well as all physician practices and outpatient clinics nationwide, would be wise to follow their lead:

1. Wash hands according to the CDC guidelines (see Chapter 7). Studies show that physicians and health care providers

wash their hands only half the time the CDC recommends for medical professionals.

2. Change smocks after seeing a patient infected with multiple antibiotic-resistant organisms.

3. Wash hands with an antimicrobial product for no less than 10 seconds before leaving an exam room, whether or not gloves were worn.

4. Screen the waiting room for patients with symptoms of infections (someone who is coughing or has draining wounds) and move them to an examining room as soon as possible.

5. Use an EPA-approved disinfectant to clean any surface the patient touches, including chairs and measurement instruments such as blood pressure cuffs.

6. Clean exam rooms when they are visibly contaminated and institute adequate procedures for the routine cleaning and disinfection of surfaces that are frequently touched.

7. Ask facilities to call your office in advance of the consult to inform you when a patient who is infected is due to arrive.

8. Prevent antibiotic resistance by refusing to prescribe an antibiotic only to satisfy a patient's clamoring for one.

[15]

Controlling the World Around You

Serious illness doesn't bother me for long because I am too
inhospitable a host.

—*Dr. Albert Schweitzer, quoted by Norman Cousins in* Anatomy of an Illness, *1979*

Many of the microbes you encounter every day are relatively harmless. In fact, they are useful because they force your immune system to react, thereby keeping it healthy and robust. This reaction is called antigenic stimulation.

Nevertheless, the World Health Organization estimates that one in every four incidents of death or disease in the world is due to an environmental problem. The number of chemicals introduced into our lives since World War II is staggering. With them arrives an alarming increase in autoimmune diseases, allergies, and infections. Of the 100,000 chemicals now in common use, 25% are thought to be toxic. Your body fat may contain residue from hundreds of different chemicals. A toxic overload can cause life-threatening diseases such as cancer and central nervous system disorders. Chemicals also weaken the immune system, inviting bacteria, viruses, fungi, and parasites to take command.

HOME SWEET HOME

Research by the University of Arizona at Tucson from May 2000 warns that these germs frequently lurk among household objects:

- Salmonella, which can thrive in human stools, is frequently spread through mutual contact with an object in the home. If a tiny amount of contaminated stool touches the hand of an infected person who then uses a phone, the next person handling it will come in contact with about 107,000 salmonella cells, of which as many as one-third will survive long enough to enter the unwitting person by transmission through the membranes of the eyes, nasal passage, or mouth.
- Rotavirus, in as small a quantity as 10,000 virus cells, can lead to infection. Telephone receivers are a preferred spot: Contact by an unwitting person can expose him or her to about 6,600 rotavirus cells, with 200 descending on a single fingertip.
- The common cold gravitates toward kitchen faucets. If nasal secretions on the hands of someone with a cold end up on a faucet, the next household member to handle the faucet can expect over 1,000 cold viruses to hitch a ride.

Washing Woes

A word of caution to those who use public laundering facilities: A study in New York demonstrated that people who share washing machines with others are more likely to get diarrhea or the common cold. Before tossing your load into the washer, run an empty cycle of ½ to 1 cup of bleach set at hot wash–hot rinse.

Common Household Hazards

SETTING	HAZARD	RECOMMENDATION
Bedroom	Inhaling dust mite allergens (on body parts and fecal matter) aggravates—and may even cause—allergies and asthma. Dust mites thrive in the damp environment created by perspiration on sheets and have plenty of human skin and scales to eat.	• Cover your mattress, box spring, pillows, and comforter with a dust mite barrier. • Wash your sheets regularly. • Try sleeping with a fresh towel placed over your pillow, and change the towel nightly. • Use an electrostatic air cleaner with the recycled air aimed at your face.
Kitchen	Research shows that kitchens—namely, kitchen sponges, sinks, and countertops—are far more contaminated than bathroom sinks and toilets. Cleaning solutions contain harmful chemicals such as crystalline silica (in cleaning powders), which can cause cancer, and butyl cellosolve (in glass cleaners), which can damage the kidneys and liver, compromising your body's ability to fend off invasion from germs.	• See Chapter 3 for food handling tips.

(continued)

(continued)

SETTING	HAZARD	RECOMMENDATION
Laundry	Pathogens can be present in undergarments if fecal matter remains, and are thus swished around from garment to garment in the washing process to the drying process. If full removal of moisture does not occur, germs will multiply.	• To prevent transmitting bacteria from garments to yourself, always wash your hands after handling wet laundry. • To avoid cross-contamination, separate items that may harbor disease-causing bacteria (undergarments and baby diapers, in particular) and wash and dry in a separate batch. Remember, just because the germs aren't visible to the naked eye does not mean they're not aboard the garment. • To disinfect the washing machine, at least once a week run an empty hot-water wash cycle with some bleach added.
Pesticide use	Pesticides contain chemicals in sufficient levels to cause physical distress in humans, including weakening of the immune system.	• A company in Nashville, Tennessee, is working on a new line of people-friendly insecticides composed of oils from cloves, cinnamon, blueberries, and other fruits and spices to attack bugs. The oils interfere with a key enzyme found only in insects. According to preliminary studies, people and animals will be able to swallow the concoction without harm.

(continued)

(continued)

SETTING	HAZARD	RECOMMENDATION
Garden	In September 2000, two cases of Legionnaires' disease, a frequently fatal form of pneumonia, were reported to have been contracted from potting soil. A few months earlier, a third case, in which the man died, was also linked to the soil. A rare bacterial strain was found in soil used by the infected people 10 days prior to their reporting symptoms. Potting soil has been blamed for outbreaks in Australia and Japan.	◆ Garden in a well-ventilated area. Repot indoor plants outside. ◆ Avoid inhaling particulate that frequently swirls up from soil during handling.
Car	What's that funny smell in your car when you turn on the air-conditioning? It could be bacteria and fungi that can trigger allergies.	◆ Let your engine run for a few minutes with only the ventilator on to dry up trapped moisture. You can also have the system flushed with an antimicrobial to help alleviate the problem.

- *Important:* As we discussed in Chapter 7, give careful thought to finishing the handwashing process by making a germ-reduced exit. While the faucet is running, wipe your hands dry, then use a clean paper towel to turn off the faucet and open the bathroom door to exit.

VENTURING INTO THE BIG, BAD WORLD

Below are just a few of the hundreds of everyday contacts that, quite literally, make us sick.

Everyday Encounters That Can Make Us Sick

SETTING	HAZARD	RECOMMENDATION
House in general; "sick house" syndrome	• Exposure to formaldehyde in low doses can cause burning of the eyes, nose, and throat, tearing, nausea, dizziness, cough, chest pain, and shortness of breath. • Chronic exposure has been associated with memory loss, menstrual irregularities, and certain cancers. Formaldehyde is used extensively in building materials and furnishings. It is also in fresh latex paint, new paper and plastic, new clothing, and some cosmetics.	• Test the formaldehyde concentration in every room with a home-testing kit.
Day care center	• Day care children are sick almost twice as much as children cared for at home. • There is so much fecal bacteria at a day care center that children usually end up with diarrhea or a stomachache sooner rather than later. • Children in full-time day care are at greater risk for upper respiratory tract infections and ear infections than	• Choose a day care center that separates children still in diapers from those who aren't. • Impress upon the staff how important you believe it is that they wash their hands after changing a diaper and that they teach children to wash their hands after using the bathroom. • Ask the staff to keep your child out of the wading pool.

(continued)

(continued)

SETTING	HAZARD	RECOMMENDATION
Day care center (cont.)	children who don't attend day care.	In addition, staff who change diapers should not handle food.
Office "sick building" syndrome	• Ozone from photocopying machines and printers, which irritates lungs and triggers allergies; markers, highlighter pens, and correction fluid that emit xylene, which causes headaches, and, in extreme cases, nerve damage. • "Sick building syndrome," a cluster of symptoms including lethargy, sore throat, stuffy nose, eye irritation, impaired memory and concentration, dizziness, nausea, skin irritation, and shortness of breath, is caused by volatile organic compounds and bioaerosols (bacteria, mold, and fungi circulating in the air supply).	• Place office equipment as far away as possible from work spaces and be sure ventilation is adequate.
Health care settings	• Studies have shown that infectious microbes are often present on stethoscopes. • More than 10 million people undergo surgical procedures involving endoscopes yearly. Flexible scopes are difficult to clean and can harbor biological debris such as dried blood, feces, and mucus. Unclean endoscopes have been responsible for the spread of infection such as tuberculosis.	• Ask your doctor, nurse, or other health care provider to swab his or her stethoscope before your examination. • Insist that your health care provider sterilize your endoscope. Disinfectant alone does not offer enough protection from infection.
Gym	• Be aware of the possibility of athlete's foot fungus on the	• Wear rubber sandals in the shower. Foam is a sign of

(continued)

SETTING	HAZARD	RECOMMENDATION
Gym (cont.)	shower floor; Pseudomonas in hot tubs/whirlpools; a rare but deadly amoeba (Naegleria fowleri) that thrives in warm water (hot tubs and heated pools).	unclean hot tubs. Examine a glass of water from the tub. If it is cloudy or discolored, stay out.
Swimming pool	• In 1997 and 1998, the water in public pools made more than 2,000 people sick. Swimming pools can easily become contaminated with the feces of young children. Chlorine does not kill all microbes!	• Do not swim if you have diarrhea. • Do not allow your children to swim if they have diarrhea. • Do not change diapers poolside. • Never swallow swimming pool water.
Hotel	• It is estimated that only about half of all hotels provide adequately clean air. In a Wall Street Journal test of air quality in nine major hotels, four had higher bacteria counts than found in a typical suburban home. Mold counts were abnormally high in some of the hotels. • Contaminated air can cause burning eyes, headaches, and dizziness and can trigger allergic reactions.	• Check for telltale signs of dampness and stuffiness before accepting a hotel room. • Avoid hotels that use vinyl wallpaper; it doesn't breathe and traps pathogens. • Look for hotels that position themselves as "environmentally smart." • Frequent travelers and companies that require employees to travel can hire an environmental consultant to assess the hotels.

TRAVEL

When we travel to exotic destinations outside our native habitat, we become unusually vulnerable to infectious disease. A new environment, complete with never-before-encountered insects, food and water, and people, can drain our immune resources and leave us vulnerable. Simple, smart precautionary measures often will help you avoid a multitude of travel-related diseases.

Avoiding Travel-Related Diseases

ILLNESS	RECOMMENDATIONS
Traveler's diarrhea	• Avoid uncooked foods (other than fruits and vegetables you peel yourself), beverages that are not bottled, and unpasteurized dairy products. • Eat well-cooked, piping-hot foods. • Do not eat food purchased from street vendors. • Use bottled water for drinking and brushing teeth. • Do not use ice cubes unless you know they were made with bottled water. • Wash hands frequently with soap and water, and always before a meal.
Respiratory infections	• Stay inside if in areas where heavy air pollution hovers, or if it is excessively humid for a prolonged period. • Consider getting a tuberculin skin test before and after travel.
Malaria, dengue, yellow fever, and other insect-borne diseases	• Keep as much skin covered as possible. • Use repellents containing diethyltoluamide (DEET) on skin and permethrin (a marigold extract) on clothes. • Check yourself for ticks immediately after being outside. • For malaria, mosquito nets (fine-meshed fabric surrounding the top and sides of a bed) may provide additional protection.
STDs	• Do not engage in sex with prostitutes. • Use condoms in all activity, including with your companion travelers.
Hepatitis B, hepatitis C, HIV, and other blood-borne infections	• Refrain from receiving piercings, tattooing, acupuncture, and other processes that break the skin surface. • Do not share razors. • Do not opt for invasive surgical or dental procedures. • Avoid contact with blood and blood products.
Animal bites and animal-transmittable diseases	• Do not pet or feed animals, and avoid all direct contact. • Check bedding for presence of hairs and visible body excretions (animal and human).
Water-related illnesses during recreational activity	• Avoid swimming or wading in nonchlorinated fresh water, especially if stagnant or still. • Follow guidelines for timetables on diving and fishing.

Source: New England Journal of Medicine, June 2000.

THE HOSPITAL

Ten percent of patients who check into a hospital will contract an infectious disease that complicates their care at best—and kills them at worst. Consider the following:

- In August 2000, legionella bacteria, which can cause a potentially fatal form of pneumonia, were discovered in the hot-water system of a hospital in the suburbs of Baltimore. While no patients were confirmed as contracting Legionnaires' disease during their stay, the hospital did report that one patient recovering at home was diagnosed with legionella infection.
- In January 2001, seven patients with blood-related malignancies being treated at the University of Iowa Hospital and Clinics developed serious infections traced to a contaminated drain in a whirlpool bathtub. The design of the drain, which closed about 1 inch below the drain's strainer, allowed uncontaminated water each time the tub was filled to become contaminated with *Pseudomonas aeruginosa*, a bacterium that can cause several ear infections as well as blood poisoning and inflammation in the eyes and heart.

Infrequent or improper handwashing by hospital personnel is now recognized as a prevailing cause of bloodstream infections in patients in health care facilities. The routine handling of catheters, intravenous lines, and breathing tubes is the most common route of transfer of germs from health care providers to patients. With the advent of such devices now being coated with antibiotics, a tiny decline has been witnessed in the rate of infections caused by hospital staff. Researchers from the Medical College of Virginia estimate that placing an alcohol dispenser at each patient bed could cut blood infection rates by 40% by offering a readily accessible way for hospital workers to disinfect their hands often.

These incidents testify to the infection risks faced by newborns in hospitals:

- In 1997 and 1998, *Pseudomonas aeruginosa* killed 16 infants in an Oklahoma City neonatal intensive care unit.
- In September 2000, researchers from New York–Presbyterian Hospital and Columbia-Presbyterian Medical Center in New York City observed a high rate of infection in infants by *P. aeruginosa* found on employees who had long fingernails or artificial nails (wraps or tips). The infants in the hospitals' care all were immunocompromised as a result of trauma, chronic disease, drug addiction, or organ transplantation, making the slightest introduction to an infectious disease life-threatening. The hospitals enacted the following regulations:

  - Health care workers are required to wash their hands at the beginning of each shift for two minutes with a hospital-grade disinfecting solution.
  - Health care workers are asked not to wear jewelry except wedding bands and wristwatches.
  - Cosmetic nail treatments are prohibited.
  - The use of water baths to heat formula has been discontinued.
  - The number of supplies kept by the patient's bedside has been reduced.

  After instituting this policy, infection was kept under control. It is estimated that *P. aeruginosa* accounts for up to 20% of all hospital infections, so these simple and inexpensive changes are effective ways in which health care providers can avert disaster.
- In January 2001, an outbreak of *Staphylococcus aureus* infections struck 31 newborns at a German hospital maternity ward. Reuse of the spatula for applying sonography gel for routine ultrasound scanning, contrary to the hospital's infection-control policy, was cited as the culprit.

DIOXIN

CDDs are a family of 75 chemically related compounds commonly known as chlorinated dioxins. The compound 2,3,7,8-TCDD (2,3,7,8-tetrachlorodibenzo-p-dioxin) is one of the most toxic and is the most studied. When released into the air, some CDDs may be transported long distances, even around the globe. When released in waste waters, some are broken down by sunlight, some evaporate into the air, but most attach to soil and settle to the bottom in sediment. CDD concentrations may build up in the food chain, resulting in measurable levels in animals.

2,3,7,8-TCDD has been shown to be very toxic in animal studies. TCDD has been classified as a Class 1 carcinogen—that is, "a known human carcinogen." It causes effects on the skin and may cause cancer in people. It has been found in at least 91 of 1,467 National Priorities List sites identified by the Environmental Protection Agency (EPA). Dioxin is the primary toxic element of agent orange and was found at the infamous toxic waste site known as Love Canal near Buffalo, New York.

The most noted health effect in people exposed to large amounts of 2,3,7,8-TCDD is chloracne. Chloracne is a severe skin disease with acne-like lesions that occur mainly on the face and upper body. Other skin effects include skin rashes, discoloration, and excessive body hair. Changes in blood and urine that may indicate liver damage also are found. Exposure to high concentrations of CDDs may induce long-term alterations in glucose metabolism and subtle changes in hormonal levels. In certain animal species, 2,3,7,8-TCDD can cause death after a single exposure. Exposure to lower levels can cause a variety of effects in animals, such as weight loss, liver damage, and endocrine disruption. In many species, 2,3,7,8-TCDD decreases the immune system's ability to fight bacteria and viruses.

You can be exposed to CDD by the following:

- Eating food, primarily meat, dairy products, and fish. This comprises more than 90% of the intake of CDDs for the general population.
- Breathing low levels in air and drinking low levels in water.
- Skin contact with certain pesticides and herbicides.
- Living near an uncontrolled hazardous waste site containing CDDs or incinerators releasing CDDs.
- Working in industries producing certain pesticides containing CDDs as impurities, working at paper and pulp mills, or operating incinerators.

Since 1976, dioxin levels in Americans have declined considerably. Nevertheless, the average daily intake is well above two federal guidelines for "safe" exposure. All American children are born with dioxin in their bodies. It crosses the placenta into growing fetuses and can be present in breast milk. Alterations in the immune system linked to dioxin include increased susceptibility to infection, abnormal T-cell levels, and increased ear infections in children. As in animals, dioxin in humans is stored in fatty tissue.

SPECIAL CONSIDERATIONS FOR THE YOUNG

With their immature immune systems, infants and children are at particularly increased risk for succumbing to an infectious disease. Toys are an outright health threat to sick babies. Researchers at the Royal Women's Hospital in Melbourne, Australia, cultured bacteria from nearly all the toys belonging to newborns in intensive care. Five of the babies became ill after being infected with the same bugs found on their toys. The team recommends that toys routinely be disinfected or destroyed.

Our natural parental instinct to protect children from all sources of potential harm may do more damage than good. A team from the University of Arizona College of Medicine has been following about 1,000 children for 15 years, monitoring respiratory function and allergens in their environment. In August 2000, the team reported that protection against asthma resulted from frequent exposure to other youngsters, but only if such contact took place in the first 6 months of life. The researchers speculate that stimulation of the immune system early in life is necessary to prevent future overreaction to allergy-inducing substances known as antigens.

BUG-BUSTING BLOCKBUSTERS

Our homes should be our castles and visitors should be invited guests—not unwelcome germs. Some fairly inexpensive yet effective measures to implement are as follows:

* Take shoes off when entering the house, or get a good mat or "hedgehog" by which the remnants of the outside world can be left at the door. The Japanese tradition of removing shoes when indoors is a lesson to be learned, especially since in summer 2000 the World Health Organization bestowed upon them the distinction of having the longest longevity in the world.
* Clean rugs with a vacuum equipped with a HEPA (high-efficiency particulate air) filter, which prevents reintroduction of debris and germs after they're collected. Steam-clean rugs at least twice a year, taking care not to drench them in either solution or water. Add a few drops of tea tree oil to the cleaning solution as a natural disinfectant.
* If you have central air-conditioning or a central forced-air heating system, install an electrostatic filter to capture debris and germs from the airflow stream. Replace the filter twice a year.

In rooms that are most often used (including the bedrooms), consider the following:

* Minimize knickknacks and objects that collect dust.
* If you experience a chronically congested nose, use a humidifier. Remember to change the water daily, and use only fresh distilled water to minimize the chances of breeding bacteria.

• In the bedrooms, encase mattresses, boxsprings, and pillows in allergy barrier covers. Change sheets weekly and wash in hot water.

Don't live in a bubble, and don't raise your child in one either. Isolation based on the reasoning that less germ exposure is better is now under question. Social contact is important for maintaining a healthy emotional state and reducing stress, which are both involved in immunity (see Chapter 17).

[16]

How Bugged Out Are You?

> The breath of life enters into the right ear and the breath of
> death enters into the left ear.
>
> —*Anonymous,* The Ebers Papyrus

The era of expanding managed care programs with its shrinking emphasis on early diagnosis mandates that each of us take control of our own health. If there is anything the preceding chapters have demonstrated, it is that much of the difference between being healthy and fit and being suddenly or persistently sick has to do with the everyday choices you make in how you live your life.

A number of diagnostic (Chapter 16) and treatment (Chapter 17) considerations are presented to help you make sense of what's eating you.

This icon indicates that the approach can be obtained from a doctor or licensed health practitioner.

This icon indicates that the approach can be done yourself, at home, with a generally low risk of complications when performed responsibly.

Parasite Checklist

Follow this checklist to monitor for common symptoms associated with a successful invasion of your body by bacteria, fungi, and viruses as well as insects, mites, worms, fleas, ticks, and protozoa:

[ ] Lethargy
[ ] Feeling hungry even after eating
[ ] Loss of appetite
[ ] Itchy nose, ears, eyes, or anus
[ ] Intestinal gas and/or bloating
[ ] Unclear thinking
[ ] Forgetfulness
[ ] Yellowish tinge to skin
[ ] Pains in the belly
[ ] Pain in the back, thigh, or stomach
[ ] Cardiac symptoms, including chest pain and/or fast heartbeat
[ ] Numbness in hands or feet
[ ] Slow reflexes
[ ] Blurry vision
[ ] Grinding teeth while asleep
[ ] Drooling while asleep
[ ] Dry lips during the day, damp lips while asleep
[ ] Bedwetting and/or incontinence
[ ] In women, menstrual problems or irregularities
[ ] In men, sexual dysfunction

 Tongue Inspection

Your tongue is a mirror of your digestive system, and you can learn a lot by observing what's coating it. From time to time, most of us develop a thin white coating on the tongue. This most often occurs when we don't drink adequate liquids, which causes tiny pieces of food to stick to the tongue. It also may result from a normal accumulation of dead cells. In both cases, the coating is harmless and can be removed by brushing the tongue or using a tongue scraper (see Chapter 9). Tongue scrapers may be mail ordered from a number of companies on the Internet. Your local drugstore may also carry them.

A thick or persistent white coating on the tongue may signal candida infection (see Chapter 5), which causes the ailment known as thrush. Thrush most often manifests as an oral infection that appears as creamy white, curd-like patches on the tongue and inside of the mouth. In adults, long-term use of antibiotics or inhaled steroids (such as those used to treat asthma) may upset the balance of microbes in the mouth, allowing an overgrowth of candida that will result in thrush. In infants, candida may exacerbate diaper rash, as this yeast grows readily on damaged skin. The infected skin is usually fiery red with lesions that may have a raised red border. Children who suck their thumbs or other fingers may occasionally develop candida

Risk Factors for Candida

- Taking antibiotics for acne for more than a month
- Ever taken broad-spectrum antibiotics for respiratory, urinary, or other infection for more than two months, or in short courses four or more times in a one-year period
- Taken cortisone-type medications (including prednisone)
- Experienced persistent vaginitis (women) or prostatitis (men) (see Chapter 5)
- Women having taken, or taking, birth-control pills
- Experienced chronic infection of the skin or nails (see Chapter 7)
- Bothered by chemicals, including perfumes, insecticides, fabric odors, tobacco smoke, and/or chemical treatments
- Cravings for sugary foods
- Cravings for yeasty carbohydrates, including breads and alcohol

around their fingernails. See a doctor for proper treatment, which usually consists of antibiotics.

A white coating on the back top of the tongue, if associated with a sore throat and a sensation of something stuck in the throat, may be a case of pharyngitis, which can be due to a bacterial or yeast invasion. See your doctor for treatment. Regular tongue cleanings (see Chapter 9) will help to reduce this buildup.

Lymph Nodes

Lymph nodes (see Chapter 2) often swell in reaction to infection. Inspect for swollen nodes as follows:

1. With fingers together, touch the flesh pads of the top of the fingers and press gently along the entire course of the neck. Relax neck muscles when doing this. Feel around to the back of the neck, up under the chin, and at the angle of the jaw.
2. A node that is enlarged due to infection often feels soft and is painful when pressure is applied to it.

pH

pH, an abbreviation for hydrogen potential, is a measure of the concentration of hydrogen ions in a liquid solution. On a scale of 0 to 14, a neutral pH is around 7. A numeric value less than 7 represents acidity; a higher value represents alkalinity. pH controls hundreds of enzymes and their function in digestion and energy production. Maintenance of acceptable pH levels in saliva, blood, and urine is necessary for the delicate balance that promotes a healthy immune system.

You can test pH at home using pH tape or testing strips that are sold in drugstores, health food stores, and home brewery shops. To test pH, do the following:

1. Tear off a 1- to 2-inch length of pH paper.
2. Collect and contain the sample: Place saliva in a clean, dry spoon; for urine, use a clean, dry glass.
3. Dip pH paper into sample.
4. Read immediately (within five seconds) by comparing to the color chart provided.

The first morning reading of saliva and urine is the most important, since both can vary widely throughout the course of the day. Measure pH before eating any food. Drink a glass of water and collect the samples after a few minutes.

To measure pH of vaginal secretions (see Chapter 5), use a swab or wooden spatula to apply a small sample to a 3- to 4-inch strip of pH paper. Distribute evenly. Wait for the color change. Normal vaginal discharge has a pH of 3.8 to 4.2. Higher values indicate infection. If your discharge tests more than 4.2, schedule an appointment with your physician so that a precise evaluation can be made.

pH Findings

- Urine pH taken first thing in the morning should be between 5.5 and 6.0.
- Saliva pH taken first thing in the morning should read 6.2 to 6.4.
- Second readings on both saliva and urine pH should be 6.4. Eating will cause these numbers to change.
- If first urine pH is higher than 6.2 (alkaline), you are likely not cleaning out waste products from the blood properly. Most often, this causes fatigue. If you also are experiencing first saliva pH less than 6.0 (acidic), you may have a toxic liver, a fatigued adrenal, or any number of digestive disorders. See the doctor to confirm your screening and institute effective treatment, which may include dietary modifications to correct your pH imbalance.

pH and Foods

Acid-forming foods:

- ♦ Meat protein, including beef, pork, fish, poultry, and eggs
- ♦ Carbohydrates, including grains, breads, and pastas
- ♦ Fats

Base-forming foods:

- ♦ Buffering products including bicarbonates

Comprehensive Digestive Stool Analysis

Offered by testing companies including Great Smokies Diagnostic Laboratory (see Resources, in Appendix B), the CDSA is an integrated battery of independent tests evaluating digestion, intestinal function, intestinal environment, and absorption. From A(eromonas) to Y(ersinia), CDSA can uncover bacteria that cause outright disease, bacteria implicated in chronic or systemic disease, and organisms that characterize an unbalanced gastrointestinal system.

BUG-BUSTING BLOCKBUSTERS

The health care industry has, in large part, been woefully lacking in providing cost-effective methods for rapid and reliable screening of illness. The techniques in this chapter are meant to be utilized as indicators within the framework of a complete preventive health care program under the supervision of a physician or licensed health care practitioner. We hope and predict that, in the years ahead, the medical establishment recognizes the profound benefits of encouraging health care providers to embrace the concept of proactively monitoring for declines in health in order to avert the much more financially costly and physically and emotionally devastating full-blown disease state.

Speak with your doctor about implementing ways to monitor changes in your health status at home. Use nonbiased educational sources of medical information—for example, the World Health Network (www.worldhealth.net). Encourage your physician to become a member of the American Academy of Anti-Aging Medicine (A4M), a not-for-profit medical society of 10,000 physicians, scientists, and health practitioners from 60 countries worldwide dedicated to the advancement of technology to detect, prevent, and treat aging-related disease and to promote research into methods to retard and optimize the human aging process.

[17]

Boost'r (Best Optimizing Options-Strategies-Treatments Reference)

> Natural forces within us are the true healers of disease.
>
> —*Hippocrates*

The goal of this chapter is to help you make sense of the wide variety of approaches that might help you prevent the odds of your falling prey to infectious disease, stimulate your immune function, or recover from illnesses resulting from invasion of pathogenic microorganisms. This listing, which is representative of currently available options as of summer 2001, does not purport to be comprehensive, and no endorsement of any particular approach is stated or implied.

Important: Review the "Please Read" section on page xix.

An approach that can be obtained from a doctor or licensed health practitioner

An approach that can be done yourself, at home, with a generally low risk of complications when performed responsibly

An approach that may have immune-stimulating properties

An approach that may have immune-healing properties

   Nutrition

Despite the availability of food and the current girth of the nation, many people suffer from suboptimal nutrition that compromises the immune system. Diet plays a role in at least 5 of the 10 leading causes of death in the United States. All the physiologic and structural functions of the body depend on nutrition. In fact, a balanced diet is the most important factor in maintaining a healthy immune system.

Nutrients Involved in the Immune System

Epithelial tissue barriers	• Vitamins A, B_2, B_3, B_6, B_{12}, folic acid, C • Iron and zinc • Protein • Essential fatty acids
T-cell immunity	• Vitamins A, B_6, folic acid, C, E • Iron, selenium, zinc • Protein • Essential fatty acids
B-cell immunity (antibodies)	• Vitamins A, B_1, B_2, B_3, B_5, B_6, folic acid, biotin, C • Protein • Essential fatty acids

Consider adding a product such as Physicians Immune Booster to your daily regimen. A proprietary blend of immune-enhancing vitamins, nutrients, and natural agents that have been demonstrated to have strong benefit in stimulating and/or supporting immunity in human and animal laboratory research, this single formula boosts the body's defense for fighting infectious attacks. Physicians Immune Booster is available at the Anti-Aging Superstore at www.anti-aging-superstore.com.

    Hydration

Water is a nutrient essential to life (see Chapter 13). Your body typically loses 2 to 3 quarts of water daily through perspiring, sneezing, breathing, urinating, defecating, and, for some women, nursing a baby. Depending on how much physical work or exercise you do and how hot or cold the temperature is, you may lose more.

The best way to monitor fluid intake is to watch the color of your urine, which should be light rather than dark. Half of all the fluids you drink should be water. Tea, coffee, milk, and juice count as fluids, but the water in foods (for example, fruits, vegetables, and soups) does not. Consider that fluid a bonus. These are general guidelines for optimal fluid intake:

- Aim for at least 8 cups of fluid a day, half of them water.
- Drink some water first thing in the morning to make up for loss of fluids during the night.
- Drink a beverage with every meal.
- Don't wait until you are thirsty; drink throughout the day.
- For every cup of caffeinated beverage you drink, consume an extra half cup of another fluid to make up for caffeine's diuretic effect.

Exercise

  Until the time of the Industrial Revolution, strenuous physical activity was an integral part of daily life in work as well as in religious, social, and cultural expression. By 1953, almost 60% of American children failed to meet even a minimum fitness standard for health (compared to less than 10% in Europe). When John Kennedy became president in 1961, he convened a conference on physical fitness and young people and established what would eventually be called the President's Council on Physical Fitness and Sports. The mid-1970s saw widespread enthusiasm for the benefits of physical activity in preventing and treating a variety of conditions that continues to this day.

One, Two, Three—Go

ONE: STRENGTH TRAINING

Strength (weight) training builds and tones muscles. Although aerobic exercise burns more calories as you are doing it, strength training builds new muscle tissue, which burns 25% more calories than any fat tissue it replaces—even when you are sitting still or asleep. If you are planning to start an aerobic exercise program, begin with some weight training to build your strength.

TWO: AEROBIC EXERCISE

Aerobic (cardiovascular) exercise helps keep your heart and lungs healthy—and burns calories, too. Even after you stop exercising, your metabolism can stay revved up for as much as an hour. The best all-around aerobic exercises are cross-country skiing, rowing, and swimming because they involve all the major muscle groups of the upper and lower body. If you have not exercised much lately, begin with 15-minute sessions of brisk walking or biking three times a week at an intensity that causes you to breathe hard—but not so hard that you can't carry on a conversation. Within six to eight weeks, you should be up to 30 minutes of aerobic activity three times a week.

(continued)

(continued)

THREE: STRETCHING

Stretching promotes flexibility and helps prevent stiffness and tension. Over time, stretching lengthens muscles and strengthens tendons and ligaments. Both yoga and tai chi are forms of stretching. Begin and end your strength training and aerobic sessions with several minutes of stretching.

GO!

Combine the following exercises for a maximum return on your investment:

- Running and yoga relieve stress.
- Running and weight training boost energy.
- Walking and weight training slim and tone.
- Aerobic dance and cycling fight boredom.
- Gardening and cycling keep you outside.
- Walking and swimming avoid high impact.
- Cross-country skiing and swimming combine the best of aerobic and anaerobic activities.

Note: Always begin an exercise program by first consulting your physician. Consider working with a professional trainer to develop a comprehensive exercise program that is right for you.

Moderate exercise boosts the function of T cells and B cells. In fact, within minutes of starting to exercise, the body's white blood cells and natural killer cells increase, and, depending on the intensity and duration of activity, they remain elevated for a few seconds to hours after exercise is completed.

It takes 12 weeks of regular exercise to become "fit"—meaning that your oxygen capacity has improved. It takes only one brisk walk, however, to improve your health—that is, to lower indicators such as blood pressure, blood sugar, and triglycerides. Exercise reduces the risk for stroke, lowers LDL (low-density lipoprotein) cholesterol and raises HDL (high-density lipoprotein), lowers the risk for sleep disorders, improves mood, boosts creativity, preserves mental acuity, and maintains muscular strength, flexibility, and balance. Regular stimulation of the immune system may have a cumulative effect.

However, high-intensity exercise can adversely affect the immune system. Overtrained athletes may be at increased risk of infection because antibodies in the blood and mucosal surfaces (such as eyes, nose, upper and lower respiratory tracts, gastrointestinal tract, and genitourinary tract) are suppressed. An open window of 3 to 72 hours after high-intensity exercise leaves the body more vulnerable to illness.

   Stress Reduction

Happy people are far less likely to get sick. Many surveys of self-perceived wellness that are correlated to quality and satisfaction of life show that happy people are less self-focused, less hostile, and less abusive: All of these characteristics, for presumably a range of biological reasons, make them less vulnerable to disease.

The concept of psychological stress was introduced in the 1930s by Hans Selye, an endocrinologist. Selye suggested that all organisms have a common biological response to negative sensory or psychological stressors. The human body can handle this response without incurring damage so long as it doesn't happen too often. But when it happens all the time, its negative effect on the body tends to accumulate and interfere with the immune system.

Researchers in a new field called psychoneuroimmunology are exploring the links between the immune system and feelings and thoughts. In several classic studies, researchers found that people under psychological stress were more likely to develop a cold when injected with a respiratory virus, more likely to have heart attacks and strokes, and less likely to produce antibodies when given a flu vaccine.

Stress Fighters: Whatever Works!

- Joining social or spiritual groups
- Having a close confidante
- Spending time with supportive friends
- Maintaining a healthy balance of food, activity, and sleep
- Having realistic expectations of yourself and others
- Journaling thoughts and feelings
- Keeping a daily gratitude journal—things, large and small, that you are thankful for
- Meditation and prayer
- Positive affirmations
- Listening to music
- Aromatherapy using essential oils such as spearmint, lavender, jasmine, frankincense, rose, neroli, chamomile, and sandalwood
- Laughing . . . a lot

   Sleep

Sleep is necessary for mental and physical restoration. It is an active state that, like diet and exercise, is critical to good health. Sleep deprivation of just 2 to 3 days can lead to serious lapses in mental function and judgment, at 4 to 5 days can cause psychosis, and at a week or more may be fatal. Studies of lab rats that were not allowed to sleep for 13 days revealed the cause of death as brain hemorrhage.

Nearly two out of three Americans get less than the recommended eight to nine hours of sleep a night. Average sleep duration has decreased from about nine hours per night in 1910 to about seven and a half hours today. Many shift workers sleep less than five hours a night.

More than 70 million people suffer from sleep deprivation caused by poor or interrupted sleep and about 50 million suffer negative health effects as a result. Some of the common reasons for sleep disruption are as follows:

- Stress and worry
- Aches and pains in the joints and muscles
- Poor-quality mattress or uncomfortable bed
- Side effects from certain medications
- For women, hot flashes or night sweats caused by hormone fluctuations

When you are asleep, your parasympathetic nervous system (PNS) is in control and your nervous system is being rejuvenated. Many important immune system processes occur as you sleep, which is why getting a lot of rest is prescribed as a treatment for so many illnesses. Given their simplicity, bed rest and deep sleep are perhaps the two most underestimated therapeutic interventions that deliver the greatest benefit for the effort spent.

Like many other body processes, sleep is influenced by circadian rhythms triggered by exposure to light and secretion of certain hormones, especially melatonin. As daylight ebbs, your pineal gland (located in the brain behind the eyes) secretes melatonin, which promotes sleep. At the same time, other body processes begin to slow down in preparation for sleep.

General Recommendations for Somnambulistic Bliss

As a frequent overseas traveler, Dr. Bob Goldman has devised a practical, tried-and-true program that often helps him and others to boost the quality of sleep. Dr. Goldman's complete program appears in *Brain Fitness* (1999, Doubleday). Seven of his favorite sleep suggestions are as follows:

1. Practice good sleep hygiene:

   - Where you sleep directly affects how well you sleep: Create a sleeping environment that is comfortable in temperature, absent of distracting lighting and sounds, and serene.
   - Don't become overstimulated: Television emits full-spectrum lighting and electromagnetic fields that can cause wakefulness and/or agitation.

• If you have allergies to airborne agents, remove plants and humidifiers (both can be sources of mold), don't let pets into your bedroom (sources of dander), and encase your mattress, boxspring, blankets, and pillows (havens for dust mites) in allergy barrier covers.

2. Eat for sleep: Starchy foods such as breads, pastas, potatoes, and milk products help promote sleep. They prompt your brain to generate the sleep-inducing neurochemical serotonin.

3. Herbs help: For some people, a modest dose of valerian root, kava, chamomile, or lavender oil speeds up the trip to dreamland.

4. Avoid certain medications: Check with your physician to verify whether any prescription and/or over-the-counter products you take may cause you difficulty in falling asleep. Blood pressure medicines, decongestants, nicotine, caffeine, diet pills, and some cold/cough remedies are frequent culprits.

5. Lower your body temperature: You reach sleep once your body temperature dips. A warm bath or shower before bedtime makes it easier for your body to cool down and the time to reach dreamland is shorter.

6. Take two: Try two baby aspirin (noncaffeinated) at bedtime when you don't feel sleepy.

7. Power nap: Just 20 minutes of restful slumber during a hectic day not only rejuvenates your thinking but can make it easier for you to sleep at night.

Consider taking a product such as PM Antistress Sleep Assist, a natural blend of medicinal herbal and nutrient ingredients shown to promote deep, restful, rejuvenative, and relaxing sleep when used at full dose. When used at low dose (one-third strength), PM Antistress Sleep Assist functions as a natural antistress calming tonic. PM Antistress Sleep Assist is available at the Anti-Aging Superstore at www.anti-agingsuperstore.com.

Sun

Daily exposure to sun exposes us to ultraviolet light (UV-A), which produces vitamin D naturally in our bodies. Vitamin D in turn helps us to produce antigens and stimulate the immune system, utilize calcium, enhance metabolism, and stabilize body temperature. Aim for 10 to 20 minutes of total-body sun exposure every day.

 Dietary Supplementation

While it is preferable that we obtain our vitamins, minerals, fatty acids, and amino acids from foods in order to optimize their synergistic action, life on the run and environmental toxins have made it difficult for our bodies to get many of the necessary nutrients from the foods we eat. Check with your doctor to determine whether you might benefit from taking a basic multivitamin, multimineral product.

Vitamins

Vitamin A Vitamin A helps protect T cells that line the body's digestive tract, skin, corneas, lungs, and bladder. It is essential for building healthy connective tissue, which is the major component of the mucous membranes in the digestive, respiratory, and urogenital tracts. When vitamin A is deficient, cancer cells have an easier time getting a foothold.

Dr. Binyamin Rothstein, an osteopathic physician in private practice in Baltimore, uses massive doses of vitamin A in an oil suspension to prevent flu and colds. "Up to 400,000 units of vitamin A is safe, except for pregnant women," Rothstein notes.

The body converts the carotenoid beta-carotene into vitamin A as needed. On its own, beta-carotene helps in the production of various immune system cells and is an antioxidant, protecting the body against free-radical damage that can suppress the immune system. Eating deep yellow fruits and vegetables will give the body the beta-carotene necessary to produce the vitamin A it needs.

B Vitamins Taken as a complex, B vitamins are available as a single supplement, with any particular nutrient(s) taken in addition and separately if medically indicated. The immune-boosting B vitamins include folic acid, pantothenic acid, pyridoxine, riboflavin, and B_{12}.

Pantothenic acid is referred to as the antistress vitamin because it is necessary for the production of adrenal hormones, cortisone, and other steroids. The biologically active form of pantothenic acid is pantetheine, which can be purchased as a supplement in tablet form.

A deficiency of pyridoxine, also known as B_6, can cause the lymph tissue to atrophy. Vitamin B_6 deficiency is common among older people, many of whom have a reduced immune response. Whole grains and greens are good sources of B_6. Supplements of just 15 milligrams daily of B_6 can have an immune-enhancing effect.

Vitamin C Thanks to Linus Pauling's work on vitamin C and the common cold, vitamin C is probably the best known of the immune-boosting nutrients. Vitamin C (1,000 to 6,000 milligrams per day) can shorten the duration of a cold and help fight secondary bacterial infections that can accompany a cold. It also reduces the infection and symptoms of other viruses such as mumps, herpes, measles, and the flu.

The adrenal glands use a lot of vitamin C in the production of stress hormones. Thus, during periods of stress, the body may need even more vitamin C than usual. At the first sign of infection, 500 to 1,000 milligrams every two hours (continued according to bowel tolerance—that is, decrease dosage at the beginning of diarrhea) may be helpful in times of stress. Check with your doctor on long-term use.

Important: In women, 10-gram doses of vitamin C daily may inactivate birth-control pills. For both men and women, high-dose vitamin C may skew the accuracy of laboratory blood tests. Before taking vitamin C, check with your doctor to determine the dosing that's right for you.

General Supplement Guidelines

NUTRIENT	DOSE
Folic acid	800 mcg
Vitamin B$_6$	10 mg
Vitamin C	500 mg
Vitamin D	400–800 IU
Vitamin E*	200–400 IU
Chromium	200–400 mcg
Copper	0.5–1.0 mg
Manganese	10–20 mg
Molybdenum	200–400 mcg
Selenium	100–200 mcg
Zinc*	15–20 mg

*Important: Studies show that very high doses of vitamin E (≥1,600 IU) and zinc (≥50 mg) can impair the immune system, so be sure to check with your doctor on your particular health needs.

Vitamin E Vitamin E is known for its potent antioxidant activity and for its positive effects on heart health, immune cells, and resistance to infection. Vitamin E supplementation increases immune response in older people.

Vitamin E includes two different compounds—tocopherols and tocotrienols—both of which have four subtypes—alpha, beta, delta, and gamma. Tocopherols and tocotrienols may work synergistically in the body. Among tocopherols, alpha and gamma are the most important. Alpha-tocopherols are thought to be the most biologically active and have been studied the most. They are found in most dietary supplements and are believed to be most effective in maintaining heart health; gamma-tocopherols come primarily from food and may be a key to fighting inflammation and strengthening the immune system.

Tocotrienols appear to fight cancer and lower cholesterol. Laboratory studies of gamma- and delta-tocotrienols indicate they fight cancer by inhibiting the Epstein-Barr virus, which seems to be implicated in cancer in some people.

Wheat germ, nuts, legumes, and vegetable oils contain all eight components of vitamin E. It is almost impossible, however, to get enough vitamin E from food alone. In supplement form, vitamin E from a natural source is more potent and is absorbed better by the body. Natural E capsules generally contain d-alpha tocopherol and/or mixed tocopherols, which are also natural. Synthetic supplements are the form dl-alpha tocopherol.

While the Recommended Daily Allowance (RDA) for vitamin E is 8 to 10 milligrams per day, 100 to 200 milligrams per day of natural vitamin E is well tolerated, safe, and documented to be clinically beneficial. Supplementation at levels greater than 1,200 milligrams daily may inhibit immunity, especially in younger people.

Coenzyme Q10 (CoQ10) There are 10 different types of coenzyme Q (CoQ). Only CoQ10 (ubiquinone) has been found in human tissue. Cells need CoQ10 to produce energy. The more energy an organ requires, the more CoQ10 it contains. Researchers believe that the level of CoQ10 in an organ may be directly related to the health of that organ. CoQ10 (30 to 100 milligrams daily) may be helpful for the following:

- Treating heart disease
- Treating high blood pressure
- Treating gum disease
- Relieving allergies and asthma by countering histamine, as well as for treating other respiratory diseases
- Treating schizophrenia
- Treating Alzheimer's disease
- Helping to heal duodenal ulcers by protecting the stomach lining

CoQ10 is found in meat (especially organ meats), eggs, spinach, broccoli, potatoes, rice, corn, rye, various nuts, sesame seeds, sardines, and mackerel. The amount of CoQ10 found in even the richest sources, however, is not enough to correct a deficiency. The liver can take other forms of CoQ and convert it to CoQ10, but this ability decreases with age. It is also available as a supplement, but be sure that you select a product that is bright yellow in dry form and has very little taste.

Minerals

Copper The body requires copper, a trace element, to mobilize and transport iron to various tissues. Thus, a deficiency in copper can result in a secondary iron deficiency. Although iron can promote oxidation, it is needed in the bone marrow for the differentiation of stem cells into various types of white blood cells. If this production is slowed, resistance to infection is compromised. Shellfish, legumes, mushrooms, nuts, and chocolate are good sources of copper. Supplementation at levels greater than 3 milligrams daily may be harmful.

Magnesium Because magnesium is involved in hundreds of enzyme reactions, a deficiency can adversely affect the immune system. The ability of immune cells to adhere to other substances requires magnesium. Nutritional experts approximate optimal daily magnesium intake by calculating 6 milligrams for every 2.2 pounds of body weight.

Methyl-Sulfonyl-Methane (MSM) MSM is organic sulfur, which occurs naturally in the body. Sulfur is found in every cell of the body and is structurally and functionally important to a number of hormones, enzymes, antibodies, and antioxidants. In the body, the highest concentrations of MSM are found in breast milk, which helps infants to build a strong immune system. Over time, MSM deficiencies occur as part of the aging process.

MSM is present in meat, fish, eggs, poultry, milk, grains, legumes, fruits, and vegetables (especially asparagus and cruciferous vegetables). Because MSM is lost in food processing and storage, dietary sources may not offer enough for therapeutic impact. At moderate levels, MSM helps to maintain healthy skin, nails, and hair. MSM may be taken daily at 250 to 2,250 milligrams per day.

Selenium In the environment, selenium is a trace mineral. But in the human body, it is an essential nutrient. In addition to its protective functions in the liver, muscles, and heart, it helps to maintain the immune system and is an important part of an antibody that fights bacterial infection. In combination with vitamin E, selenium has an anti-inflammatory effect and may fight various types of cancer. It is also a key ingredient in the antioxidant enzyme glutathione. Studies suggest that selenium and glutathione may play a key role in slowing the spread of HIV infection in the body.

Selenium is found in seafood, whole grains, meat, egg yolks, chicken, milk, and garlic. Supplementation at levels greater than 800 micrograms a day may be toxic.

Zinc One of the most important nutrients for a healthy immune system, zinc is a vital ingredient in a number of enzymes essential to the immune response. Zinc has been shown to increase the activity of natural killer cells and to boost the production of antibodies in response to infections. It can hasten the healing of wounds and may have some antiviral properties as well. Lozenges containing zinc as the active ingredient may be useful in shortening the duration of colds (see Chapter 6). Zinc plays a role in the hormones that ensure antibody production.

Zinc is found in meat, eggs, poultry, and seafood. Supplementation at levels greater than 80 milligrams daily may suppress immunity.

Amino Acids

Arginine An essential amino acid, arginine's greatest potential is in the area of heart health. Arginine boosts nitric oxide, which relaxes blood vessels, keeps arteries flexible, and stimulates the pituitary gland to release growth hormone (see the section on human growth hormone).

Glutamine The most abundant amino acid in muscles and blood, glutamine provides fuel for various cells of the immune system and is a critical component in wound repair. For the overstressed and for athletes who are overtrained—and thus immunosuppressed—glutamine helps prevent infection. The body can make glutamine but may not make enough when under stress.

Glutathione Glutathione, a powerful antioxidant, helps the liver detoxify effectively and is necessary for DNA (deoxyribonucleic acid) production and repair. Glutathione also helps recycle other antioxidants such as vitamins C and E. Glutathione replenishment may be important therapy for people with AIDS.

Fatty Acids

Omega-3 Fatty Acids Omega-3 fatty acids, found primarily in fish oils, seem to have a powerful effect on the immune system. Potent anti-inflammatory agents, omega-3s help curb an overactive immune system and thus are helpful in the treatment of autoimmune diseases such as rheumatoid arthritis, chronic inflammatory bowel disease, and psoriasis. Omega-3s are also effective in curbing the inflammatory response to severe burns, sepsis, systemic inflammatory response syndrome (SIRS), and asthma. Eat fish several times a week for naturally occurring omega-3s and the nutrients that accompany them. Use canola oil in cooking and salad dressings. Fish oil capsules should be taken only with guidance from a qualified nutritionist.

Hormones

Dehydroepiandrosterone (DHEA) DHEA has been dubbed the "mother of all hormones." It is the most abundant steroid in the human body and is involved in the manufacture of the hormones testosterone, estrogen, progesterone, and corticosterone. The decline of DHEA with age parallels that of human growth hormone, so by age 65, your body makes only 10 to 20% of what it did at age 20.

DHEA appears to be a potent immune system booster. Dr. Raymond Daynes, head of the division of cell biology and immunology at the University of Utah at Salt Lake City, found that it rejuvenated many measurements of immune function in mice, including the production of T cells and other immune factors, which decline with age. In mice with viral encephalitis, DHEA eased some symptoms, reduced the death rate, and postponed both the onsets of the disease and death. Older people do not respond as well to vaccines as younger people. But when Daynes gave old mice vaccines laced with DHEA, their ability to mount defenses against such diseases as hepatitis B, influenza, diphtheria, and tetanus equaled that of a young animal. The animals he placed on DHEA replacement therapy, according to Daynes, also looked "far, far healthier in their later months."

DHEA may also be beneficial in autoimmune disease, where the body's immune system attacks its own tissue as though it were a foreign invader. In a clinical trial of 57 women with the autoimmune disease systemic lupus erythematosus, researchers at Stanford University Hospital in California found that DHEA relieved symptoms such as skin rashes, joint pain, headaches, and fatigue. Many also reported a higher tolerance for exercise and better concentration.

Human Growth Hormone (HGH) HGH is secreted by the pituitary gland. HGH decreases with age at the rate of about 14% per decade after age 30. In addition to assisting in DNA repair and rejuvenating the immune system, HGH replacement decreases fat tissue and increases lean tissue, increases bone density, promotes heart health, and improves mood.

Injectable HGH is the only form of growth hormone replacement with scientific studies validating its efficacy. Nonprescription alternatives range from amino acid HGH boosters (combinations of arginine, lysine, glutamine, and ornithine) to oral sprays and homeopathic remedies that purport to contain HGH. Inspect independent studies (be skeptical if none are available) evaluating these products before purchasing them.

Melatonin Melatonin is produced in the dark during sleep. Levels wane near daybreak, as bright light signals the production cycle to shut down. It is secreted by the pineal gland, a small organ set behind and between the eyes that governs the sleep-wake cycle and, in animals, seasonal rhythms of migration, mating, and hibernation. In the human population, melatonin levels are highest in children.

Melatonin stimulates the thymus, a key organ of the immune system involved in the production of disease-fighting T cells (see Chapter 2). Melatonin boosts the immune system, lowers elevated cholesterol, and may be useful in preventing and treating cancer.

Thymic Protein A Thymic protein A is one of about 30 proteins produced by the thymus gland to program immature white blood cells produced in the bone marrow. Thymic protein A programs and refreshes T-4 helper cells so that they are able to carry out their function of regulating the immune system and keeping it in balance. Because the thymus gland shrinks with age, however, it becomes less efficient in preparing T-4 cells. Strengthening the immune system with thymic protein A is believed to lead to increased stamina, energy, and ability to ward off infections, from colds and flu to hepatitis and HIV.

Other Vital Agents

Alpha-Lipoic Acid Alpha-lipoic acid (or, simply lipoic acid) is a powerful antioxidant. Scientists believe that it plays a role in "turning off" genes that can cause cancer when exposed to carcinogens such as radiation and free radicals. It is also thought to work closely with vitamins C and E, recycling them to be more effective. The body uses lipoic acid to produce energy and makes only enough to fulfill this basic metabolic need. In Germany, lipoic acid is given by prescription to treat long-term complications of diabetes. Alpha-lipoic acid supplements may be taken daily at 20 to 50 milligrams per day.

Apple Cider Vinegar Vinegar supplements, available as 500 milligrams of dried vinegar in tablet form, are a natural source of acetic acid. Apple cider vinegar creates an internal pH environment that bugs can't stand. Its use in oral form is an extension of its well-documented efficacy as a vaginal douche against yeast infections. Proponents of apple cider vinegar suggest the following:

- The acetic acid and butyric acid contained in vinegar support gastrointestinal (GI) health by producing friendly bifido bacteria.
- Vinegar has both antiseptic and antibiotic properties, and can be helpful in treating sore throats, cuts, wounds, digestive problems, and gum infection.
- Vinegar may reverse hardening of the arteries by dissolving calcium deposits in arteries.
- Vinegar may break up gallstones and kidney stones by dissolving calcium deposits.
- Vinegar may destroy human herpesvirus-6 (HHV-6), both A and B strains, within a few weeks.

In the event that taking liquid apple cider vinegar is cumbersome or inconvenient, vinegar tablets, 500 milligrams each (equivalent to 1 tablespoon of liquid vinegar), are available from health food stores.

Carotenoids More than 600 carotenoids have been isolated in plants—so far. In addition to beta-carotene (see section on vitamin A), carotenoids include phytochemicals (plant chemicals) such as alpha- and gamma-carotene, lutein, zeaxanthin, and lycopene. Supplements do not contain all the carotenoids naturally occurring in a variety of fruits and vegetables. Try to eat at least five servings of fruits and vegetables daily.

Colostrum Within hours after giving birth, human and animal mothers secrete colostrum as a prelude to breast milk. It gives newborns a "vaccination" of antibodies, immune system protection, and growth factors. While two types are available, whole colostrum is preferred over defatted colostrum because fat is necessary to assist in transporting colostrum protein into the bloodstream. See also the sections on lactoferrin and transfer factors.

Enzymes Enzymes drive every chemical reaction in the body and there are thousands of them at work—more than 20 are involved in food digestion. Supplemental plant-based enzymes, which replace naturally occurring food enzymes destroyed during processing and cooking, increase the level of digestion in the upper GI tract so that less undigested food passes into the colon and more nutrients are available for absorption.

Lactobacillus Acidophilus As many as 30% of people taking an antibiotic will develop diarrhea because the drug creates an imbalance in natural intestinal flora (see Chapter 4). Of those, about a third will go on to develop colitis (inflammation of the colon). *Lactobacillus acidophilus* in two 8-ounce servings of yogurt per day can reduce the rate of antibiotic-induced diarrhea by half. *Lactobacillus acidophilus* also may prevent frequent occurrences of vaginal candidiasis (yeast infection; see Chapter 5).

Lactoferrin A protein found in breast milk, lactoferrin helps combat infection during the critical period when the infant's immune system is not yet fully functional. Lactoferrin is most abundant in colostrum ("first milk"). During inflammatory reactions, certain immune cells release lactoferrin into the blood and tissues as a defense against infection. Lactoferrin reduces swelling and facilitates circulation around injury sites. It also regulates iron in the digestive tract, thus helping to maintain the balance of helpful bacteria and harmful bacteria that need iron to grow. See also the section on colostrum.

Nicotinamide Adenine Dinucleotide (NADH) NADH, which occurs naturally in meat, is present in all cells and assists in metabolism and in breaking down food. It is effective in treating chronic fatigue syndrome, perhaps because it stimulates production of adenosine triphosphate (ATP), which gives the body energy. When metabolism is slowed by cutting calories, NADH is freed up and is able to support a protein that influences the lifespan of cells.

Polyphenols A plant chemical found in both green and black tea, polyphenols are strong antioxidants. Although most of the research on tea has been done in the laboratory and on animals, there is strong evidence that tea offers positive health benefits to humans. Herbal teas do not contain polyphenols in any significant amount.

Transfer Factors As small messenger molecules, transfer factors conduct immune recognition signals between immune cells. In doing so, they help "educate" young immune cells about present or potential danger. The most abundant source of transfer factors is colostrum, the "first milk" of humans and other animals such as cows. Transfer factors have been used to treat bacterial and viral infections, parasites, autoimmune disease, and fungal disease. See also the section on colostrum.

Whey Protein As a derivative of milk production, the amino acids in whey proteins are closely related to those required by the human body. Whey proteins also have proportionately more sulfur-containing amino acids and contain a relative surplus of a variety of essential amino acids. In particular, whey protein contains about 2.5% cysteine, a sulfur amino acid known to increase the cellular level of glutathione, a potent antioxidant.

The proteins in whey are widely recognized for their high biological value. A high biological value indicates a sufficient amount of protein absorbed and retained by the muscles in relation to the amount consumed. Inasmuch as protein is intimately involved in anabolism (protein synthesis and muscle growth), whey protein may be the best candidate for maximizing muscle growth. It also features one of the highest profiles of branched-chain amino acids (BCAA) compared to other protein sources. Those on diets high in BCAA demonstrate greater signs of muscle preservation when the body is in a catabolic state (breakdown of muscle tissue). Severe metabolic stresses such as sepsis, major operations, burns, strenuous exercise, and certainly fending off infection are associated with accelerated muscle catabolism.

Among various forms available (concentrate, peptides, hydrolysate, etc.), whey protein isolate is considered superior by many because of its purity, high glutathione content, and increased bioavailability.

Important: Whey may be contraindicated if you have milk allergies.

Herbal Remedies

Since the Dietary Supplement Health and Education Act of 1994 removed medicinal herbs from the strictly regulated drug category, herbal products have become commonplace in numerous retail outlets selling over-the-counter drugs or personal care products. Sales of nutritional herbs are estimated to be as high as $14 billion. More often than not, however, the marketing of herbal products is way ahead of the science. It becomes the consumer's own obligation to carefully assess claims, verify the sources, and determine who—slick marketers or scientists with feet on the ground—is touting the product and can substantiate it.

There are hundreds of herbs with thousands of indications for preventing and treating disease. Follow package directions on dosing.

Buyer Beware

Look for a USP designation on the label of herbal products. This designation indicates that the product meets five quality standards set for supplements by the United States Pharmacopeia: disintegration, dissolution, potency, purity, and expiration date. Don't be fooled by products that claim to be "laboratory tested" or "quality assured." These words mean very little without the USP approval.

The active constituents in herbs vary depending on the conditions in which the plant was grown, the plant's level of maturity when harvested, how the plant is dried, and how it is stored. In pharmaceuticals, standardizing—that is, conducting assays and then adjusting potency to a given standard—controls these variables. With the public becoming more interested in herbs and more discriminating in choosing products, standardization is becoming more prevalent in herbal preparations. Some manufacturers standardize their herbal products to contain a consistent level of certain marker compounds. A marker compound may be an herbal product's active ingredient.

Acemannan

See the section on aloe vera.

Active Hemicellulose Compound (AHCC)

This extract, which comes from the hybridization of several types of Japanese mushrooms (mainly shiitake) that are grown in rice bran, has been shown to be a powerful stimulator of the immune system's natural killer cells. The mushrooms are chopped up and "opened" with an enzyme that releases alpha-glucan. Clinical research supports AHCC's effectiveness in fighting various cancers, hepatitis, and diabetes.

Alkylglycerols (AKGs)

AKGs are fats that stimulate the immune system. They are found in human breast milk, cow's milk, and the livers of most animals and fish. Shark liver contains an exceptionally high level of AKGs. Alkylglycerols are considered critical to the development of a healthy immune system in children. They are vital to the production and stimulation of white and red blood cells. Animal studies suggest that AKGs may inhibit cancer growth and may help protect healthy tissue from the effects of radiation therapy.

Aloe Vera

The healing power of aloe vera is well known. Many people keep an aloe vera plant handy so that they can use the gel of its leaves to soothe and treat burns. Less well known is the fact that aloe's sap and leaf rind also contain a healing compound called acemannan as well as fatty acids, enzymes, pain-killing compounds, anti-inflammatories, and antiseptics. Traditionally, sap and leaf rind were not used in commercially available aloe vera products because they also included a

Top Anti-Infective, Anti-Inflammatory Herbs

HERB	ACTION/INDICATIONS
Aloe gel (mucilage)	Externally, helps heal minor wounds and burns; internally, acts as antibacterial and anti-inflammatory
Arnica	Reduces inflammation and pain of bruises, aches, and sprains
Bearberry (uva ursi leaves)	Acts as antibacterial and anti-inflammatory for urinary tract infection
Calendula (marigold)	Acts as anti-inflammatory and healing agent for skin and mucous membrane wounds
Chamomile (German)	Acts as anti-inflammatory and healing agent for skin and mucous membrane wounds; taken internally, as an anti-inflammatory in the GI tract and anti-infective for minor illness
Cranberry	Helps prevent infection by creating environment in which bacteria cannot cling to walls of urinary tract
Echinacea	Taken internally, acts as immune stimulant; inhibits symptoms of minor viral/bacterial infections; used externally to treat hard-to-heal superficial wounds
Garlic	Acts as immune stimulant; in large doses, may be used to treat bacterial, viral, fungal, yeast, and parasite infections
Goldenrod (European)	Increases urine volume by promoting blood flow in kidneys; used to treat inflammation of kidney and bladder
Licorice root	Helps relieve chronic inflammation of peptic ulcer and gastritis caused by *Helicobacter pylori* bacteria; may stimulate immune system to fight staphylococcus and streptococcus infections
Melissa (balm)	Used in treatment of cold sores resulting from infection with herpes simplex type 1 virus
Milk thistle fruit/ seed (silymarin)	Assists in treatment of chronic inflammatory liver disease
Peppermint	Antibacterial
Tea tree	Antimicrobial; useful in treating skin infections and toenail fungus/mold/yeast
Willow bark	Anti-inflammatory

laxative called aloin. Now, however, aloin can be removed from the mix, allowing all the beneficial components of the aloe plant to be used.

Arabinogalactan (AG)

AG is a phytochemical extracted from the timber of the larch tree. The immune-enhancing herb echinacea also contains AG, as do leeks, carrots, radishes, pears, wheat, red wine, and tomatoes. AG increases the activity of natural killer cells and other immune system components.

Astragalus

In traditional Chinese medicine, the astragalus root is used to promote wound healing and enhance the immune system by boosting the activity of white blood cells. Studies suggest that the herb, used nasally or orally, also might protect against the common cold and flu.

Bee Products

Honey Used as a skin treatment, honey prevents infection and speeds healing by starving existing bacteria and shielding against new bacteria.

Pollen Bee pollen is essentially the male seed of a flower blossom that has been collected by bees and to which bees add certain digestive enzymes. Analysis of bee pollen shows it typically contains a wealth of nutrients utilized by the human body, including the following:

VITAMINS	MINERALS	ENZYMES/ COENZYMES	PROTEINS/ AMINO ACIDS
Provitamin A	Calcium	Amylase	Isoleucine
B₁ Thiamine	Phosphorous	Diastase	Leucine

(continued)

(continued)

VITAMINS	MINERALS	ENZYMES/ COENZYMES	PROTEINS/ AMINO ACIDS
B_2 Riboflavin	Potassium	Saccharase	Lysine
B_3 Niacin	Sulfur	Pectase	Methionine
B_6 Pyridoxine	Sodium	Phosphotase	Phenylalanine
Pantothenic acid	Chlorine	Catalase	Threonine
Biotin	Magnesium	Disphorase	Tryptophan
B_{12} Cyanocobalamin	Iron	Cozymase	Valine
Folic acid	Choline	Manganese	Cytochrome systems
Inositol	Copper	Lactic dehydrogenase	Histidine
Vitamin C	Zinc	24-Oxidoreductase	Cystine
Vitamin E	Silicon	21-Transferase	Tyrosine
	Molybdenum	33-Hydrolase	Alanine
Vitamin K	Boron	11-Lyase	Aspartic acid
Rutin	Titanium	5-Isomerase	Glutamic acid
Pro-vitamin A	Pepsin	Hydroxyproline	Proline
		Trypsin	Serine

Propolis Consisting mostly of tree resins, propolis is used by honey bees to seal the cracks and openings in hives. Propolis is rich in anti-inflammatory, antioxidant flavonoids. It also contains terpenoids, which have antibacterial, antifungal, and antibiotic effects. For acute internal infections, propolis can be taken along with regularly prescribed medications. Propolis is an effective salve for wounds, especially in combination with honey, and in dry powder form may be sprinkled onto mouth sores as a therapeutic dressing.

Royal Jelly Secreted from glands on the bee's head, royal jelly is used to feed bee larvae for three days. The queen bee, however, eats royal jelly exclusively and it is believed to account for her fertility and her relatively long life (five to seven years vs. seven to eight weeks for worker bees). Royal jelly contains collagen and several vitamins and is thought to be an anti-inflammatory.

Beta 1,3/1,6 Glucan

Derived from baker's yeast and young rye plants, beta 1,3/1,6 glucan helps the immune system fight bacterial, viral, fungal, and parasitic pathogens by activating key immune cells known as macrophages. Taken before and after surgery, beta 1,3/1,6 glucan has been shown to help reduce infection. It also appears to enhance the activity of conventional antibiotic therapy.

Black Currant Seed Oil

According to a study published in February 2000 by researchers at Tufts University in Boston, 4.5 grams of black currant seed oil daily was able to promote cell-mediated immune function. It is rich in gamma-linoleic acid, which other studies have shown stimulates production of an anti-inflammatory hormone (prostaglandin-1).

Cranberry

Research indicates that regular consumption of cranberry juice reduces bacteria associated with urinary tract infection. Condensed tannins (proanthocyanidins) in cranberries prevent *Escherichia coli* from adhering to the walls of the kidneys, bladder, and urethra. When bacteria cannot adhere to tissue, they are washed out of the urinary tract during urination.

Echinacea

An herb native to North America, echinacea (purple cone flower) is an important component of Native American medicine, traditionally used as both an anti-inflammatory and an antiseptic, especially for skin problems. In recent years, echinacea has been studied for its antiviral, immune-boosting, and antibody-producing properties. Echinacea increases the production of white blood cells and helps them move into the circulatory system more quickly. Currently, one of the most popular uses for echinacea is to relieve the symptoms and shorten the duration of the common cold. Whether echinacea can prevent colds is a matter of some debate.

Echinacea products vary widely and often include other ingredients such as zinc and goldenseal. There are three different types of echinacea *(E. purpurea, E. pallida,* and *E. angustifolia),* and various formulations contain different parts of the plant (leaves, flowers, roots). Studies indicate that the best results occur in people who use a liquid or tincture form, rather than a pill or capsule.

Elderberry

Every part of the elder tree has a food or medicinal purpose. For centuries, the elderberry has been used to treat colds and flu. Scientists believe that antioxidant flavonoids found in the elderberry fight viral infection.

Garlic

Garlic, a member of the onion family, has been used medicinally for centuries. By 1500 B.C., the Egyptians had identified 22 different uses for garlic, ranging from treating headaches to general physical weakness. Garlic has been proven effective against a number of fungal infections, including yeast infections. Allicin, the antibacterial agent in garlic, accounts for the infection-fighting power of the herb. During World War II, garlic was used as an antimicrobial agent for soldiers' wounds.

Garlic is also considered to be a cholesterol- and triglyceride-lowering agent. It helps reduce hypertension and increases circulation. Garlic enhances the immune system and may help in preventing certain cancers, especially those of the colon and stomach. For infection fighting, consume three or four chopped, crushed, or chewed cloves per day, or, in supplement form (1.3% allicin), 600 to 900 milligrams divided into two to three doses daily.

Aged garlic extract is aged in alcohol for 20 months, which is thought to convert allicin and other unstable sulfur-based compounds in raw garlic into more stable and effective substances. Aged garlic extract is available in liquid, capsules, and tablets.

Ginseng

Ginseng helps to regulate blood pressure and maintain blood glucose levels; a traditional use is in the control of diabetes. Several studies have shown that ginseng supports the thymus and spleen, and therefore boosts the immune system. Ginseng also appears to have anti-cancer potential; a recent study found that a ginseng extract had potent antioxidant effects, acting as a scavenger of free radicals. Korean researchers recently found that people who regularly used ginseng had a dramatically reduced risk of developing cancer of the ovaries, pancreas, and stomach.

Goldenseal

An anti-inflammatory and antibiotic agent, goldenseal is effective against bacteria and fungi. It also appears to stimulate the activity of macrophages, the immune cells that attack harmful bacteria. Goldenseal can be made into a paste and applied directly to the skin to treat impetigo, ringworm, and other skin infections.

Important: Goldenseal may be contraindicated if you are allergic to ragweed.

Grapefruit Seed Extract (GSE)

Research has demonstrated that grapefruit seed extract can be effective in treating candidiasis, including *Candida albicans* vaginitis. Study subjects douched every 12 hours for three days using a weak solution of GSE (5 drops per 8 ounces of distilled water). Researchers also have had positive results using GSE as an antimicrobial on food and as a deep cleanser for skin. Added to toothpaste and mouthwash, GSE may protect against viral and bacterial infection in the mouth.

Inositol Hexaphosphate (IP6)

Found in the germ of the bran portion of whole grains (especially whole-kernel corn) and in legumes, IP6 is an antioxidant thought to prevent tumor development by controlling cell development, and it may assist in the treatment of existing cancer by helping natural killer cells to enter cancer cells. IP6 also may be beneficial in the treatment of kidney stones, cardiovascular disease, and liver disease. It should be taken under the direction of a qualified health professional.

Licorice

The herb's natural sweetness and flavor (it is 50 times sweeter than sugar) are due to its high content of glycyrrhizin. Glycyrrhizin is also responsible for most of licorice's medicinal properties, including its ability to reduce inflammation, soothe throat tissues, and reduce allergy symptoms.

The ulcer-healing compounds in licorice are thought to be flavonoids. They apparently work by promoting the overall health of the gastrointestinal system rather than reducing the secretion of stomach acid that triggers ulcers. Additional compounds with therapeutic effects include sterols and gums.

In people with high blood pressure, deglycyrrhizinated licorice

(DGL) products cause fewer side effects and are much safer for long-term use than glycyrrhizin-containing licorice.

MGN-3

Thought by some experts to be the most powerful immune system booster available, MGN-3 is produced by integrating an extract from the outer shell of rice bran with extracts from three different types of mushrooms: shiitake, kawaratake, and suehirotake. In Japan, extracts of these mushrooms are leading prescription treatments for cancer. MGN-3 boosts the activity of natural killer cells, T cells, and B cells. Cancer patients have used MGN-3 both as a treatment and to lessen the toxicity of conventional therapies and improve their effectiveness. MGN-3 also has been used successfully, though to a lesser extent, with AIDS patients and patients with hepatitis B and C.

Milk Thistle

See the section on silymarin.

Mushrooms

There are more than 100,000 varieties of mushrooms, some 700 of which are edible. In laboratory tests (mostly in Japan and China), about 50 species have been confirmed to have some medicinal properties. Mushrooms are available in various forms, including whole, dried, powdered, tinctures, capsules, tablets, and tea. Most edible mushrooms are rich in vitamins, minerals, fiber, and amino acids.

Maitake Known in Japan as the "dancing mushroom," the maitake (*Grifola frondosa*) mushroom is called the "hen of the woods" by American mushroom hunters. D fraction, an extract from maitake mushrooms, is marketed in the United States and Japan as a dietary supplement. It has been shown to stimulate the production and effectiveness of immune cells. It protects healthy cells from cancer, helps prevent the spread of cancer (metastasis), and slows tumor growth.

Unlike other mushroom extracts, D fraction is effective not only by injection but orally as well. Two other fractions, X and ES, have been used to lessen the side effects of chemotherapy.

As an HIV/AIDS treatment, maitake may help prevent the destruction of T cells. In animal studies, maitake have lowered blood pressure and glucose levels. Maitake mushrooms, fresh or preserved, taste good and can be used in a variety of food preparations. Maitake tea, juice, powder, and granules are available. A liquid extract of maitake D fraction is available to health professionals.

Reishi Long used in Chinese medicine, reishi mushrooms have been shown to lower blood pressure, cholesterol, and triglycerides. Researchers are exploring the potential impact of reishi on cancer.

Shiitake The shiitake *(Lentinus edodes)* mushroom has been revered in Asia for centuries, both as a food and as a medicine. Its most studied active ingredient is lentinan. Shiitake can be used for all diseases involving immune system depression, including allergies, yeast infections, AIDS, and cancer. Using the whole mushroom, rather than isolated components, takes advantage of shiitake's many benefits.

Olive Leaf Extract

A staple of folk medicine for centuries, olive leaves have been steeped for tea or chopped up as a salad ingredient. Olive leaf extract is recognized for its ability to fight viral and bacterial infections. The plant chemical oleuropein interferes with the production of amino acids essential to bacteria and viruses. Studies have indicated that olive leaf extract kills antibiotic-resistant *Staphylococcus aureus,* and may be useful in fighting HIV and AIDS. Oleuropein is also considered a strong antioxidant.

Rye Extract

Rich in vitamins, minerals, enzymes, and phytochemicals such as lignans, isoflavones, and beta-1,3-glucan, rye extract is available in drops, creams, gels, and sprays to treat colds and flu, rashes, wounds, burns, fatigue, teeth and gums, and cold sores.

Saponins

Saponins are plant chemicals found in soybeans, chickpeas, asparagus, tomatoes, potatoes, and oats. In nature, saponins appear to act as antibiotics that protect plants from microbes. In humans, saponins might fight cancer and infection.

Shark Liver Oil

See the section on alkylglycerols.

Silymarin

An extract of milk thistle, silymarin is composed of phytochemicals called flavonoids. It prevents liver damage by acting as an antioxidant. Silymarin enhances the detoxification action of the liver by increasing the level of glutathione. The higher the liver's glutathione level, the greater the liver's capacity to detoxify the body. Silymarin can protect against chemical poisoning from alcoholism and workplace chemicals. It can be used to treat acne and psoriasis, and helps protect the lining of the gastrointestinal tract (gastric mucosa), which prevents pathogens from entering the bloodstream. Silymarin combined with phosphatidylcholine (a component of lecithin) appears to be absorbed better by the body.

St. John's Wort

In June 2000, German researchers announced results of a study demonstrating the value of St. John's wort—an herb widely taken to combat depression—in fighting bacteria. Researchers from the University of Freilburg found that low concentrations of hyperforin, the active ingredient in St. John's wort, inhibited the growth of several types of bacteria, including *Staphylococcus aureus* and *Corynebacterium diphtheria*. Particularly noteworthy is the ability of hyperforin to inhibit bacteria (meticillin-resistant *S. aureus*) that are resistant to penicillin and other antibiotics.

Tea Tree Oil

A 0.5% solution of tea tree oil has been shown to kill 60 strains of antibiotic-resistant *Staphylococcus aureus*. For more about tea tree oil, see the section on essential oils at the end of this chapter.

Important Considerations with Use of Herbal Products

People who might be especially vulnerable to adverse side effects from herbal products include pregnant women and their fetuses, lactating women, infants, the elderly, and people taking prescription medications.

The American Society of Anesthesiologists recommends that patients planning surgery stop taking herbal preparations at least two to three weeks prior to surgery to avoid adverse reactions to anesthesia. The following common herbs can interact dangerously with anesthesia:

- St. John's wort may intensify the effect of anesthesia and narcotics.
- Ginkgo biloba can interfere with blood clotting.
- Ginseng has been associated with hypertension and tachycardia.

When Herbal Remedies and Drugs Don't Mix

Herbal products are not classified as medications by the Food and Drug Administration, so information regarding their potential interaction with drugs is limited and based largely on anecdotal reports or assumptions based on known mechanisms of action—that is, if we know how the herb works in the body, we can make some assumptions about how it might interfere with a certain drug.

Check with your pharmacist for drug-herb interactions before adding either a drug or an herb to your regimen.

Uva Ursi

A small evergreen shrub found in the northern United States and Europe, uva ursi's most active component is arbutin, found in its leaves and at one time marketed as a urinary antiseptic and diuretic. Historically, uva ursi has been used to treat bladder and kidney infections, kidney stones, and bronchitis. When given alone, arbutin is broken down by intestinal bacteria almost completely before it can have any effect. Other components in the uva ursi plant, however, prevent this degradation.

 Ileocecal Bowel Massage

Ileocecal bowel massage seeks to help open the ileocecal valve (ICV) located between the small and large intestines. When this valve is not functioning properly, waste material accumulates in the small intestine, where it becomes toxic. ICV massage consists of the following steps:

1. Place a hot water bottle or warm compress on the abdomen for 10 minutes.
2. Rub the abdomen, slowly and deeply massaging in a circular motion. Begin in the lower right quadrant, pressing deeply, kneading the abdominal contents in a firm but not

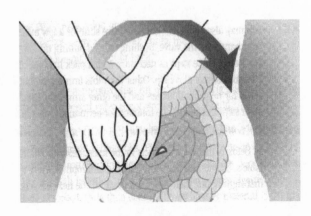

Source: Reprinted from
R. Klatz and R. Goldman,
7 Anti-Aging Secrets,
ESM Publishers, 1996.

uncomfortably vigorous manner. Continue for two to five minutes.

3. Done correctly and completely, you should feel a gurgling sensation that confirms you've opened the ICV valve and toxins are flowing out of your GI system as normal. ICV massage can also alleviate most pain associated with trapped gas in the intestine and colon.

    Detoxification

Detoxification is a natural process by which the body rids itself of an accumulation of internal and external toxins—such as free radicals, metabolic waste, industrial chemicals, pesticides, food additives, heavy metals, drug residues, and various other pollutants—that interfere with the body's ability to absorb nutrients and protect itself from infection.

Today, we are exposed to many pollutants, including petrochemical residues that the kidneys cannot flush out, contaminants in the food chain, and everyday products such as cosmetics and dry-cleaning agents—just to name a few. We also have changed the nature of our food supply, adding preservatives and other chemicals that interfere with optimal nutrition. In addition, we have ever-increasing levels of stress that challenge our well-being.

As a result, we can no longer rely on the body's natural abilities to detoxify itself. We are far more vulnerable to what experts call toxic bioaccumulation, as well as the damaged detox system, suppressed immunity, infection, mental sluggishness, and fatigue that accompany it.

Many nutrition experts recommend detoxifying twice a year—for example, once or twice during spring and fall. Weekend detoxification plans are also available. Here are some general guidelines on detox therapy:

• Keep warm during detoxification. Cold is a stressor to the body. A sauna or steam bath can drive toxins from the body via perspiration.

- Get plenty of rest. Your body needs all its energy for eliminating accumulated toxins.
- Eat wholesome, unprocessed foods to give your liver a rest from processing pesticides and food additives.
- Take your time when eating. Choose a comfortable position, chew food well, and relax for a few minutes before and after a meal.
- Drink lots of clear, pure, natural water to flush the intestines, liver, and kidneys—at least eight glasses each day. Make two of those glasses hot water with the juice of a half lemon added. Twelve glasses of distilled sterile water (see Chapter 13) or water from fruit and vegetable juices is even better.

Some Tips on How to Detox

Water and juice fasts used to be the favored methods for detoxification. Proponents maintained that with the stress of digestion removed, the body is better able to rid itself of accumulated toxins. Fasting for more than two or three days, however, should be done only under the care of a knowledgeable health care practitioner, especially if you have preexisting liver, kidney, metabolic, or cardiovascular disease. Although short fasts can be tremendously helpful and cleansing, longer fasts (more than four days) can weaken muscles and organs and cause metabolism to slow down. In addition, fasting drains the body of glutathione, an antioxidant critical to detoxification, and the toxins released by fasting can overwhelm the liver's cleansing ability.

Current thinking acknowledges that detoxification is dependent upon good nutrition. By nourishing the body with lean protein, high-fiber complex carbohydrates, and essential fats, the intestinal tract, liver, and kidneys get the support they need to do their jobs.

Important: People who have heart disease, cancer, diabetes, hypothyroidism, eating disorders, or extreme fatigue, are underweight or recovering from surgery, or women who are pregnant or lactating, should avoid aggressive fasting detoxification programs.

- Avoid beverages that have been processed—for example, soft drinks, alcohol, tea, and, especially, coffee.
- Take a multivitamin and mineral supplement as well as an acidophilus supplement daily.
- Take a supplement especially designed for liver support. Supplements may include the antioxidant glutathione or certain liver-protecting herbs such as dandelion root or milk thistle (see the section on immune boosters at the end of this chapter).
- Exercise moderately to encourage the detox process. Stretching exercises, yoga, and brisk walking several times daily are particularly helpful to encourage lymph circulation.
- Use a loofa or dry brush to remove dead skin cells, thus helping toxins to escape. Dry brushing also stimulates the lymphatic system.
- Try lymphatic massage or trampoline jumping (rebounding) to boost lymphatic circulation.
- Consider aromatherapy, breathing, relaxing, and meditation to assist the detox process.
- Remember that excessive detoxification—that is, going to extremes with fasting, laxatives, enemas, colonics, diuretics, and exercise—can be just as harmful as no detox at all.

   Colonic Irrigation

In the 1920s and 1930s, colonic therapies were common in the United States. Ever since Princess Diana let it be known that she underwent colonic irrigation on a regular basis, the procedure has had a resurgence in popularity as a way to do the following:

- Release toxins
- Restore the normal balance of intestinal microorganisms
- Stimulate the immune system

- Aid in tightening leaky gut syndrome
- Restore pH balance in the colon
- Restore intestinal muscle tone
- Remove intestinal parasites without use of heavy drugs
- Adjunctive for weight loss

Some proponents of colonic therapy maintain that the cleansing process is helpful to organs near the colon (such as the uterus, ovaries, prostate, bladder, and spine) because it relieves pressure caused by a distorted colon.

Consider Colonics Carefully

Colonic irrigation is controversial. It can be addictive in that it creates a dependence of your system on the procedure, since it can destroy the natural balance of bacteria in your colon. If not performed properly, it can be dangerous. The procedure cleans 5 feet of colon, whereas a household enema cleans only the lower 8 to 12 inches. In a typical irrigation procedure, the therapist guides an applicator into the anus. Filtered water and various herbal remedies are gradually introduced into the colon and then released, taking fecal material and toxins away with them. A session usually lasts about 30 to 60 minutes, but one session may not be enough to restore balance.

When choosing a colonic irrigation therapist, be sure that he or she is properly trained and that the facility and equipment are clean. Disposable applicators and tubing should be used. Be sure to ask potential therapists to explain how their machines are kept sterile and how and when they are tested for sterility. Ideally, you will be treated using a totally disposable set of tubing, applicators, and equipment plugged into a disposable water unit, eliminating the potential for cross-contamination from a previous client to you.

Certain people should avoid colonic irrigation, including those suffering from ulcerative colitis, diverticulitis, Crohn's disease, severe hemorrhoids, and tumors of the large intestine or rectum.

Intestinal Cleansing

Intestinal cleansing is generally considered a safer type of colonic therapy. Its proponents suggest that the colon be cleansed twice a year. The process, which may take 4 to 12 weeks, begins with an adjustment to the diet that includes limiting consumption of refined flour products, cheese, and meats. Some practitioners also suggest that their patients drink as much as 2 quarts of lemon water or plain water daily separate from meals for up to a week.

Upon completing these preparations, the patient is given a series of supplements that include components such as fiber, various herbs, acidophilus, chlorophyll or the juice of green leafy vegetables, aloe vera juice, and an abundance of water. The precise components used depend on the practitioner. Some practitioners also recommend a weekly, biweekly, or daily enema to be given after a natural bowel movement. (When used as part of a short-term cleansing program, enemas probably are not harmful; however, they should not be used over a long period of time. Enemas can become psychologically addictive and can create physical dependence.)

Toxin Elimination Bath

Bathe away the bad stuff by treating yourself to a bath containing Epsom salts, which contain magnesium—that's deficient in many of us—and baking soda, which is a pH-balancing agent. Follow these directions:

1. Run a bath as hot as you can tolerate.
2. Pour in a 1-pound bag of Epsom salts and a 1-pound box of bicarbonate of soda.
3. Use a natural loofa to open up your pores by gently scrubbing the solution all over your body.

Proper Breathing

Breathing is a science. We breathe 20,000 times a day, and it's vital that every breath we take be done properly. Nostril breathing is far superior to mouth breathing, which should be avoided. Nostrils filter and purify the air before it enters our respiratory system. Try this technique:

1. Sit upright in a chair, feet on the floor, knees together, spine straight, shoulders aligned.
2. Relax both mentally and physically.
3. Slowly inhale through your nose and fill your belly with air. Place one hand on the abdomen and one on the chest and check that you're not moving your chest, only your abdomen.
4. Pause when the inhalation is completed. Inhale a little more air, and hold in the breath for 20 seconds.
5. Slowly exhale through your mouth. Squeeze as much air out as you can.
6. Relax the body again.
7. Repeat for a total of 10 breaths.
8. Sit in the chair quietly for 10 minutes.
9. Repeat this process four to six times a day.

    Chest Percussion

Chest percussion is a Western adaptation of the hitting method of the Tao system of traditional Chinese medicine. Vibrations that are created and deliberate can effectively break up thick secretions commonly associated with respiratory infections. With a firm but gentle strike of the palm side of a cupped hand, move along the center of the upper rib cage downward to the bottom of the rib cage, tapping 10 to 12 times every 4 or so inches apart. The cupping delivers a maximal vibration that penetrates the chest cavity, bronchial tree, and the depths of the lungs, loosening thick mucus secretions. The action of the cilia (tiny hairs that direct the flow of air and sputum) will clear the loosened mucus and restore a fuller breathing capacity.

Similar rapid but low-intensity cupping over the sternum is useful in stimulating the thymus (see Chapter 2), an important organ of immunity.

Important: Do not use chest percussion if you are experiencing chest pain, have fractured ribs, are experiencing an irregular pulse, or have a tendency to bleed (or are taking blood thinners).

 Acupuncture

Acupuncture is one of many types of treatment modalities of traditional Chinese medicine. Though the underlying mechanism is not understood, acupuncture works by stimulating points on the surface of the body that affect bodily processes or, in some cases, specific systems. Most often the treatment is used to enhance the effectiveness of Western medical therapies for a variety of chronic conditions. Pain management is one of its most popular uses. Acupuncture can assist in treatment of diseases such as chronic hepatitis not simply by reducing symptoms but by boosting the immune system to fight the infection. Research suggests that acupuncture works by increasing the level of interferon, a key immune system messenger hormone.

 Colloidal Silver

Often called the penicillin of alternative medicine, colloidal silver (CS) disables the enzymes that bacteria, parasites, viruses, and fungi rely on to use oxygen. Unable to breathe, the organisms die and are eliminated from the body. CS delivers the kiss of death to at least 650 disease organisms. In addition, microorganisms cannot develop a resistance to it.

CS may sound like something very high-tech, but in fact it has been used for several thousand years. In ancient Greece and Rome, people stored water and wine in silver urns to retard the growth of bacteria. During the bubonic plague in Europe, children of wealthy families sucked on silver spoons to preserve their health—thus the phrase "born with a silver spoon in your mouth." American pioneer families put silver dollars in fresh milk to keep it from spoiling.

Silver-based products were the most commonly used antimicrobials until the late 1930s, when convenient, inexpensive antibiotic drugs were introduced and silver-based products all but disappeared. Two holdovers are the silver nitrate eyedrops given to newborns to prevent infection and the silver-based ointments used to treat severe burns.

Lately, silver's antimicrobial properties have been rediscovered. Clinical research has uncovered no adverse effects from properly prepared colloidal silver, nor have there been any reported cases of CS-drug interaction. Among the conditions CS has controlled are severe burns, acne, boils, candida and yeast infections, chronic fatigue syndrome, digestive problems and colitis, ear and sinus infections, herpes, shingles, lupus, malaria, viral and fungal infections, blood parasites, rheumatoid arthritis, and ringworm. CS also has been effective in treating cancer and AIDS if used at a certain point in the disease

Tips on Using Colloidal Silver

- The recommended dosage of CS depends upon the concentration of the product you are using, which is expressed as parts per million (ppm). Concentrations range from 5 ppm to 500 ppm. In general, the greater the ppm, the larger the CS particle size. This variable is important because it takes a smaller particle size to kill a virus than a bacterium. Some companies have developed technology that allows increased ppm while preserving a smaller particle size.
- CS can be taken internally in a small amount of distilled drinking water. It also can be applied topically to cuts and open sores and can be inhaled or sprayed using an atomizer.

FDA Position Statement on CS

In February 1997, the U.S. FDA issued the following statement: "The use of colloidal silver–containing products constitutes a potentially serious public health concern. . . . The consumption of silver by humans may result in argyria— a permanent ashen-gray or blue discoloration of the skin, conjunctiva [eye], and internal organs. . . . Colloidal silver–containing products have never been approved by the FDA for treatment of animal disease in any animal species."

cycle when infected cells have reverted to a more primitive way of using oxygen.

Important: Do not use CS for prolonged periods of time (more than seven consecutive days).

   Homeopathy

Based on the principle that "like cures like," the word *homeopathy* is a combination of Greek words meaning "similar disease." Samuel Hahnemann, a German physician practicing in the late 1700s, developed a theory based on the three principles that subsequently formed the foundation of the homeopathic tradition: (1) the law of similars; (2) the minimum dose; and (3) the single remedy. It is an approach that treats disease by administering minute, highly diluted quantities of an agent (typically on the order of 10^{-6} to 10^{-10} and beyond), on the premise that such dosing will evoke the same symptoms in the ill person (to build tolerance) as the disease when given to a healthy individual.

Some homeopathic remedies are so dilute that no molecules of the proposed healing substance remain. Homeopathic practitioners believe that the substance has left its "imprint," a spirit-like essence, on the solution, to enable stimulation of the body.

The FDA regulates homeopathic remedies and allows the approach great latitude as follows:

- Manufacturers of homeopathic remedies are deferred from submitting new drug applications to the FDA.
- Homeopathic remedies are exempt from good manufacturing practice requirements relating to expiration dating and testing of finished product for identity and strength.
- Homeopathic products are permitted to contain more than 10% alcohol (the limit on conventional drugs), by FDA exemption.

Over the past several years, the FDA has issued 12 warning letters to homeopathic marketers. The primary violation cited was the marketing of prescription homeopathic drugs (claiming to treat a serious disease and not administered for self-limiting, minor health problems). Additional infractions included violations of minimum safety standards on packaging, the overgeneralization of a health claim, and the incorrect marketing of vitamins and phytonutrients as homeopathic remedies.

The American Medical Association, the American Academy of Pediatrics, and the research journals *The Lancet* and the *British Medical Journal* have not given their nod of acceptance to homeopathy. It is strongly recommended that those seeking a homeopathic practitioner check on the status of their practitioner's state licensing.

   Hyperthermia

Aspirin is most often prescribed to lower a fever associated with infection or inflammation. Some medical experts believe, however, that the body's fever mechanism has evolved over millions of years as an adaptive response to infection and as such is one of the body's most powerful defenses against disease.

In fact, the use of heat for healing—where a body temperature above 98.6°F is deliberately induced, a process known as hyperthermia—is clearly documented in human history. Over 5,000 years ago, Egyptians immersed people in hot oil, and the use of hot springs was

Err on the Safe Side

Do not be tempted to "starve" a fever. For every 1° rise in body temperature, there is an estimated 7% increase in the rate at which your body burns calories (metabolism) just to carry out basic functions such as breathing and pumping blood.

Adults should see a doctor right away if any of the following applies:

+ Fever is 103°F or higher.
+ Fever is prolonged.
+ Fever is accompanied by recurrent shaking or chills.
+ There are no apparent symptoms except a temperature exceeding 101°F that lasts for more than three days.
+ There are no apparent symptoms except a low-grade fever lasting several weeks.
+ There has been known exposure to an infectious disease.
+ Fever is accompanied by severe headache, stiff neck, swelling of throat, or confusion/disorientation.

first documented in the Book of Genesis in the Bible. Hyperthermia is gaining in popularity today as a therapeutic approach. In the hyperthermia procedure, the body is exposed to temperatures up to 106°F. When heat is applied, the blood vessels in normal tissues open up (dilate), dissipating the heat and cooling the cell environment.

When heat is applied to a tumor, however, vital nutrients and oxygen are cut off, causing the tumor's vascular system to collapse. Elevated temperature appears to shrink tumors and has been shown to speed the secretion of antibacterial chemicals, enhance the activity of interferon (the body's first-line defense against viruses), and boost T-cell proliferation. Hyperthermia also can help release toxins from fat cells, which makes it a useful detoxification method.

Hyperthermia has been shown to lower disease and death rates in animals with bacterial and viral infections. Consequently, researchers are taking a close look at hyperthermia as a treatment for HIV/AIDS.

Hot Do-It-Yourself Alternatives

Hot-water bottles and baths, saunas, and steam baths are less complicated forms of hyperthermia treatment that you can prescribe for yourself for acute and chronic viral infections and chronic fatigue syndrome—as long as you do not abuse them. In addition, when your body temperature is slightly elevated due to an infection, consider skipping the aspirin, acetaminophen, ibuprofen, and any other fever-lowering medications, thus giving your body an opportunity to use the fever for its natural purpose—to kill or reduce the numbers of invading viruses and bacteria and to sweat pathogens out of the body. If your temperature exceeds 103°F, however, call for immediate medical attention.

The therapy is not without controversy. Some researchers have successfully treated infection by raising the body temperature of patients as high as 106°F (with 100% humidity) for 10 hours; in other studies, however, some patients have experienced severe side effects and even death.

There are three basic types of hyperthermia. Heating just a small portion of the body is called local hyperthermia and is sometimes used to treat upper respiratory infections or wounds. Regional hyperthermia refers to heating a larger area such as an arm or a leg. Whole-body hyperthermia is used as a cancer treatment. The heat selectively kills heat-sensitive malignancies.

High-tech hyperthermia therapies involving application of electromagnetic energy, high-energy sound waves, infrared heat, or removing blood, heating it, and returning it to the body must be done under the direction of an experienced health-care practitioner.

People who have anemia, heart disease, diabetes, seizure disorders, or tuberculosis should be extremely careful when using hyperthermia therapy, as should pregnant women. The very old and the very young, who may have trouble regulating body temperature, should avoid hyperthermia unless under a physician's close supervision.

Lymphatic Pump

The immunologic response to infection or vaccine is generated in the lymph nodes. Lymphatic fluid from tissue or from an injection site is channeled by the lymphatic vessels to the lymph nodes where T cells and B cells are activated. The lymphatic pump is a manipulative technique developed by osteopathic physicians and performed by D.O.'s and health professionals. The objective is to facilitate the movement of lymphatic fluid through the body's natural filtration system. It has proven to be remarkably effective at stimulating immunity and helping to reduce the discomfort of any condition in which thick mucus buildup hinders clear breathing.

 ## Therapeutic Massage

Research suggests that medical massage can strengthen the immune system, relieve pain, reduce damaging stress hormones, and alleviate symptoms of depression and anxiety. Massage also has been linked to reducing inflammation, helping people with asthma breathe easier, alleviating chronic fatigue and migraines, and easing the symptoms of irritable bowel syndrome. Scientists speculate that massage accomplishes all of this by improving circulation, boosting the flow of lymph, flushing out lactic acid, and stimulating the release of endorphins.

 ## Oxygen Therapy

Oxygen therapy refers to a range of treatments that can be categorized into two basic groups: *oxygenation,* or oxygen to the blood, and *oxidation,* a chemical process in which an electrically charged particle (electron) is split off from a molecule (which may or may not be an oxygen molecule).

Oxygenation

Among the essentials needed to support life, oxygen is probably the one we think about least. Unfortunately, the air isn't as pure as it once

Potential Uses of Oxygen Therapy

* Jump-starting the body's antioxidant defenses and ability to fight free radicals
* Boosting metabolism and counteracting the hypoxia (low oxygen level) that leads to sluggish cell activity and oxidative stress
* Improving the efficiency of hemoglobin in transporting oxygen around the body
* Improving blood flow by helping to keep cell membranes flexible
* Detoxifying and fighting infection by destroying bacteria, viruses, parasites, and fungi that thrive in low-oxygen environments and don't have the antioxidant resources to fight back

Benefits specific to hyperbaric oxygen are as follows:

* Reversing carbon monoxide poisoning by displacing the lethal gas with oxygen
* Stimulating the regrowth of damaged tissues in burns, crush injuries, and radiation

Some speculative benefits of hyperbaric oxygen include the following:

* Killing cancer cells and reducing toxic symptoms associated with chemotherapy
* Relieving fatigue and numbness associated with AIDS
* Increasing resistance to opportunistic infections in people with AIDS
* Treating tissue damaged by stroke
* Relieving the symptoms of multiple sclerosis
* Detoxifying from drug addiction and alcoholism

was and our bodies may not be as efficient at using it as they once were.

When the body's cells become low in oxygen, a snowball effect occurs. Cellular processes become less efficient, causing even lower oxygen levels and creating the ideal home for bacteria, viruses, parasites, and fungi that thrive in low-oxygen environments. Robbed of oxygen and further weakened by invaders, cells cannot produce a critical substance known as adenosine triphosphate (ATP). Without ATP, the door is wide open to fatigue, disease, immune imbalance, and a host of other conditions associated with aging. The only way to break this cycle is to give the body more oxygen over an extended period of time. The secret is knowing how much and for how long.

Oxygen can be administered in a number of ways—orally, rectally, vaginally, by vein, by artery, through inhalation, or via skin absorption. Hyperbaric oxygen therapy (100% oxygen delivered under high pressure) is familiar to most people as a treatment for deep-sea divers who, having surfaced too quickly, suffer from decompression sickness (the bends). It also can be used to treat a number of conditions that benefit from an oxygen-rich environment.

Oxidation

More often than not, we try to counteract the damage oxidation can cause by using *antioxidants*. But oxidation isn't always a bad thing. In fact, the body functions best in a state of oxidative balance. When infection or environmental stress challenges this balance, the body may need an oxidation wake-up call. Because of the potential for damage, however, oxidative therapies are controversial and must be administered by a qualified professional. Oxidative therapies include hydrogen peroxide, ultraviolet blood irradiation, and ozone.

Hydrogen Peroxide Hydrogen peroxide is known to most people as a topical antiseptic or as an ingredient in mouthwash and toothpaste. It is composed of two hydrogen atoms and two oxygen atoms (H_2O_2). Proponents of H_2O_2 therapy believe it can be used in baths, nasal sprays, douches, colonics, and enemas. Binyamin Rothstein, D.O., a

Baltimore-based osteopathic physician in private practice, gives his patients a very dilute concentration of hydrogen peroxide intravenously over a 1½- to 3-hour period. "This therapy must be done carefully because it introduces very potent free radicals into the body," Rothstein explains. "Done the right way, it stimulates powerful antioxidant reactions. Hydrogen peroxide therapy is especially helpful in treating chronic and acute bronchitis, emphysema, sinusitis, and chronic fatigue syndrome."

Rothstein says the number of treatments needed varies with each patient. Generally, he prescribes 10 treatments over three weeks, then phases out treatments slowly. "One of the remarkable effects of this therapy," Rothstein notes, "is its potential effect on stroke. Hydrogen peroxide seems to wake up the dormant tissue surrounding tissue killed by stroke. This therapy has positive effects whether it's applied 10 days or 10 years after a stroke occurs."

Other conditions that may be improved with peroxide therapy include cancer, heart disease, shingles, chronic obstructive pulmonary disease, candidiasis, and influenza.

Ultraviolet Blood Irradiation (UVI) Blood irradiation may sound high-tech, but it has been around since the 1930s, when it was administered to thousands as a reliable and effective method to treat polio and sepsis. Lately, it has been making a comeback. The therapy involves placing a small amount of blood in a UVI machine, where a special wavelength of ultraviolet light kills viruses and bacteria. The treated blood is then reintroduced into the body. Ultraviolet blood irradiation introduces ultraviolet energy into the bloodstream, which is thought to produce small amounts of ozone from the oxygen circulating in the blood.

"Some experts believe this therapy works like a vaccine," Rothstein explains. "Others believe it stimulates the immune system or transfers UV energy into the body. I believe it's a combination of vaccine-like action and immune system stimulation."

Rothstein recommends UVI therapy for all types of hepatitis (especially hepatitis C), chronic fatigue syndrome, and any kind of acute infection. Three treatments are usually enough, but each person will have his or her unique needs. "For a bad cold, I'll use peroxide therapy," he says. "UVI is too heavy-duty. Some practitioners use both therapies together. I don't," he continues. "Sometimes I do add a vitamin C and glutathione by intravenous drip therapy."

Proponents of UVI therapy claim it can do the following:

- Destroy/inhibit the growth of bacteria
- Enhance the immune system's ability to fight infection
- Increase oxygenation of the blood
- Increase cell permeability
- Successfully treat conditions such as viral infection, pneumonia, wound infections, septicemia, inflammatory processes (pancreatitis, bursitis, etc.), autoimmune diseases, immune deficiencies, and peripheral vascular disease

Ozone Ozone therapy combines oxygenation and oxidation. Ozone (O_3) contains three oxygen atoms and is less stable than oxygen, which contains only two. When ozone enters the body, one of the atoms breaks away, creating an oxygen molecule (oxygenation). The extra oxygen atom then becomes an oxidizing agent (oxidation). Medical-grade ozone is made from pure oxygen. It is usually administered by drawing blood (about 1 pint), mixing it with ozone, and reinfusing it. Ozone therapy is widely used in Europe but is not yet sanctioned by the Food and Drug Administration for use in the United States.

Because of the pressure inherent in treatment, people with a history of middle ear infection, emphysema, or spontaneous pneumonia should avoid hyperbaric oxygen therapy.

    Essential Oils

In this section, Anne Vermilye, M.S., C.H.T., C.M.T., who has been in private practice since 1991 and holds a master's degree in phar-

*macology, shares her expertise on the scientific and therapeutic uti-
lization of medicinal essential oils. Ms. Vermilye practices in Mill
Valley, California.*

When administered properly, in many cases essential oils can be an
effective alternative to antibiotic drugs. Essential oils are some of the
most powerful antibacterial agents known. Essential oil therapy has
been part of the mainstream European health care system for 120
years.

Medicinally applied pure essential oils are extremely beneficial
in every area of health and complement all health care treatments.
It is important to use pure, unadulterated essential oils that have
not been stored in clear glass or near light or heat. Essential oil
therapy has some contraindications and must be administered
responsibly, but essential oils have no toxic side effects and are generally broad-spectrum—that is, they benefit multiple areas of the
body at once.

Therapeutic Oils

OIL	POTENTIAL THERAPEUTIC EFFECT
Bay laurel *Pimenta racemosa* and *Laurus nobilis*	• Stimulating to the circulation of lymphatic fluids and dermal tissues • Alleviates pain of swollen lymph nodes when they are fighting germs • Strengthens immune system
Chamomile, German *Matricaria chamomilla*	• Acts as an anti-inflammatory and antiulcerative, and neutralizes toxic bacterial metabolic wastes
Chamomile, Roman *Anthemis nobilis* and *Chamaemelum nobile*	• Strengthens and cleanses liver and spleen • Stimulates production of white blood cells • Has antibiotic and antiseptic properties

(continued)

(continued)

OIL	POTENTIAL THERAPEUTIC EFFECT
Clove bud *Syzygium* *aromaticum*	• Strong antiseptic, antiviral, antifungal, and analgesic • Stimulating to circulatory and nervous systems
Elemi *Canarium* *iuzonicum*	• Stimulates thymus gland
Eucalyptus *Eucalyptus* *radiata*	• Acts as an antiviral and antiseptic
Ginger *Officinale*	• Stimulates immune system • Internally, beneficial for intestinal ailments
Helichrysum *Helichrysum* *italicum* (also known as everlast and immortelle)	• Acts as a powerful anti-inflammatory and antioxidant • Promotes new cell growth • Stimulates liver and regulates cholesterol
Lavender *Lavandula vera*	• Acts as an anti-inflammatory • Most broad-spectrum of all healing essential oils
Niaouli *Melaleuca* *quinquenervia* *viridiflora* (MQV)	• Boosts immune system • Acts as an antiseptic
Neroli *Citrus aurantium* *ssp. aurantium*	• Relieves stress and calms emotional trauma
Oregano *Origanum vulgare*	• Acts as an antiviral and broad-spectrum antibiotic • Considered a potent analgesic
Palmarosa *Cymbopogon* *martinii*	• Generates new cell growth • Acts as an antiseptic and antiviral

(continued)

(continued)

OIL	POTENTIAL THERAPEUTIC EFFECT
Ravensara aromatica *Cinnamomum camphora*	• Made from distilling eucalyptus and clove-scented leaves • Acts as a detoxifying agent
Rosemary *Rosmarinus officinalis verbenon*	• Stimulates the nerves • Acts as a potent antiseptic
Tea tree *Malaleuca alternifolia*	• Acts as an antiviral, antibacterial, and antifungal
Thyme *Thymus vulgaris linalol, Thymus vulgaris thujanol-4,* and *Thymus vulgaris carvocrol*	• Acts as an antiviral, antibacterial, and antiseptic • Considered a good broad-spectrum oil

Essential oils attack the whole pathogen, not just a specific aspect of the organism. This is commonly thought to be why pathogens do not become resistant to the effects of essential oils.

The correct use of medicinal essential oils is best delivered by a trained and licensed expert. He or she will instruct you on proper application via inhalation, skin application, and baths.

BUG-BUSTING BLOCKBUSTERS

To summarize, the leading nutrients for immune function include the following.

The A List of Immune Boosters	
Vitamin C	• Offers general immune support. • Levels may be compromised when body is under stress from infection, chronic disease, or surgery.
Vitamin E	• Acts as an immune system stimulant, especially for older people. • Has antioxidant effect on oxidized fats and cholesterol. • Protects cell membranes and DNA from free-radical damage.
Selenium	• Supports body's detoxification system. • Antioxidant effect may benefit cardiovascular system and protect against cancer.
Vitamin A	• Supports normal cell reproduction and reduces infection rate. • Keeps body's first line of defense—skin, lungs, and linings of mouth and throat—healthy. • Protects against pollutants and other irritants.
Beta-carotene	• Converts to vitamin A, but has different antioxidant effect. • Stimulates T cells. • Enhances communication between immune cells.
Zinc	• Supports T and B cells. • Can improve antibody response to vaccines. • Helps in healing.
Echinacea	• Increases ability to fight infection. • Stimulates T cells.
Elderberry	• Eases fever and muscle aches of the flu and other respiratory infections.
Maitake	• Most powerful immune system booster of all medicinal mushrooms.

(continued)

(continued)	
Garlic	• Prevents growth of harmful bacteria, fungi, and viruses. • Increases lymphocytes and natural killer cells.
Lactobacillus acidophilus	• Reintroduces friendly bacteria to the colon. • Acts as a mild antibiotic.
CoQ10	• Increases antibodies. • Enhances heart function. • Helps lower blood pressure.

[18]

Sage Advice on Bug Busting

Your heaviest artillery will be your will to live.
Keep that big gun going.

—*Norman Cousins,* Anatomy of an Illness, *1979*

LESSONS LEARNED: IMPLICATIONS FOR PERSONAL FREEDOMS

While the saying goes that "curiosity killed the cat," we contend that "complacency kills humans." Satisfied for decades with the performance of antibiotics and vaccines, apportionment of public health budgets worldwide have been dramatically cut back. All of us are now mired in the muck that has been created by managed care: The one-on-one physician-patient relationship has been abandoned in a climate of cost-containing, cost-cutting medical care. To compound the problem, a climate of government interference is deliberately exclusionary toward innovative medicine. Incorrectly, physicians and health practitioners are labeled as experimental if they dare to think outside the lines drawn by conventional care. As history well documents, it is through innovation and experimentation that nearly all great advances in medicine originate.

Despite the United States spending more than any other nation per capita on health care, 40 to 50 million Americans are uninsured and without access to quality health care. In the era of HMO (health maintenance organization) medicine, with health care dollars in the hands of bureaucrats and administrators, the profession of being a primary health care physician has been relegated to rote treatment of symptoms of illness, rather than prevention from full-blown disease states. It is necessary that every health care consumer be an educated patient. You must ask questions, and, if necessary, challenge the system to fight for your medical rights.

Since we began writing this book, the world has become a much more dangerous place. The incidents that took place on September 11, 2001, and subsequently are difficult reminders that each of us must be cognizant of the potential for infectious disease. Indeed, infectious disease is a powerful variable in your ability to lead a long and healthy life. As we have seen throughout this book, infectious disease can kill you not only quickly; it can also kill you slowly. Or it can rob you of an active, satisfying lifestyle. It is within your power to prevent infectious disease from affecting the length and quality of your life. Take control of your health destiny today.

Appendix A

Infection Facts

The top infectious diseases in the U.S. are as follows:

1. AIDS
2. Lyme disease
3. Meningococcal infections
4. *Escherichia coli*
5. Malaria

—R. S. Wurman, "Understanding USA" at www.understandingusa.com

The cold-causing rhinovirus can live for 2 hours on the skin's surface.
—T. Zoellner, "Where the Germs Are,"
Men's Health, September 1999, p. 123

Up to 40% of the germs on a phone receiver can rub onto the next user's hands.
—"Bugged Phones," *New Scientist*, May 27, 2000

It takes a full five minutes of washing to flush out 99% of the most dangerous bacteria from the hands.
—G. Williams, "Your Mother Was Right,"
Discover, December 1999

The school-age child averages 4 colds per year, and each cold lasts 14 days. This translates to an excess of 164 million lost school days annually among kindergarten through 12th grade students in public schools.
> —Centers for Disease Control and Prevention, reported in
> "Study Finds Hand Sanitizers Reduce Illness-Related
> Absenteeism in Schools," October 23, 2000

The numbers of *Staphylococcus aureus* bacteria can double every 20 minutes and enjoy a good meal of an open cut.
> —T. Zoellner, "Where the Germs Are,"
> *Men's Health*, September 1999, p. 123

Flu leads to about 20,000 deaths and 110,000 hospitalizations each year in the U.S.
> —Reported by CNN.com, September 28, 2000

During the seven weeks of peak incidence of flu during the 1999–2000 season, about 77% of American households were affected.
> —*Vitamin Retailer,* September 2000

In an average year, influenza is associated with 20,000 to 30,000 deaths nationwide.
> —*Vitamin Retailer,* September 2000

Nose blowing produces a rapid change in pressure in a short period of time. If you have a cold, blowing your nose may lodge virus-laden mucus deep into the sinuses. By providing germs with a safe hideout, nose blowing may increase the duration and discomfort of colds. Neither sneezing nor coughing have the same intense effect.
> —"Don't Blow It," *New Scientist,* September 10, 1999

In the United States, we spend each year an average of $3,925 per person on health care—the highest per capita in the world.
> —R. S. Wurman, "Understanding USA" at
> www.understandingusa.com

A grand total of 160,000 Americans die to infectious diseases as the underlying cause of death.
> —Centers for Disease Control and Prevention, "Keep the Germs Away"
> fact sheet at www.cdc.gov

A phone survey of 10,000 people found that 1 in 4 believes taking antibiotics will shorten the duration of a cold, and 1 in 2 expects a prescription for antibiotics if a cold is serious enough for them to seek medical attention.
> —J. V. Eng, presentation at International Conference on
> Emerging Infectious Diseases, July 2000

In 1954, 2 million pounds of antibiotics were produced in the U.S. In 2000, the figure exceed[ed] 50 million pounds.
> —Centers for Disease Control and Prevention, "Antibiotic Resistance"
> fact sheet at www.cdc.gov

Humans consume 235 million doses of antibiotics annually.
> —Centers for Disease Control and Prevention, "Antibiotic Resistance"
> fact sheet at www.cdc.gov

An estimated 50 million of the 150 million antibiotic prescriptions written by American physicians are unwarranted.
> —M. D. Pinkowish, M. Cohen, S. Levy, and P. Mead,
> "Infectious Diseases: Still Emerging in 1998,"
> Patient Care, August 15, 1998

Manufacturers of vaccines receive more than $1 billion in the U.S., $3 billion worldwide. The total will likely increase to $7 billion within the next 2–3 years.
> —R. Neustaedter, "Vaccines: Does Your Child Really
> Need Them?" Let's Live, April 2000, p. 46

At least 65 million people—more than one in five Americans—are believed to be infected with a viral STD other than HIV.
> —www.plannedparenthood.org

Only one in five women are using birth control methods that effectively protect them from both pregnancy and sexually transmitted diseases.
> —"Survey: Young Women Not Acting Smart in Bedroom,"
> reported at www.newsstream.com, October 2000

Of the 15 million people in the U.S. who contract STDs, around 3,750,000—one quarter—are teenagers.
> —www.plannedparenthood.org

In 2000, candida treatment stood at a market worth $2.5 billion per year.
—*BusinessWeek,* October 9, 2000

As a group, men between 20–24 years old suffer some of the higher rates of gonorrhea.
—www.plannedparenthood.org

80% of people with an STD experience no noticeable symptoms.
—B. Moscicki et al., "The Use and Limitations of Endocervical Gram Stains," *American Journal of Obstetrics and Gynecology,* 157:1, July 1987

One third of the foreign residents in North Carolina have recently tested positive to tuberculosis infection.
—S. Young, presentation at International Conference on Emerging Infectious Diseases, July 2000

In New Jersey, from 1992 to 1998, vancomycin-resistant enterococci have increased five-fold.
—L. C. Wu, presentation at International Conference on Emerging Infectious Diseases, July 2000

You are at risk for cryptosporidium infection if you've recently swum in a public pool, visited a farm, or traveled—even out of your resident state.
—L. Wilcox, presentation at International Conference on Emerging Infectious Diseases, July 2000

Staphylococcus, enterococcus, and streptococcus are implicated as a leading factor in causing many of the 90,000 Americans to die of hospital-acquired antibiotic-resistant infections.
—B. I. Koerner, "Return of a Killer," *U.S. News and World Report,* November 2, 1998

The in-hospital cost of hospital-acquired infections resulting from 6 common kinds of resistant bacteria is $1.3 billion per year (1992 dollars).
—"HHS Press Release—Antimicrobial Resistance," U.S. Department of Health and Human Services, January 18, 2001

People receiving bone marrow transplants have markedly less infection with the fungus Aspergillus if they use HEPA filters to clean the air they breathe.
—T. G. M. Bauters, presentation at International Conference on
Emerging Infectious Diseases, July 2000

In a one-year period in the U.S., an estimated 225 million cases of acute diarrhea occur. Nearly 20% require doctor's care and 5 million require hospitalization.
—B. Imhoff, presentation at International Conference on
Emerging Infectious Diseases, July 2000

Fewer Americans are ordering rare and medium-rare hamburgers in restaurants. The decrease translates to 5% fewer cases of E. coli, amounting to savings in medical costs and lost productivity of $7.4 million a year. The concern over food-borne illnesses was cited in 7 out of 10 surveyed.
—Reported by Orlando Sentinel, October 30, 2000

Barbecued pork has been implicated as a vehicle for Salmonella infection in Georgia. Scientists suspect the failure to reach proper internal temperature during cooking.
—C. Rebmann, presentation at International Conference on
Emerging Infectious Diseases, July 2000

As much as 40% of chickens in grocery stores are contaminated with antibiotic-resistant Campylobacter jejuni. The most common bacterial cause of bacterial illness, C. jejuni infects an estimated 2.4 million people each year.
—S. Rossiter, presentation at International Conference on
Emerging Infectious Diseases, July 2000

5,000 Americans became ill with antibiotic-resistant Campylobacter infection after eating chicken.
—K. Hollinger, presentation at International Conference on
Emerging Infectious Diseases, July 2000

Yearly, the U.S. can expect an influx of:

- 16.7 million farm animals, mostly livestock and poultry
- 20 million wild animals to be brought in, primarily for the exotic pet trade
- 1.75 million illegal aliens to enter
—J. Ginsburg, "Bioinvasion,"
BusinessWeek, September 11, 2000

Food-Borne Infections in the U.S., 1988–1997

PATHOGEN	CAUSE OF OUTBREAK	LOCATION, YEAR
Hepatitis A	Frozen strawberries	Michigan, 1997
Salmonella serotype Typhimurium DT104	Farm visit	Nebraska, 1996
Cyclospora cayentanensis	Guatemalan raspberries	Multistate and Canada, 1996
Salmon enteritidis PT4	Egg-containing foods	California, 1995
S. enteritidis	Mass-distributed ice cream	Multistate, 1995
Norwalk-like virus	Gulf Coast oysters	Louisiana, 1994
Escherichia coli O157:H7	Fast-food hamburgers	Multistate, 1993
E. coli O157:H7	Raw apple cider	Massachusetts, 1991
Vibrio cholerae O1, El Tor	Thai coconut milk	Maryland, 1991
Trichinella spiralis	Undercooked pork	Iowa, 1990
Salmonella chester	Sliced cantaloupe	Multistate, 1989
Yersinia enterocolitica	Pork chitterlings	Georgia, 1988

Source: Adapted from S.F. Altekruse, M.L. Cohen, and D.L. Swerdlow, "Emerging Food-borne Diseases," Emerging Infectious Diseases, 1997;3:285–293.

Among adults age 35–44, 48% have gingivitis, and 22% have destructive gum disease. In children age 5–17, tooth decay is 5 times as common as asthma and 7 times as common as hayfever.

—Centers for Disease Control and Prevention/Oral Health Resources, "Oral Health 2000" fact sheet at www.cdc.gov/nccdphp/oh/sgr2000-fs1.htm

Around the world, 2,900 people died from tuberculosis in 1997.

—R. S. Wurman, "Understanding USA" at
www.understandingusa.com

Up to 2% of the world's 16 million tuberculosis sufferers have multi-drug resistant strains. In parts of Russia and China, as well as Estonia and Latvia, more than 10% of TB patients are treatment-resistant.

—Reported at ABCNews.com, June 12, 2000

In Russia, the cases of syphilis have risen 40-fold since the collapse of the Soviet Union.

—Associated Press, June 28, 2000

The first influenza outbreak of the 1999–2000 season in Ireland was brought to the U.S. by a church group on a group tour in Ireland.

—J. F. Perz, presentation at International Conference on Emerging Infectious Diseases, July 2000

In Japan, there is a high correlation of neurological damage, in addition to death, with a particular strain of influenza (H3N2).

—T. Morishima, presentation at International Conference on Emerging Infectious Diseases, July 2000

A compulsory program of measles/mumps/rubella (MMR) vaccine in the Italian armed forces significantly reduced the incidence of both measles and rubella, but not mumps.

—R. D'Amelio, presentation at International Conference on Emerging Infectious Diseases, July 2000

Malaria kills 2.6 million people a year, 70% of whom are children.

—Associated Press, June 28, 2000

Malaria is resistant to the top medication 80% of the time.

—Reported by ABCNews.com, June 12, 2000

The U.S. Office of Technology Assessment estimates that 130,000 to 3 million deaths could occur following the release of 100 kilograms of aerosolized anthrax over Washington, D.C., making the attack as lethal as a hydrogen bomb.

—Reported by MSNBC, October 3, 2000

Among the eccentric habits of the reclusive American tycoon Howard Hughes was an insistence on severing contact with acquaintances for months—even years—should they become sick. Hughes' germ phobia reached an all-time high in 1958, when he took residence in the Beverly Hills Hotel sitting buck naked in his self-designated germ-free zone, shielding himself from direct contact with the outside world by handling objects with clumps of tissue.

—G. Hamilton, "Let Them Eat Dirt,"
New Scientist, July 18, 1998

In 1946, the U.S. Centers for Disease Control and Prevention (U.S. CDC) was founded as the "Communicable Disease Center." Its subsequent name change was a response to the observation that any and all diseases are preventable, and a revised mission to identify and manage health risks on a public health scale was instituted.

—G. D. Lundberg, *Journal of the American Medical Association,*
CDC Morbidity and Mortality Weekly Report, March 3, 1999;
48(LMRK); vii–viii

Worldwide, life expectancy has increased dramatically during the last decade of the 20th century. But in celebrating our extra years we must recognize that increased longevity without quality of life is an empty prize: health expectancy is more important than life expectancy.

—Dr. Hiroshi Nakajima, director-general of WHO,
World Health Report, 1997

Appendix B

Resources/For More Information

General

American Academy of Anti-Aging Medicine/The World Health Network
   773-528-4333
   www.worldhealth.net

CDC Health A–Z
   http://www.cdc.gov/health/diseases.htm

Griffith, H. W. *Complete Guide to Symptoms, Illness and Surgery.* Putnam Berkeley Group, 1995.

Klatz, R. *New Anti-Aging Secrets for Maximum Lifespan.* Sports Tech Labs, 2000.

Konlee, M., *How to Reverse Immune Dysfunction,* 8th ed. Keep Hope Alive, Ltd., 1999.

Murray, M., and Pizzorno, J. *Encyclopedia of Natural Medicine,* 2nd ed. Prima Health, 1997.

National Foundation for Infectious Diseases
   www.nfid.org

Vanderhaeghe, L. R., and Bouic, P. J. D. *The Immune System Cure: Nature's Way to Super-Powered Health.* Prentice Hall Canada, 1999.

Preface

ConsumerLab.com
   www.ConsumerLab.com

1: It's a Bug's Life

All the Virology on the WWW
  www.virology.net
ProMed-Mail: Program for Monitoring Emerging Diseases
  www.healthner.org/programs/promed.html

2: Sworn to Defend, Protect, and Serve

Autoimmune Related Disease Association (AARDA)
  800-598-4668

3: You Are What You Eat

Centers for Disease Control and Prevention
  888-MY-ULCER
Center for Science in the Public Interest
  www.cspinet.org
Food and Drug Administration Consumer Information Line
  800-532-4440
Food and Drug Administration Food Information Line
  800-FDA-4010
Fox, N. *It Was Probably Something You Ate: A Practical Guide to Avoiding and Surviving Food-Borne Illness.* New York: Penguin Books, 1999.
National Food Safety Initiative
  http://vm.cfsan.fda.gov/~dms/fs-toc.html
United States Department of Agriculture (USDA)
  www.fsis.usda.gov
United States Department of Agriculture Meat and Poultry Hotline
  800-535-4555

4: Digestion, Immunity, and Parasites

Keep Hope Alive Limited
  www.keephope.net

5: Bladder, Kidneys, and Genitourinary Complaints

Crook, W., Brodsky, J., and Crook, C. *The Yeast Connection: A Medical Breakthrough.* New York: Vintage, 1986.

6: The Breath of Life: The Respiratory System

American Lung Association
    800-586-4872
    www.lungsusa.org
Cleaning the Air: Asthma and Indoor Air Exposure, National Academy Press.
    800-624-6242
National Asthma Education and Prevention Program
    301-592-8573
    www.nhlbi.nih.gov
U.S. Centers for Disease Control and Prevention (CDC), National Center for
    Infectious Diseases, Division of Viral and Rickettsial Diseases, Influenza
    Branch
    www.cdc.gov/ncidod/diseases/flu/weekly.htm
    Pneumococcal Disease Web Site
    www.cdc.gov/ncidod/dbmd/diseaseinfo/streppneum_a.htm
World Health Organization
    www.who.ch/emc

7: More Than Skin Deep

Fine, K. 14 Common first-aid procedures, *Complete Home Medical Guide from
    the Columbia University College of Physicians and Surgeons* at
    http://cpmcnet.columbia.edu/texts/guide/toc/toc14.html.
Seaton, K. *Life Health and Longevity.* Scientific Hygiene Inc., 1994.

8: ABCs of Hepatitis

Advisory Committee on Blood Safety and Availability, HHS Office of
    HIV/AIDS Policy
    202-690-5560
    www.hhs.gov/bloodsafety
American Liver Foundation
    800-GO LIVER
    www.liverfoundation.org
Hepatitis Foundation International
    973-239-1035 or 800-891-0707
    www.hepfi.org

HepC Connection
   303-860-0800 or 800-522-HEPC
   www.hepc-connection.org
National Digestive Diseases Information Clearinghouse
   301-654-3810
   www.niddk.nih.gov

10: STD Fundamentals

American Association for Chronic Fatigue Syndrome
   206-521-1932
   www.weber.u.washington.edu/~dedra/aacfs1.html
American Social Health Association
   800-230-6039
   http://www.ashastd.org
CFIDS Association of America
   800-442-3437
   www.cfids.org
Herpes Network
   www.herpes.net/index.html
Home Access Health (at-home HIV test kit)
   www.homeaccess.com
Keep Hope Alive, Limited
   www.keephope.net
   262-548-4344
National AIDS Hotline
   800-342-2437
National Herpes Hotline
   919-361-8488
Planned Parenthood
   www.plannedparenthood.org
   1-800-230-PLAN
U.S. Centers for Disease Control and Prevention (CDC), Division of Viral
   Diseases
   404-639-1338 or 888-232-3228
   www.cdc.gov/ncidod/diseases/cfs/cfshome.htm
U.S. Centers for Disease Control and Prevention (CDC) National AIDS
   Hotline
   800-342-AIDS

U.S. Centers for Disease Control and Prevention (CDC) National Prevention
   Information Network
   800-458-5231
U.S. Centers for Disease Control and Prevention (CDC) National STD Hotline
   800-227-8922

11: Pets Our Pets Don't Need: Zoonotic Diseases

American Lyme Disease Foundation
   www.aldf.com
   914-277-6970
National Institute of Allergy and Infectious Diseases
   www.niaid.nih.gov.factsheets/rabies.htm
U.S. Centers for Disease Control, Division of Parasitic Diseases/Animals
   http://www.cdc.gov/ncidod/dpd/parasiticpathways/animals.htm

12: Immunization

American Academy of Pediatrics
   www.aap.org/family/parents/immunize.htm
Immunization Action Coalition
   www.immunize.org
National Network for Immunization Information
   www.immunizationinfo.org
National Vaccine Information Center
   800-909-SHOT
   www.909shot.com
U.S. Centers for Disease Control and Prevention (CDC) National
   Immunization Program
   800-232-2522
   www.cdc.gov/nip/pdf/child-schedule.pdf
Vaccine Adverse Event Reporting System
   800-822-7967 (24 hours)
   www.fda.gov/cber/vaers.html
   www.cdc.nip/VAERS.html

13: The Elixir of Life: Water

International Bottled Water Association
   703-683-5213
   www.bottledwater.org

14: Who Says
Cleanliness Is Next to Godliness?

Alliance for the Prudent Use of Antibiotics
617-636-0966
http://www.healthsci.tufts.edu/apua/home.html
Division of Bacterial and Mycotic Diseases/National Center for Infectious
Diseases/Centers for Disease Control and Prevention
http://www.cdc.gov/ncidod/dbmd/antibioticresistance/
Wash Up America/National Hygiene Foundation
888-247-5900

15: Controlling the World Around You

EPA Scientific Advisory Board
202-260-8414
International Association for Medical Assistance to Travelers
716-754-4883
Travel Information for Older Americans
http://travel.state.gov/olderamericans.html
Travel Warnings
202-647-5225
http://travel.state.gov
Travelers hotline
888-232-3228

16: How Bugged Out Are You?

Great Smokies Diagnostic Laboratory
800-522-4762
www.gsdl.com

17: BOOST'R
(Best Optimizing Options-Strategies-Treatments
Reference)

American Botanical Council
512-331-8868
www.herbalgram.org

Food and Drug Administration's MEDWATCH
    800-332-1088
Herb Research Foundation
    303-449-2265
    www.herbs.org
Pacific Institute of Aromatherapy
    415-479-9121
    www.pacificinstituteofaromatherapy.com

Appendix C

References

1: It's a Bug's Life

Arnon, S., et al., for the Working Group on Civilian Biodefense. Botulinum toxin as a biological weapon: Medical and public health management. *Journal of the American Medical Association* 2001; 285: 1059–1070.

Dennis, D., et al., for the Working Group on Civilian Biodefense. Tularemia as a biological weapon: Medical and public health management. *Journal of the American Medical Association* 2001; 285: 2763–2773.

Fulginiti, V. A. The millennium in infectious diseases: Focus on the last century, 1900–2000, *Medscape General Medicine,* March 31, 2000.

Garrett, L. *The Coming Plague.* New York: Penguin, 1994.

Ginsburg, J. Mad cow: The U.S. is not immune, *Business Week,* Jan. 29, 2001.

Hacker, S. M., and Roaten, S. P. Strategies for managing bacterial skin infections, *Patient Care,* Sept. 15, 1999, pp. 53–58.

Henderson, D., et al., for the Working Group on Civilian Biodefense. Smallpox as a biological weapon: Medical and public health management. *Journal of the American Medical Association* 1999; 281: 2127–2137.

Inglesby, T., et al., for the Working Group on Civilian Biodefense. Plague as a biological weapon: Medical and public health management. *Journal of the American Medical Association* 2000; 283: 2281–2290.

International notes update: Human plague—India, 1994, *Mortality and Morbidity Weekly Report* 1994; 43 (39): 722–723.

Johnson, K. R. Mycobacterium tuberculosis transmitted to worker at medical waste treatment plant, *Journal of the American Medical Association* 2000;284:1682–1688.

Lawton, S. C. A medical guide to bioterrorism. 2001.

Microbes implicated in heart disease, *Science News,* vol. 158, Aug. 19, 2000, p. 120.

Ross, P. E. Do germs cause cancer? *Forbes,* Nov. 15, 1999, pp. 199–208.

Viral hemorrhagic fevers: fact sheet. CDC Disease Information—Special Pathogens Branch, at www.cdc.gov/ncidod/dvrd/spd/mnpages/ dispages/vhf.htm.

What are nanobacteria? Available at www.nanobaclabs.com.

2: Sworn to Defend, Protect, and Serve

Candon, P. Thymus tissue transplant restores immune function, *Medical Tribune,* Nov. 4, 1999, p. 21.

Lane, I. W. *Immune Power.* Garden City Park, N.Y.: Avery Publishing Group, 1999.

Seaton, K. Allergies, infection & stress, Advanced Health Products, 1998.

Survival of the fittest, and oldest, *The Economist,* June 3, 2000.

Understanding the Immune System, National Institutes of Health Publication No. 93–529, Bethesda, Md., January 1993.

Zuliani, G., Romagnoni, F., Soattin, L., Leoci, V., Volpato, S., and Fellin, R. Predictors of two-year mortality in older nursing home residents. The IRA study. Istituto di Riposo per Anziani, *Aging (Milano)* 2001; 13(1): 3–7.

3: You Are What You Eat

Acheson, D. W., and Levinson, R. K. *Safe Eating.* New York: Dell Publishing, 1998.

Armitage, K., Brooks, J. T., Jones, T. F., et al. Microbes on the menu: Recognizing foodborne illness, *Patient Care,* June 15, 2000.

Broadhurst, C. L. Bee products: Medicine from the hive, *Nutrition Science News,* August 1999.

Prier, R., and Solnick, J. V. Foodborne and waterborne infections, *Postgraduate Medicine* April 2000; 107(4): 245–252.

Taormina, R., Beuchat, L. R., and Slutsker, L. Infections associated with eating seed sprouts: An international concern, *Emerging Infectious Diseases* 1999; 5(5): 626–634.

4: Digestion, Immunity, and Parasites

Gibson, G. R., and Roberfroid, M. B. *Dietary Modulation of the Human Colonic Microbiota: Introducing the Concept of Prebiotics.* American Institute of Nutrition, 1995.

Lee, W. H. *The Friendly Bacteria.* New Canaan, Conn.: Keats Publishing, 1988.

Mathis, S. Colostrum: Not just for newborns, *Let's Live,* September 2000, pp. 49–52.

Mindell, E. *Probiotics: Nature's Internal Healers.* Garden City Park, N.Y.: Avery Publishing Group, 1998.

Rosenberg, R. *Probiotics: Continuing Education Module.* Kenmore, Wash.: New Hope Natural Media (with Bastyr University), 1999.

Seinela, L., and Ahvenaien, J. Aspirin contributes to ulcer disease in elderly patients with *H. pylori* infection, *Gerontology* 2000; 46:271–275.

Should you take supplements of "friendly" bacteria? *Tufts University Health & Nutrition Newsletter*, September 2000.

Wolfson, D. A probiotics primer, *Nutrition Science News,* June 1999; 4(6): 276–278.

5: Bladder, Kidneys, and Genitourinary Complaints

Armitage, K. B., Bologna, R. A., Horbach, N. S., et al. Best approaches to recurrent UTI, *Patient Care,* June 15, 1999, pp. 38–69.

Baken, L., Koutsky, L., Kuypurs, J., et al. Genital human papillomavirus infection among male and female sex partners: Prevalence and type-specific concordance, *Journal of Infectious Diseases* 1995; 171:429–432.

Baker, B. *E. coli* UTI isolates show new resistance, *Family Practice News,* Jan. 15, 1999, p. 32.

Centers for Disease Control and Prevention. Chlamydia supplement: Sexually transmitted infections and vaginitis. National Institute of Allergy and Infectious Diseases, National Institutes of Health, Bethesda, Md., August 1992.

Clark, H. R. *The Cure for All Diseases.* San Diego, Calif.: New Century Press, 1995.

Ferenczy, A. Epidemiology and clinical pathophysiology of *Condylomata acuminata, American Journal of Obstetrics and Gynecology* 1995; 172:1331–1339.

Fitzherbert, J. Genital herpes and zinc, *Medical Journal,* August 1, 1979, p. 399.

Gottlieb, B., editor-in-chief. *New Choices in Natural Healing.* Emmaus, Pa.: Rodale Press, 1995.

Habib, F. K., Ross, M., Lewenstein, A., et al. Identification of a prostate inhibitory substance in a pollen extract, *Prostate,* March 1995; 26(3):133–139.

Heidrich, F., Berg, A., and Bergman, J. Clothing factors and vaginitis, *Journal of Family Practice* 1984;19:491–494.

Hilton, E., Isenberg, H., Alperstein, P., et al. Ingestion of yogurt containing

Lactobacillus acidophilus as prophylaxis for candidal vaginitis, *Annals of Internal Medicine* 1992; 116:353–357.

Jojanovic, R., Congema, E., and Nguyen, H. Antifungal agents vs. boric acid for treating chronic mycotic vulvovaginitis, *Journal of Reproductive Medicine* 1991; 36:593–596.

Lewin, D. J. The herpesvirus, *National Institute of Health Resources Journal*, September 7, 1995; 7:49–53.

Lininger, S. W., Jr., editor-in-chief, et al. *The National Pharmacy*, 2nd ed. Rocklin, Calif.: Prima Publishing, 1999.

MacDonald, R., Ishani, A., Rutka, I., and Wilt, T. J. A systematic review of Cernilton for the treatment of benign prostatic hyperplasia, *British Journal of Urology* May 2000; 85(7): 836–841.

Marti, J. E., et al. *Alternative Health Medicine Encyclopedia*. Detroit, Mich.: Visible Ink Press, 1995.

Orenstein, R., and Wong, E. B. Urinary tract infections in adults, *American Family Physician* 1999; 59(5):1225–1234.

Pitchford, P. *Healing with Whole Foods*. Berkeley, Calif.: North Atlantic Books, 1993.

Policar, M. S. Genital tract infections: How best to treat trichomoniasis, bacterial vaginosis, and Candida infection, *Consultant,* August 1996; 36: 1769.

Reynolds, T., ed. Alternative therapies and women's health, *National Women's Health Report* 1995; 17(3):4.

Seltanoff, J. *Natural Healing.* New York: Warner Books, 1988.

Sherrard, J. *National Guideline for the Management of Trichomoniasis Vaginalis.* Radcliff Infirmary, Oxford, England, May 12, 2000.

Sweet, R. *The Vaginitis Report,* vol. 1, *The Encyclopedia of Natural Remedies.* Pleasant Grove, Utah: Woodland Publishing, 1995.

Tenney, L. *The Encyclopedia of Natural Remedies.* Pleasant Grove, Utah: Woodland Publishing, 1995.

Weisberg, M., and Summers, P. Patient self-diagnosis of vulvovaginal candidiasis, *Female Patient* 1996; 21:60–64.

Weiss, R. F. *Herbal Medicine.* Beaconsfield, England: Beaconsfield Publishers, 1988.

Wichel, M., and Bisset, N. G., eds. *Herbal Drugs and Phytopharmaceuticals.* Stuttgart, N.J.: Medpharm Scientific Publishers, 1994.

Wolner-Hanssen, P., Kreiger, J. N., Stevens, C. E., et al. Clinical manifestations of vaginal trichomoniasis, *Journal of the American Medical Association* 1989; 264: 571–576.

Woznicki, K. *Antimicrobial Agents and Chemotherapy.* Interscience Conference on Antimicrobial Agents and Chemotherapy, San Diego, February 1999.

6: The Breath of Life: The Respiratory System

Bullock, C. Chronic infectious sinusitis linked to allergies, *Medical Tribune,* Dec. 7, 1995:1.

Devitt, M. Meningitis vaccine under scrutiny in UK, *Dynamic Chiropractic,* Oct. 16, 2000.

Dolin R. Prevention and treatment of influenza, *UpToDate,* July 2000.

Evans, R. Environmental control and immunotherapy for allergic disease, *Journal Allergy and Clinical Immunology* 1992; 90: 462–468.

Fungus implicated as cause of chronic sinusitis, *Patient Care,* Nov. 30, 1999, p. 7.

Glezen, W. P., Mostow, S. R., Schaffner, W., with McCarthy, R. The revolution in influenza care, *Patient Care,* Oct. 30, 2000, pp. 22–41.

How green was my sputum, *Family Practice News,* August 1, 2000, p. 16.

Indoor allergens and asthma, *Journal of the American Medical Association,* Feb. 16, 2000; 283(7): 875.

Influenza '99: New antiviral approved, flu shot season begins, *Geriatrics,* Sept. 1999; 54(9).

Kaiser, L. The role of neuraminidase inhibitors in influenza, *Second International Symposium on Influenza and Other Respiratory Viruses,* December 12, 1999.

Kenyon, T. A., et al. Transmission of multidrug-resistant *Mycobacterium tuberculosis* during a long airplane flight, *New England Journal of Medicine* 1996; 334:933–938.

Laino, C. *H. pylori* implicated in allergies, *Medical Tribune.*

MacDonald, R., Ishani, A., Rutka, I., and Wilt, T. J. A systematic review of Cernilton for the treatment of benign prostatic hyperplasia, *British Journal of Urology,* May 2000; 85(7): 836–841 and March 24, 1994; 1.

Marcus, A. Brain disease scare, reported by www.healthscout.com, Oct. 28, 2000.

Maudlin, R. Influenza vaccine, 1999–2000, *Modern Medicine,* Nov. 1999; 67:58–59.

Mayell, H. Global warning: Tuberculosis on the rampage, Environmental News Network, April 30, 2000.

National Women's Health Report: The Women's Guide to Influenza, National Women's Health Resource Center, December 1999.

Neuzil, K. Advances in influenza treatment and control, 38th Annual Meeting of the Infectious Diseases Society of America, 2000.

Noll, D. R., Shores, J. H., Gamber, R. G., et al. Benefits of osteopathic manipulative treatment for hospitalized elderly patients with pneumonia, *Journal of the American Osteopathic Association* 2000; 100(12):776–782.

Osterhaus, A. D. M. E., et al. Dutch researchers identify influenza B virus in seals, *Science,* May 12, 2000; 288: 1051–1053.

Rennard, B. O., Ertl, R. F., Gossman, G. L., Robbins, R. A., and Rennard, S. I. Chicken soup inhibits neutrophil chemotaxis in vitro. *Chest* 2000; 118(4): 1150–1157.

Risk of recurrent MI reduced by 67% after influenza vaccination, *Family Practice News,* April 13, 2000, p. 5.

Too few diabetics are immunized against flu and pneumonia, *Modern Medicine,* August 1997; 65:40.

Tuberculosis risk on aircraft, Centers for Disease Control and Prevention National Center for Infectious Diseases: Travelers' Health, at www.cdc.gov/travel/tb_risk.htm.

7: More Than Skin Deep

Bykowski, M. Be aggressive when treating dog and cat bites to forestall infection, *Family Practice News,* July 1, 1999, p. 29.

Decker, M. D. *Eikenella corrodens, Infection Control,* Jan. 1986;7(1):36–41.

Donohue, M. Reports of superlice may really be reinfestation, *Family Practice News,* May 1, 2000, p. 24.

Hacker, S. M., and Roaten, S. P. Strategies for managing bacterial skin infections, *Patient Care*, Sept. 15, 1999, pp. 53–58.

Press Release, Study finds hand sanitizers reduce illness-related absenteeism in schools, distributed by Internetwire.com, Oct. 23, 2000.

Rayan, G. M., Downard, D., Cahill, S., and Flournow, D. J. A comparison of human and animal mouth flora, *Journal of the Oklahoma State Medical Association*, Oct. 1991; 84(10): 510–515.

Smith, P. F., Meadowcroft, A. M., and May, D. B. Treating mammalian bite wounds, *J Clin Pharm Ther*, Apr. 2000;25(2):85–99.

Uganda's Ebola death toll rises to 92, at cnn.com, November 6, 2000.

Update on Superficial Fungal Infections: A Postgraduate Medicine Special Report, McGraw Hill Companies, July 1999.

Vukovic, L. Home remedies, *Natural Health*, September 2000, p. 61.

Wirthlin Worldwide for American Society for Microbiology. Handwashing study: A survey of handwashing behavior, September 2000.

8: ABCs of Hepatitis

Berkson, B. M. A conservative triple antioxidant approach to the treatment of hepatitis C. Combination of alpha lipoic acid (thioctic acid), silymarin, and selenium: Three case histories. *Medizinische Klinik* 1999;15(94):84–89.

Carithers, R. L. American Association Study of Liver Diseases Practice Guidelines: Liver transplantation, *Liver Transplantation,* Jan. 2000; 6(1):122–35.

Hancin, B. Hepatitis C infection is an STD in 20% of patients, *Family Practice News,* Dec. 1, 1999, p. 28.

Hepatitis C: An uncertain prognosis, *Health News* 2000;6(3):1–2.

Hepatitis fact sheets from National Center for Infectious Diseases, U.S. Centers for Disease Control and Prevention, available at www.cdc.gov/ncidod/diseases/hepatitis.

Hepatitis from A to E, Hepatitis Branch, U.S. Centers for Disease Control and Prevention, April 2000.

Revelle, M. Progress in blood supply safety, *FDA Consumer Magazine,* May 1995.

9: Oral Infections

Improving oral health fact sheet, at CDC Oral Health Resources, http://www.cdc.gov/nccdphp/oh/htm.

Loos, K. What is the most effective tothpaste? at http://www.smiledoc.com/dentist/tothpast.html.

McBrice, D. R. Management of aphthous ulcers, *American Family Physician,* July 1, 2000;62(1):149–154.

Oral Health Resources, Centers for Disease Control and Prevention, at http://www.cdc.gov/nccdphp/oh.

10: STD Fundamentals

Arens, M., and Travis, S. Zinc salts inactivate clinical isolates of herpes simplex virus in vitro, *Journal of Clinical Microbiology* 2000;38:1758–1762.

Gonorrhea on the rise, *Family Practice News,* August 1, 2000, p. 16.

HIV: Past, present, and future, *Postgraduate Medicine,* April 2000;107(4):109–113.

Konlee, M. *How to Reverse Immune Dysfunction,* 8th ed. West Allis, Wisc.: Keep Hope Alive, 1999.

McFarlane, M., Bull, S., and Rietmeijer, C. A. The Internet as a newly emerging risk environment for sexually transmitted diseases, *Journal of the American Medical Association,* July 26, 2000;284(4):443–446.

Motluk, A. Rub on the rioja, *New Scientist,* Sept. 23, 2000.

Public Health Service guidelines for the management of health-care worker exposures to HIV and recommendations for postexposure prophylaxis, *CDC Morbidity and Mortality Weekly Report,* May 15, 1998;47(RR-7), pp. 1–28.

11: Pets Our Pets Don't Need: Zoonotic Diseases

Animals—zoonotic diseases fact sheet, U.S. Centers for Disease Control and Prevention, at http://www.cdc.gov/ncidod/dpd/parasiticpathways/animals.htm.

Lewis, C. New vaccine targets Lyme disease, *FDA Consumer Magazine,* May–June 1999, pp. 99–134.

Lyme disease fact sheet, U.S. Centers for Disease Control and Prevention, at http://www.cdc.gov/ncidod/dvbid/lymeinfo.htm.

Marcus, L. Wilderness-acquired zooneses, in P. Auerbach (ed.), *Wilderness Medicine,* 4th ed. St. Louis, Mo.: Mosby, 2001.

Terkeltaub, R. A. Lyme disease 2000, *Geriatrics,* July 2000;55(7):34–47.

12: Immunization

Devit, M. Rotavirus vaccine may trigger juvenile diabetes, *Dynamic Chiropractic,* Sept. 18, 2000.

Haroff, L. Vaccine jitters, *Time,* September 13, 1999, pp. 64–65.

Obesity linked to cold-like virus, reported at biospace.com, July 27, 2000.

Stone, A. Anthrax vaccines won't be stopped, *USA Today,* Feb. 23, 2000.

13: The Elixir of Life: Water

International Bottled Water Association, www.bottledwater.org.

14: Who Says
Cleanliness Is Next to Godliness?

Cordell, R., Pickering, L., Waggoner-Fountain, L., et al. Common infections in child care, *Patient Care,* Aug. 15, 1998, pp. 60–86.

Levy, S. B. The challenge of antibiotic resistance, *Scientific American,* March 1998, p. 48.

Niederman, M. S., Skerrett, S. J., Yamauchi, S. K., et al. Antibiotics or not? *Patient Care,* Jan. 15, 1998, pp. 60–89.

Oliwenstein, L. Antibacterial backlash, *Women's Day Health for Women,* Summer 1999, pp. 66–67.

Pal, S. Bacterial resistance increases in the 1990s, *Pharmacist,* December 1999, p. 12.

Prevent antibiotic resistance by washing your hands thoroughly, *Modern Medicine,* August 1997; 65:22.

Roderick, K. Antibacterial soap dangers, reported at www.thirdage.com, Sept. 11, 2000.

Schorr, M. Clean freaks, reported by www.abcnews.com, Sept. 7, 2000.

Wu, C. Beyond vancomycin, *Science News,* April 24, 1999;155:268–269.

15: Controlling the World Around You

Carpenter, S. Modern hygiene's dirty tricks, *Science News,* August 14, 1999;156:106–110.

Conlin, M. Is your office killing you, *BusinessWeek,* June 5, 2000, pp. 114–130.

Germ exposure may be good for kids, *AP Health News,* reported at www. thirdage.com, August 25, 2000.

Legionella bacteria found at Baltimore County hospital, reported at www.cnn.com, August 26, 2000.

Mercola, J. M. Current health news you can use, *Townsend Letter for Doctors and Patients,* May 1999, p. 34.

Potentially fatal germs under fingernails of hospital personnel should be eradicated, study says, reported at www.cnn.com, September 7, 2000.

Ryan, E. T., and Kain, K. C. Health advice and immunizations for travelers, *New England Journal of Medicine,* June 8, 2000;342(23):1716–1726.

Schaffner, W. Travel medicine: The road to good health, *Patient Care,* Sept. 15, 1998, pp. 112–144.

ToxFAQs, from Agency for Toxic Substances and Disease Registry, http://www.atsdr.cdc.gov/toxfaq.html.

Zoler, M. L. Spike in invasive group A strep spreading in households, *Family Practice News,* September 1, 2000, p. 121.

16: How Bugged Out Are You?

Greenberg, C. *Biological Terrain,* August 1999.

Konlee, M. *How to Reverse Immune Dysfunction,* 8th ed. West Allis, Wisc.: Keep Hope Alive, 1999.

The lymph system, at www.testuniverse.com, September 9, 2000.

Vanderhaeghe, L. R., and Bouic, P. J. D. *The Immune System Cure: Nature's Way to Super-Powered Health,* Prentice Hall Canada, 1999.

17: BOOST'R (Best Optimizing Options-Strategies-Treatments Reference)

Schnaubelt, K. *Advanced Aromatherapy: The Science of Essential Oil Therapy.* Rochester, Vt.: Traditions International, 1998.

Smucker, J. M. Colloidal silver, an internal FDA memo, February 28, 1997, available at http://vm.cfsan.fda.gov/~ear/mi-97-3.html.

Stehlin, I. Homeopathy: Real medicine or empty promises? U.S. Food and Drug Administration, at www.fda.gov/fdac/features/0906_home.html.

18: Sage Advice on Bug Busting

American Association for World Health. *Emerging Infectious Diseases: Reduce the Risk,* 1997.

Klatz, R. *New Anti-Aging Secrets for Maximum Lifespan,* STL, 2000. To obtain a copy, call American Academy of Anti-Aging Medicine at 773-528-4333 or visit www.worldhealth.net.

Reuter's Medical News. World leaders declare war on disease, September 29, 2000.

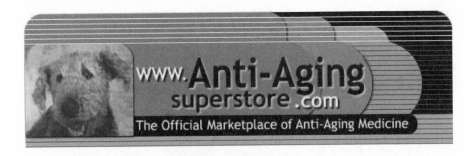

PRODUCTS FOR YOUR PERSONAL BUG-BUSTING REGIMEN
AVAILABLE EXCLUSIVELY AT THE ANTI-AGING SUPERSTORE
WWW.ANTI-AGINGSUPERSTORE.COM

Natural Maxi-Cleanse Disinfectant Soap™—Improves efficacy of handwashing. Containing a blend of unique natural disinfectant agents in a fortified soap, this product is shown by laboratory testing to remove 99% of all germs from hands. All-natural antibacterial ingredients.

Physicians Immune Booster™—Boosts the body's defense for fighting infectious attacks. A proprietary blend of immune-enhancing vitamins, nutrients, and natural agents that have been demonstrated to have strong benefit in stimulating and/or supporting immunity in human and animal laboratory research.

PM Antistress Sleep Assist™—A natural blend of medicinal herbal and nutrient ingredients shown to promote deep, restful, rejuvenative, and relaxing sleep when used at full dose. When used at low dose (one-third strength), PM Antistress Sleep Assist functions as a natural antistress calming tonic.

Saf-T-Sex-Lube™—Containing a number of natural antibiotic and antiseptic ingredients. A long-lasting sexual aid lubricant that may help protect against STDs by preventing skin irritation, bruising, cuts, abrasions, and scrapes that would allow bacteria to have access to capillary blood vessels. Most STDs will not penetrate intact skin: Saf-T-Sex-Lube protects skin with skin-healing agents and a long-lasting, highly efficient skin lubricant that actually forms a protective coating atop the skin.

Also available . . .
R. Klatz, *New Anti-Aging Secrets for Maximum Lifespan* (2000).
R. Goldman with R. Klatz (and Lisa Berger), *Brain Fitness* (1999).
R. Klatz (with Carol Kahn), *Grow Young with HGH* (1998).
R. Klatz and R. Goldman, *Stopping the Clock* (1996).
R. Klatz and R. Goldman, *7 Anti-Aging Secrets* (1996).

These products are not intended to diagnose, prevent, treat, or cure any disease or illness. These statements have not been evaluated by the FDA, and no claims on efficacy are made.

About Dr. Klatz and Dr. Goldman

DR. RONALD M. KLATZ is a leading authority in the new clinical science of anti-aging medicine. The founder and president of the American Academy of Anti-Aging Medicine, a not-for-profit public foundation, he has pioneered the exploration of new therapies for the treatment and prevention of age-related degenerative diseases and oversees educational programs for more than 10,000 physicians and scientists from 60 countries.

Other accomplishments include co-founding the National Academy of Sports Medicine, an internationally recognized educational institution, and serving as a director of Life Science Holdings (LSH), a biomedical company dedicated to the research and development of organ transplant and other advanced medical technologies. Dr. Klatz is the inventor, developer, or administrator of more than 100 scientific patents. In 1993 he was awarded the Gold Medal in Science for Brain Resuscitation Technology, and in 1994 he was honored with the Grand Prize in Medicine for Brain Cooling Technology.

A best-selling author and editor, Dr. Klatz served as senior medical editor of *Longevity* magazine and a contributing editor to the *Archives of Gerontology and Geriatrics,* and was a syndicated columnist with Pioneer Press, a division of Time-Life Inc. He is the author of *Ten Weeks to a Younger You, Brain Fitness, Hormones of Youth, Grow Young with HGH, Seven Anti-Aging Secrets, Advances in Anti-Aging, Stopping the Clock, Death in the Locker Room / Drugs & Sports, The E Factor, The Life Extension Weight Loss Program,* and *Deprenyl—The Anti-Aging Drug.* Dr. Klatz has been a co-host of the national Fox Network television series *Anti-Aging Update,* is a regular presenter at scientific conferences, and has appeared on dozens of national and international television and radio broadcasts.

Dr. Klatz is a graduate of Florida Technological University, the College of Osteopathic Medicine and Surgery (Des Moines, Iowa), and the University of Central America Health Sciences School of Medicine. He is board certified in family practice and sports medicine. He maintains an academic research post at Oklahoma State University as clinical assistant professor in the Department of Medicine, and serves as professor at Central America Health Sciences University. A consultant to the biotechnology industry and a respected adviser to several members of the U.S. Congress and others on Capitol Hill, Dr. Klatz devotes much of his time to research and to the development of advanced biosciences for the benefit of humanity.

DR. ROBERT M. GOLDMAN founded the National Academy of Sports Medicine (international president), the American Academy of Anti-Aging Medicine (chairman of the board), and the High Technology Research Institute. He has served as a senior fellow at the Lincoln Filene Center, Tufts University, and as an affiliate at the Philosophy of Education Research Center, Graduate School of Education, Harvard University. He is clinical assistant professor of medicine at Oklahoma State University's Department of Medicine and is a professor in the Department of Internal Medicine at the Central America Health Sciences University School of Medicine. He is a fellow of the American Academy of Sports Physicians and a board diplomat in sports medicine and anti-aging medicine.

Dr. Goldman received his B.S. from Brooklyn College in New York. He received his M.D. from the Central America Health Sciences University School of Medicine, a government-sanctioned, Ministry of Health–approved, and World Health Organization–listed medical university. He received his doctor of osteopathic medicine and surgery (D.O.) degree from CCOM/MidWestern University.

Dr. Goldman co-founded and serves as chairman of the board of Life Science Holdings, a biomedical research company with more than 150 medical patents under development in the areas of brain resuscitation, trauma and emergency medicine, organ transplant, and blood-preservation technologies. He has overseen cooperative research agreement development programs with such prominent institutions as the American National Red Cross, NASA, the Department of Defense, and the FDA's Center for Devices and Radiological Health. As an inventor, Dr. Goldman was awarded the Gold Medal for Science (1993), the Grand Prize for Medicine (1994), the Humanitarian Award (1995), and the Business Development Award (1996).

A black belt in karate and a world-champion athlete with over 20 world strength records, in 1995 Dr. Goldman was awarded the Healthy American Fitness Leader Award from the President's Council on Physical Fitness and Sports and the U.S. Chamber of Commerce.

Dr. Goldman is chairman of the International Medical Commission overseeing sports medicine committees in more than 176 nations. He has served as a special adviser to the President's Council on Physical Fitness and Sports. Aside from the numerous books he has authored, Dr. Goldman has contributed to hundreds of published articles and has made many international media appearances. He visits an average of 20 countries annually to promote brain research and sports medicine programs.

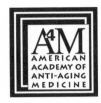

SOCIETY-WIDE BENEFITS OF LONGEVITY:
THE IMPACT OF ANTI-AGING MEDICINE
DR. RONALD KLATZ, PRESIDENT &
DR. ROBERT GOLDMAN, CHAIRMAN
AMERICAN ACADEMY OF ANTI-AGING MEDICINE

Globally, human life expectancy is on the rise. Recently, Kevin Murphy and Robert Topel of the University of Chicago Business School calculated the value of these extra years of life.[1] Assigning a value per-life of $5 million (extrapolated from accident payouts by insurers), Murphy and Topel calculated what the six years' gain in average life expectancy during 1970–1990 alone were worth across the total U.S. population. Their analysis concluded that the increase in life expectancy over the twenty-year period was worth a whopping $57 trillion in 1992 dollars. Converted into a yearly evaluation, the Murphy and Topel study assigned a *$2.4 trillion a year value on longevity for the U.S. alone.*

Focusing in on the potential financial gain if the leading causes of death were to be eradicated, Murphy and Topel estimate that eliminating deaths from *heart disease* would generate an economic value of *$48 trillion,* curing *cancer* would be worth *$47 trillion.* All totaled, Murphy and Topel argue that *reducing the death* rate from either heart disease or cancer by 20% would be worth around *$10 trillion* to Americans—more than one year's U.S. Gross Domestic Product.

Anti-aging medicine is a medical specialty founded on the application of advanced scientific and medical technologies for the early detection, prevention, treatment, and reversal of age-related diseases. It is a health-care model promoting innovative science and research to prolong the healthy life span in humans. Certainly, until we eradicate the age-related decline in health that leads to many of us becoming dependent and disabled in our older years, society will bear increasing financial costs to sustain the older population. Old-age dependency rates will rise in every major world region during the next twenty-five years. In the absence of scientific solutions that halt the onset of the degenerative diseases of aging, the elderly support burden in the year 2025 will be 50% larger than that in 1998.[2]

The benefits of longevity are wide-ranging, thanks in large part to the **eight years of leadership in the fast-growing clinical specialty founded, and led by, the American Academy of Anti-Aging Medicine** (A4M, Chicago, IL; www.worldhealth.net). Contact us for free information that can improve your life and the lives of your loved ones.

1. Murphy, K., and Topel, R. The health effect, *The Economist,* June 1, 2000.
2. Sixty-five plus in the United States, United States Census Bureau Statistical Brief by Economics and Statistics Administration, U.S. Department of Commerce, May 1995.

Visit The World Health Network, www.worldhealth.net—
the Internet's leading anti-aging portal and source for information on aging intervention

RETURN THIS INTEREST INDICATOR TO RECEIVE INFORMATION

NAME (first, middle, last):_____

PROFESSIONAL DESIGNATION(S): [ ]M.D. [ ]D.O. [ ]Ph.D. [ ] R.Ph. other: _____

MAILING ADDRESS: _____ (street)

_____(city/state/zip/country)

TELEPHONE: _____ FAX: _____

E-MAIL ADDRESS: _____

I AM INTERESTED IN:

[ ] Establishing membership in the A4M as: [ ] individual   [ ] organization

[ ] Board Certification in anti-aging medicine

[ ] Free subscription to *Anti-Aging Medical News,* the trend-setting industry publication

[ ] Free subscription to *The Report of the Medical Committee on Aging Research & Education,* a scholarly review of the latest clinical, research, and public policy developments in human longevity

[ ] Free subscription to A4M's electronic newsletters (provide e-mail address above)

FAX TO THE AMERICAN ACADEMY OF
ANTI-AGING MEDICINE AT: (773) 528-5390 or
MAIL TO: A4M ~ 2415 North Greenview Ave. ~ Chicago, IL 60614 USA

Consumers for **E**ducation, **A**wareness, and **S**afety of **E**ateries is a public safety campaign that advocates the consistent and thorough implementation of proper hygiene and sanitation techniques at dining establishments.

Each year, more than 75 million citizens in the United States become ill from food poisoning; of these, 325,000 require hospitalization, and 5,000 die.

Established in 2000 by the American Academy of Anti-Aging Medicine (A4M, Chicago, IL), CEASE encourages restaurant patrons to alert establishment owners and managers of flagrant hygiene and sanitation violations that, left uncorrected, may result in anything from discomfort to death.

CEASE urges you, the recipient, to take actions on the observations contained in this Notice.

CEASE! LIVES DEPEND ON IT!

C onsumers for
E ducation,
A wareness, and
S afety of
E ateries

From a Member of:
Consumers for
Education,
Awareness, and
Safety of
Eateries

Submitted to
Owner/Manager
on Duty

ATTENTION:
OWNER OR FOOD SERVICE MANAGER
OF THIS ESTABLISHMENT

URGENT AND CONFIDENTIAL

OPEN IMMEDIATELY
YOUR PROMPT RESPONSE IS REQUESTED

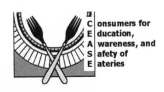

C onsumers for
E ducation,
A wareness, and
S afety of
E ateries

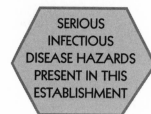

SERIOUS
INFECTIOUS
DISEASE HAZARDS
PRESENT IN THIS
ESTABLISHMENT

PUBLIC HEALTH VIOLATION
OFFICIAL NOTICE

Better Business Bureau
office with jurisdiction
is being notified

Date Issued: _____

Establishment: _____

Located at: _____

Cc: Better Business Bureau

Dear Sir or Madam:

I am a consumer who has found just cause to be concerned about my health, and the health of others who frequent this establishment. Today I observed the following:

[ ] Bathroom is unclean and untidy

[ ] Bathroom does not have: [ ] soap   [ ] toilet paper   [ ] hand towels/(operational) drying unit

[ ] Staff uses same cloth/sponge to clean several tables without rinsing in between

[ ] Staff does not use disinfectant to clean tables

[ ] Staff that cleans tables doesn't wash hands before setting table

[ ] Staff that appears to have a cold was allowed to handle food and utensils

[ ] Meat(s) was/were served bloody/runny

[ ] Rancid: [ ] dairy product   [ ] fish   [ ] meat   [ ] poultry

[ ] Moldy: [ ] vegetables   [ ] fruits   [ ] breads

[ ] Cross-contamination observed (raw meats/fish/poultry with raw fruit/vegetables)

[ ] Food(s) to be served hot was/were lukewarm/cold upon my being served

[ ] Food(s) to be served cold was/were lukewarm/hot upon my being served

[ ] Sneeze guard does not adequately cover the self-serve bar(s)

[ ] My food was not prepared to my special ordering requests

[ ] Observed kitchen staff not using gloves to prepare/cook food

[ ] Observed kitchen staff handling food and nonfood items with same gloves/unwashed hands

[ ] No current board of health inspection report visibly posted

[ ] OTHER: _____

_____

_____

Index